Bodies Politic

PICTURING HISTORY

Series Editors
Peter Burke, Sander L. Gilman, Ludmilla Jordanova, Roy Porter,
†Bob Scribner (1995–8)

In the same series

Health and Illness
Images of Difference
SANDER L. GILMAN

Men in Black
JOHN HARVEY

Dismembering the Male
Men's Bodies, Britain and the Great War
JOANNA BOURKE

The Feminine Ideal
MARIANNE THESANDER

The Destruction of Art
*Iconoclasm and Vandalism since
the French Revolution*
DARIO GAMBONI

Trading Territories
Mapping the Early Modern World
JERRY BROTTON

Landscape and Englishness
DAVID MATLESS

Global Interests
Renaissance Art between East and West
LISA JARDINE AND JERRY BROTTON

Eyes of Love
*The Gaze in English and French Painting
and Novels 1840–1900*
STEPHEN KERN

Pictures and Visuality in Early
Modern China
CRAIG CLUNAS

Maps and Politics
JEREMY BLACK

Mirror in Parchment
*The Luttrell Psalter and the Making
of Medieval England*
MICHAEL CAMILLE

Picturing Empire
*Photography and the Visualization of
the British Empire*
JAMES RYAN

The Thief, the Cross and the Wheel
*Pain and the Spectacle of Punishment in
Medieval and Renaissance Europe*
MITCHELL B. MERBACK

'Down with the Crown'
*British Anti-monarchism and Debates about
Royalty since 1790*
ANTONY TAYLOR

The Jewish Self-Image
*American and British Perspectives,
1881–1939*
MICHAEL BERKOWITZ

Picturing Tropical Nature
NANCY LEYS STEPAN

Representing the Republic
Mapping the United States 1600–1900
JOHN RENNIE SHORT

Eyewitnessing
The Uses of Images as Historical Evidence
PETER BURKE

Bodies Politic

Disease, Death and Doctors in Britain, 1650–1900

Roy Porter

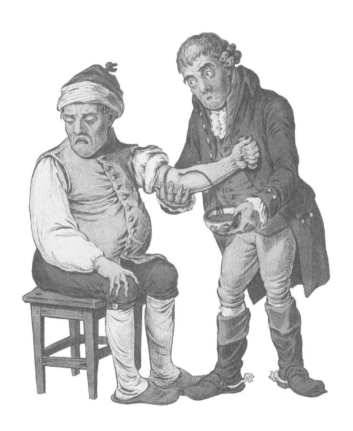

REAKTION BOOKS

To Natsu, again
        the love of my life

Published by Reaktion Books Ltd
79 Farringdon Road, London EC1M 3JU, UK

www.reaktionbooks.co.uk

First published 2001

Colour printed by Balding & Mansell Limited, Norwich
Printed and bound in Great Britain by Butler & Tanner, Frome, Somerset

British Library Cataloguing in Publication Data

Porter, Roy, 1946–
    Bodies politic – disease, death and doctors in Britain,
    1650–1900. – (Picturing history)
    1. Medicine – Great Britain – Pictorial works 2. Medicine –
    Great Britain – Pictorial works – History 3. Medical
    personnel – Great Britain – Pictorial works
    I. Title
    610.9'41

    ISBN 1 86189 094 X

Contents

'What is the use of a book', thought Alice, 'without pictures or conversations?'

LEWIS CARROLL, *Alice's Adventures in Wonderland* (1892)

These Papers are delivered to a Set of artists very dextrous in finding out the mysterious Meanings of Words, Syllables, and Letters. For Instance, they can decypher a Close-stool to signify a Privy-Council; a Flock of Geese, a Senate; a lame Dog, an Invader; the Plague, a standing Army; a Buzard, a Minister; the Gout, a High Priest; a Gibbet, a Secretary of State; a Chamber pot, a Committee of Grandees; a Sieve, a Court Lady; a Broom, a Revolution; a Mouse-trap, an Employment; a bottomless Pit, the Treasury; a Sink, a C—t; a Cap and Bells, a Favourite; a broken Reed, a Court of Justice; an empty Tun, a General; a running Sore, the Administration.

JONATHAN SWIFT, *Gulliver's Travels* (1726)

Most people waste time and health for nothing; one compiles the commonest sort of things, another repeats what has already been said a hundred times, a third busies himself with totally useless research; this one is killing himself over the most frivolous compositions, that one composes utterly boring works – and none think of the harm they are doing to themselves or the little profit that the public will draw from it.

S.-A.-A.-D. TISSOT, *De la santé des gens de lettres* (1768)

Acknowledgements

Over the last few months, drafts of this book have been read by Janet Browne, Chris Lawrence, Fiona MacDonald, Clare Spark, Christine Stevenson, Jane Walsh and Andrew Wear. To all those friends and colleagues I am deeply grateful for their perceptive comments and candid criticism. Drawing upon the fabulous resources of the Iconographical Collection of the Wellcome Library, Andrea Meyer-Ludowisy has lent invaluable help with picture research, and with extraordinary generosity Michèle Stokes gave up months of her time to aid me in researching aspects of this book: much of Chapter 10 in particular is based on her work. Over the years, I have also learned an enormous amount from those whose pioneering scholarship long ago tackled the problems which I have now belatedly addressed, above all John Brewer, Sander Gilman, Ludmilla Jordanova, Ronald Paulson, George Rousseau, Barbara Stafford and Peter Wagner.

Most of the work for this book was undertaken during the happy years I spent at the Wellcome Institute for the History of Medicine in London, disbanded last year. I am delighted to acknowledge the enormous support given to me by members of the staff, notably my secretaries, first Frieda Houser and then Rebecca Baker, and Caroline Overy and Sharon Messenger as research assistants (and, in the final stages, Jane Henderson). Retyping of the seemingly endless drafts has been done by the tireless and unfailing Sheila Lawler. Thanks also to Jed Lawler for coming to the rescue of a computer illiterate. My thanks also to Helen Kemp, who proved an excellent copy-editor, and to Jane Henderson for the index.

Preface

This book arose out of a flash of professional awakening some years ago. Having been a historian all my working life, it dawned upon me that I had never seriously examined images or grappled with visual evidence.

Though shocking, the belatedness of my recognition of this blindspot should come as no surprise. For we historians have always been Gutenberg's children, trapped in webs of words. We pore over written sources, back our arguments with verbal evidence, communicate our findings in prose – and demand the last word. The fact that writing on paper (or tomorrow, the website) forms our raw materials and the tools of our trade amounts, for the most part, to sound sense, for it reflects a key truth about the recorded past: making history has meant getting yourself written into it. The pen may never truly have been mightier than the sword – such authorial delusions of grandeur! – but it has routinely been near the right hand of the mighty. The elites most scholars study have been commemorated in documentation, through scribes and inscriptions, ledgers and letters, and ultimately elegies, obituaries and obelisks. In the Beginning was the Word and, ever since that *incipit*, in myriad ways ours has been and remains a logocentric world, dominated by the 'peoples of the book' and their philosophy of 'write is might'.

Indeed cultural snobberies have disparaged the *merely* visual. Appearances deceive, we say; beauty is but skin deep, appealing to the eye not mind; and what are pictures but beguiling shadows that flicker on the cave wall, mere simulacra or travesties of truth?[1] Down the centuries the distrust of 'appearances' and 'show' enjoined by Platonism and by Judaeo-Calvinism's iconoclastic sledgehammer has commanded great authority, notably in the abominating of idolatry. The acclaimed superiority of the word has reinforced further preferences: spirit over soma, reason over the senses, book over body; and in their turn all such value judgments have underwritten (or undermined) received truths and social hierarchies, not least the ascendancy of literate men (the 'phallic pen') over painted ladies.[2] Even today, reading a book is widely held to be 'better' than watching television or (telling phrase) going to the pictures; and academe still pooh-poohs vulgar 'coffee-table' books, ones (like this?) prettied up with illustrations. These are, admittedly, complex questions, not helped by simplistic sermonizing.[3] Suffice to say, however, that, swayed by such prejudices, historians (I include myself) still suffer from a curious and even wilful myopia – one supported by publishers' accountants who fear pictures as pricey. These prejudices it is one of the designs of the 'Picturing History' series to overcome.

This epiphany prompted a desire to delve at long last into a corner of 'my' historical patch that I had hitherto neglected. For a couple of decades I had been raking over the medical world of the 'long eighteenth century' in Britain – patients and practitioners, healing practices, teachings about the body in sickness and in health; but I had confined myself to texts. What, I now pondered, would images reveal? Would they illustrate and reinforce the standard stories? Or suggest alternative or conflicting 'readings'? If every picture tells a story, what tales would the available images tell? How were healing and associated body practices portrayed and performed in that world we have lost?

The challenge laid down by such questions seemed particularly apt. For reasons both cultural and technological, that long eighteenth century brought a great surge in the making of images of all sorts, be they illustrations of novels or chapbooks, topographical engravings, sporting prints, technical drawings, satirical squibs, anatomical atlases, trade cards, or that ubiquitous taste for face-painting so despised by William Blake[4] – all to the accompaniment of high hopes amongst champions of modernity that prints no less than talk and texts would serve to spread the light. Unlike their Netherlandish colleagues, English artists began to address medical topics in any numbers only in the eighteenth century.[5]

I did not get far before being struck by the folly of even contemplating treating graphic evidence in splendid isolation from other kinds – a grotesque repetition of my earlier short-sightedness, only this time in reverse! The visual and the verbal, my preliminary spadework made abundantly clear, were two sides of the same cultural coin: Georgian satirical prints, for instance, were awash with words, while many of the pictures of medical scenes I was now scanning were illustrative of poems, plays or novels (illus. 1).[6]

Images were not routinely produced, independently of writing, so as to get through to those who could not read. Typical, rather, at every level of graphic sophistication, were the presence and interplay of word and image. It was a conjunction which was sometimes tacit: thus

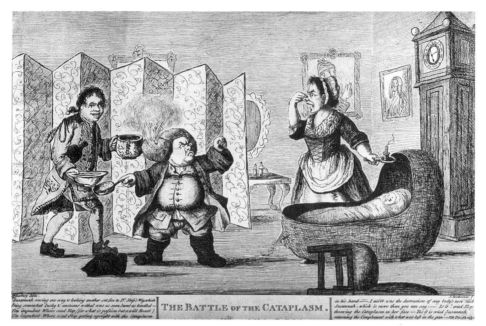

1 James Bretherton, 'THE BATTLE OF THE CATAPLASM', 1773, etching after Henry William Bunbury.
The captioning continues: 'Susannah rowing one way & looking another set fire to D^r.
Slop's Wig, which being somewhat bushy & unctuous withal was soon burnt as kindled –You
impudent Whore cried Slop (for what is passion but a wild Beast) You impudent Whore cried
Slop getting upright with the Cataplasm in his hand – I never was the destruction of any body's
nose' said Susannah, 'which is more than you can say'; – Is it? cried Slop, throwing the
Cataplasm in her face –Yes it is cried Susannah returning the Compliment with what was left in
the pan' (Laurence Sterne, *The Life and Opinions of Tristram Shandy* [London, 1761]). In the
chaos surrounding the botched birth of Tristram, the servant Susannah sets the obstetrician Dr
Slop's wig alight; he throws a cataplasm, or poultice, in her face. The etching is nearly contem-
poraneous with the novel; in the print, the incident is, in effect, turned into a scene in a play.

history painting in the grand manner did not generally carry with it, in
so many words, a running commentary, keying in the heroic or mytho-
logical figures; yet those engaged in the fine arts habitually gave their
paintings or pieces of sculpture titles, mottoes, tags and literary quotations, and cultural allusions suffuse their *oeuvre*. And the combination
of the verbal and visual is routine, as with broadsheet ballads, illustrated novels and bibles, trade advertisements and funeral monuments,
to name but a few genres.[7]

My project thus turned in short order from a putative picture
gallery into a knot of questions about the production and meaning of
corporeal and medical representations within media fusing the verbal
and visual. It also became quite clear to me – as long before to other
scholars – that the point of interrogating visual evidence must be to
enrich our grasp of cultural representation, not in expectation that

graphic material, be it conversation pieces, statues, engravings from surgical handbooks, etc., would open privileged windows upon a hidden past.[8] The graphic evidence analysed below never remotely approximates to unedited closed–circuit television tapes, fortuitously preserved in the midden of time and giving unmediated access to yesterday's concealed realities. The pictures of physicians and parables of patients here offered are emphatically not polaroids of the world we have lost, but rather figures in a landscape, characters strutting on cultural stages. They are embodiments, in form and content alike, of discursive practices and aesthetic expectations, governed by moral tropes and comic conventions, to be approached hermeneutically. Be they verbal or visual, all facts are artefacts. What follows is, indeed, a study of the real thing – provided that it is accepted that representations are realities.[9]

I should also make it clear that this book has no pretensions to be a work of art history: I leave questions of the interpretation of images in terms of the practice of art itself to those more trained than I and blessed with a better eye. My interest in visual material lies in contextualizing it within the wider cultural pool.

A word, lastly, as to how this book builds on my previous writings. Between them, four earlier books, two jointly authored with Dorothy Porter, investigated the relations of sick (and mad) people with their healers in early modern England, teasing out attitudes and actions as recorded in letters, diaries, journals and autobiographies.[10] In this work, by contrast, it is stereotypes and images, visual and verbal, which comprise the core subject matter – models of patients and practitioners created for general consumption, media constructs and public identities. Unorthodox medicine gets its due in this book, I trust, though for greater coverage of this topic see the second, illustrated, edition of my account of that subject, recently published under the new title of *Quacks: Fakers and Charlatans in English Medicine*.[11]

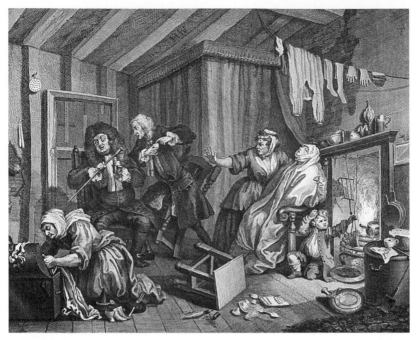

2 William Hogarth, *A Harlot's Progress*, pl. 5, 1732, engraving with etching.

Next to the fire, and wrapped in 'sweating blankets', Moll Hackabout nears death as two doctors (identified as Richard Rock and Jean Misaubin) argue. Strewn on the floor are various popular remedies for venereal disease. Teeth were loosened with mercury as part of the 'salivation cure' for syphilis, and several of Moll's teeth rest on a piece of paper bearing Dr Rock's name. One woman helps Moll; the other begins a premature search for grave-clothing. Rock was further referred to by Hogarth in his 'The March to Finchley' and 'The Four Times of the Day, Morning'.

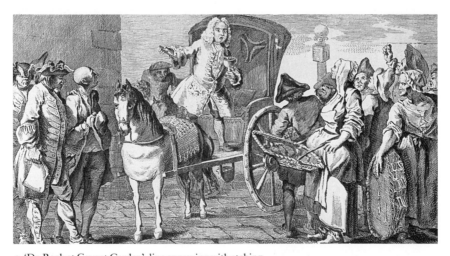

3 'Dr. Rock at Covent Garden', line engraving with etching.

A man carries a pile of books entitled 'Dr Rocks 52 ways', and a pregnant woman sells 'gin' ('Public Spirit').

1 Introductory: Framing the Picture

Art historians have drawn attention to the fondness of eighteenth-century artists for mining their compositions with textual codes and hints.[1] Take the fifth plate of William Hogarth's *A Harlot's Progress* series, which features two arrogant physicians, resplendent in their wigs, buckled shoes, lace cuffs and canes, locking horns in altercation, whilst the blanket-wrapped syphilitic heroine Moll Hackabout is expiring even as they squabble (illus. 2). Who are those asses? Debate has been spirited, especially regarding the puffed-up fellow tapping a vial of his medicine with the end of his cane. Is he Joshua ('Spot') Ward, the age's most courtly quack?[2] Or Dr Richard Rock, as most suppose, partly on the grounds that, to the right, atop the coal scuttle by the spittoon, lies a paper lettered 'Dr Rock' containing some of Moll's teeth, which have fallen out presumably as a side effect of Rock's much-touted mercurial syphilis cure. By the table, which has been knocked over, another handout pronounces 'PRACTICAL SCHEME ANODYNE NECKLACE', a medicine popular for teething toddlers, but also for that 'secret disease';[3] while round and about the mantelpiece lie bowls, medicine bottles and a clyster bag.

Notorious for his 'Incomparable Electuary' (the 'only venereal antidote'), which was also trumpeted as his 'anti-venereal, grand, specifick pill', Rock, born in 1690, was quite a celebrity, his image appearing frequently in prints (illus. 3). 'This great man, short of stature, is fat, and waddles as he walks', so Goldsmith described him:

> He is usually drawn at the top of his own bills sitting in his armchair, holding a little bottle between his finger and thumb, and surrounded with rotten teeth, nippers, pills, packets and gallipots. No man can promise fairer than he; for, as he observes, 'Be your disorder never so far gone, be under no uneasiness, make yourself quite easy; I can cure you'.

Engravers and essayists certainly expected to wring a laugh out of allusions to Rock and a handful of other high-profile quacks, who in turn knew how to get their names about.[4]

The irascible fellow springing up from his chair to vindicate his pills is generally identified as the notorious Dr Jean Misaubin. He also crops up, it is believed, in the third plate of Hogarth's *Marriage A-la-Mode* in the guise of 'Monr De la Pillule', old, squat, bow-legged and toothless (illus. 4). The house visited by Viscount Squanderfield, the poxy peer who is the anti-hero of that sequence, is taken to be Misaubin's residence at 96 St Martin's Lane, Covent Garden, here rendered by Hogarth festooned with medical paraphernalia: anatomical specimens, Egyptian mummies, a narwhal tusk, a barber's shaving basin, a pair of bizarre machines, a urine flask, a hydrocephalic child's head, broken combs, a spear, shield and lance, and various other telltale signs of tawdry medical and social showiness.[5]

If the identification is right, Hogarth was having one of his sly digs at the pretensions of physicians. His premises certainly carry the whiff of a quack, but the grotesquely conceited Misaubin – in *Tom Jones* Henry Fielding tells us that 'he used to say that the proper direction to him was, "To Dr Misaubin, in the World"' – was in fact a 'regular' physician, a French university graduate who in 1719 had been admitted a licentiate of the Royal College of Physicians.[6] As ever shuffling appear-

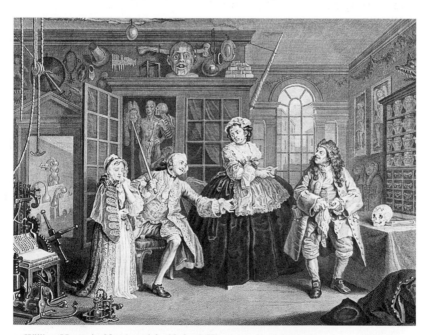

4 William Hogarth, *Marriage A-la-Mode*, pl. III, 1745, coloured aquatint.
    In the 'museum' of the quack doctor Jean Misaubin (see illus. 2), Viscount Squanderfield holds out a pill box, probably containing a patent venereal-disease treatment, to a young girl. The machinery includes a dislocated-limb-straightener. The traditional apothecaries' crocodile lurks in the eaves.

ance and reality, Hogarth invites us to infer that it is ostentatious regulars who are the true charlatans. His verbal/visual puns thus provoke many reflections: there is far more to the prints than meets the eye.

Book titles, mottos, captions and other bits and pieces of writing are frequently planted in prints, at first sight to clue the viewer in on the artist's message, if actually to sow doubt through visual punning, jarring juxtapositions and double meanings.[7] Take George Cruikshank's 'The Blue Devils—!!' (illus. 35). Sitting by a grate empty save for a long bill, a depressed gentleman clad in nightgown, cap and slippers is beleaguered by various devils: a bailiff serves him a writ; a hangman drapes a noose around his neck; a demon obligingly offers him a cut-throat razor. At his feet a minuscule beadle escorts three women, heavy with child, and, ushered by a skeletal physician, an undertaker scurries towards him, ominously bearing a coffin. On the wall, pictures of shipwrecks, fires and the hero being hounded by a harridan round off the tale of torment. By the chair lies a book, *Ennui*, while two others rest upon the shelf, *The Miseries of Human Life* and *Domestic Medicine*.

This is a picture packed with symptoms inviting the diagnostic gaze. Why has the gentleman been saddled with such harbingers of disaster as a hangman and a bailiff? And what are we to make of the books? Two have titles that seem self-explanatory. *Ennui* is a novel by Maria Edgeworth; while James Beresford's *The Miseries of Human Life* facetiously chronicles mankind's follies through conversations between Mr Samuel Sensitive and Mr Timothy Testy, whingeing on about the trials and tribulations of life.

But what of the third? The physician William Buchan had published his *Domestic Medicine* in 1769 by way of a manifesto for rational healthiness. Though himself an Edinburgh-trained regular, Buchan denounced the restrictive practices and mystifications of his own profession and aspired to 'lay open' medicine to all, espousing a bold medical populism as his contribution to democratic knowledge and the rights of man. For far too long had healing been monopolized and perverted by a medical cabal; health lay within everyone's grasp if only the sick would abandon the exorbitant rigmaroles of faculty-bound polypharmacy and opt for self-help, simple treatments, plain diet, hygiene and temperance.

Domestic Medicine proved hugely popular, remaining in print for 90 years; the two books every Scottish croft housed, they said, were Buchan and the Bible.[8] In principle, then, the wretch bedevilled by the blues should have viewed it as reassuring, a talisman of good health. Cruikshank, however, insinuates the very reverse: reading medical books may, in truth, be one of the blunders that have turned this fellow into a gloomy hypochondriac about to slit his throat. Indeed, medical writings themselves warned how readily reading such works could prove pathological.[9] If that be so, well might the anxious viewer ponder: is it also dangerous to pore over prints like 'The Blue Devils—!!'? Are admonitions bad for you? Should we be warned about health warnings? (You have been warned!)

If books are often planted in prints, so as to produce comically subversive palimpsests of meanings, hingeing on infinite regressions, the converse happens too. In 1768, the popular actor-manager Samuel Foote staged a farce entitled *The Devil Upon Two Sticks*.[10] Its Molièrian targets, no strangers to the Georgian boards, were the asinine pomposities of medicine and the law. Its action culminates in an incident which (however hard to imagine nowadays!) evidently tickled London's theatregoers: a street demo staged in 1767 by the Licentiates (rank and file) of the Royal College of Physicians, in protest against the power monopoly enjoyed within that august institution by its Fellows, the inner elite (illus. 36).[11] One scene in Foote's play features a knot of lawyers and practitioners poring over a sheet of paper:

> SQUIB … such a print, poys! just fresh from the plate; Feel it; so wet you may wring it.
>
> JULEP And pray, good doctor, what is the subject?
>
> SQUIB Subject? Gad take me, a trimmer! this will make some folks that we know look about them; Hey, Julep, don't you think this will sting?
>
> JULEP I profess I don't understand it.
>
> SQUIB No? Why, zounds, it is as plain as a pikestaff; in your own way too, you blockhead! Can't you see? Read the title, you rogue! But, perhaps you can't without spectacles. Let me see; ay, 'The State-Quacks; or, Britannia dying.' You take it?
>
> JULEP Very well.
>
> SQUIB There you see her stretched along on a pallet; you may know she is Britannia, by the shield and spear at the head of her bed.
>
> APOZEM Very plain; for all the world like the wrong side of a halfpenny.
>
> SQUIB Well said, little Apozem! You have discernment I see. Her disease is a lethargy; you see how sick she is, by holding her hand to her head; don't you see that?
>
> JULEP I do, I do.
>
> SQUIB Well then, look at that figure there upon her left hand.
>
> JULEP Which!
>
> SQUIB Why he that holds a draught to her mouth.

JULEP What, the man with the phial?

SQUIB Ay, he, with the phial: That is supposed to be ... [whispers] offering her laudanum, to lull her faster asleep.

JULEP Laudanum! a noble medicine when administered properly; I remember once, in a locked jaw ...

SQUIB Damn your lock'd jaw! hold your prating you puppy! I wish your jaws were lock'd! Pox take him, I have forgot what I was going to ... Apozem, where did I leave off?

APOZEM You left off at faster asleep.

SQUIB True; I was at faster asleep. Well then, you see that thin figure there with the meagre chaps; he with the straw in his hand?

APOZEM Very plain.

SQUIB He is supposed to be ... [whispers] You take me.

JULEP Ay, ay.

SQUIB Who rouses Britannia, by tickling her nose with that straw; she starts, and with a jerk ... [starting, strikes Julep.] I beg pardon! ... and with a jerk knocks the bottle of laudanum out of his hand; and so, by that there mans, you see, Britannia is delivered from death.

JULEP Ay, ay.

SQUIB Hey! you swallow the satire : Pretty bitter I think?

JULEP I can't say that I quite understand ... that is ... a ... a ...

SQUIB Not understand? then what a fool am I to throw away my time on a dunce! I shall miss too the reading a new pamphlet in Red-Lyon-Square; and at six I must be at Serjeant's-Inn, to justify bail for a couple of journey-men printers.

APOZEM But, Dr Squib, you seem to have forgot the case of the College, your brethren.

SQUIB I have no time to attend their trifling squabbles: The nation! the nation! Mr Apozem, engrosses my care.[12]

I have not been able to find a print titled 'The State-Quacks; or, Britannia Dying' which precisely corresponds to Foote's description.[13] Many, however, broadly depicted the sort of scene here mentioned, a symbolic Britannia languishing, diseased, neglected or poisoned by false doctors (read: politicians), though perhaps ultimately rescued by a heroic one. Along these lines a Gillray engraving of 1804, 'BRITANNIA Between DEATH and the DOCTOR'S' (illus. 38), showed the nation being treated, or rather mistreated, by its doctors, that is, statesmen.[14] Crowing over Henry Addington's ignominious exit from office, Gillray implied that the former prime minister's nostrums ('Composing Draft') had left the wan Britannia on the brink of the grave – death being personified as the arch-enemy Napoleon, then preparing an invasion. The body politic is rescued only by the return of her one-time chief physician, Pitt the Younger, represented booting Addington (himself a doctor's son) out of the House, while also trampling over Charles James Fox's bloated body. Pitt brandishes, like a lantern, a flask of 'Constitutional Restorative', while *The Art of Restoring Health* (another text-within-a-print) pokes out of his pocket. Lying discarded on the ground are 'Whig Pills' (actually dice, Fox being a notorious gamester; the Whigs are a gamble), and in Fox's raised hand, alongside bogus remedies, is some 'Republican Balsam'.[15]

Foote's comic cameo, and the questions it prompts, serves as my curtain-raiser. Mention of a print called 'The State-Quacks' was surely enough in itself to have pricked up the ears of Georgian theatre-goers tuned in to news, gossip and rumour.[16] One conventional representative device is inscribed humorously by Foote within another; not, in this case, the archetypal 'play within a play' but the 'print within a play'. The laugh is on the prating Welsh lawyer Squib and the apothecaries Julep and Apozem as they bicker with each other over its hieroglyphics – just as the likes of Rock and Misaubin would proverbially bicker over their diagnoses and remedies while patients passed away under their very noses. Since fathoming the meanings of such prints and similar cultural productions is the business of this book, the last laugh may well be on its author – and his readers: are we all Squibs and Juleps? *De te fabula narratur.*

The spat over the print's meaning brings home, of course, the imbe-cilities of professionals: if they can't even read a print, why should anyone feel confident doctors can diagnose a disease? How absurd that this crew of short-sighted and self-righteous wranglers should plume themselves for being sage statesmen, privy to the *arcana imperii* and proud that their own deciphering of the prints proves what good citizen they are! The doctors teased in Foote's farce are (as will be seen in later chapters) stage versions of those who were endlessly ribbed in the prints and novels of the day.

Through addressing Cruikshank's cartoons, Foote's farce and much other comparable material, this book raises questions about the portrayal of matters corporeal and medical in post-Restoration England. What symbolic significance did medicine carry? And how did the body and healing practices in turn supply metaphorical commentary upon the wider worlds of politics and the body politic? Major developments in health and society were making such issues matters of moment.

In the early modern centuries no one could afford to ignore the darts of disease. Every soul walked in the shadow of death – indeed even to be in the land of the living was the survivor's privilege, for so many had already fallen, notably in infancy and childhood. The Restoration brought the worst outbreak of plague for 300 years, with one in eight Londoners dying in 1665-6 alone. That menace happened to retreat, but appalling epidemics of smallpox and other fevers continued to mow down tens of thousands each year, and so-called 'new diseases' like rickets and diphtheria were worsening.[17] Newly delivered mothers died from puerperal fever; dysenteric fevers decimated the very young, and up to two-fifths of all children perished before they reached their fifth year. Teenagers fell to smallpox, while gout, rheumatism and respiratory complaints racked the old.[18] The rise of seaports and industrial towns bred new 'filth diseases', and tuberculosis, that 'white plague', became a dire urban killer.[19] Not least, the Georgian era grew notorious for those nervous, hysterical and mental disorders styled the 'English Malady', giving the island its reputation as Europe's madness and suicide epicentre.[20] 'Sick – Sick – Sick ... O Sick – Sick – Spew', protested Garrick to his brother George in 1767; 'Sick! Sick! Sick! Sick!', came the literary echo in Laurence Sterne's *Tristram Shandy*. Small wonder.[21]

Medicine, furthermore, was credited with scant power to guard against such threats – the healer's art seemed a paper shield (illus. 37). Drawing on the legacy of Hippocrates and Galen, and building on centuries of experience, 'learned medicine' prided itself upon its clinical acuity and still set great store by its philosophy of managing health through the regulation of diet and exercise. Its therapeutic rationale lay in expelling toxic substances from the body – by purging, sweating, vomiting and the ritual of bloodletting, performed by barber-surgeons – aiming thereby to restore 'balance' and fortify the constitution. Scores of medicaments were used, from herbal 'simples' to chemical, mineral and metallic preparations laced with antimony, mercury and other poisonous ingredients. Some were useful palliatives, and many 'worked', in the sense of bringing about predicted and dramatic effects like purging and vomiting. But very few 'worked' as antibiotics do, that is by destroying the (as yet utterly unknown) micro-organisms responsible for infections. Overall, medicine's powers to save lives had barely advanced since antiquity. Nor could surgery do much more. Surgeons admittedly performed useful external procedures, dressing wounds, lancing boils, fitting trusses, pulling teeth and, as just mentioned, letting blood. Experience had taught, however, that all but the most simple incisions or fractures turned septic or gangrenous; hence operations were limited in scope yet, even so, frequently brought complications, always painful, sometimes lethal.

In such circumstances, small wonder that the medical profession elicited mixed feelings. Radicals in the Civil War era (1642-60) held that healing had been perverted by the corrupt clique dominating London's Royal College of Physicians, chartered in 1518. By curbing membership and policing metropolitan practice, the College's oligarchy, critics avowed, was blocking newer, better, or cheaper approaches to healing, including those advocated by the Swiss iconoclast and torcher of Avicenna's texts, Paracelsus. Physicians, complained the religious firebrand Lodowick Muggleton, were 'the greatest cheats in the world'.[22] Similar criticisms long continued.

English medicine assuredly had no cause for complacency. The shortcomings of Oxford and Cambridge were underscored by the fact that the top physicians had trained abroad, mainly in France and Italy though later in the Dutch Republic. Outside the capital, the university-trained doctor was the exception before the eighteenth century; most practitioners had gained their skills by apprenticeship and consequently lacked formal anatomical or scientific training.[23]

Above all, critics denied that doctors did much good. The complacent physician parroting his Greek aphorisms was an easy butt; and the toll of the 'English sweat' in Tudor times, the successive waves of bubonic plague, which peaked in 1665, or the endless fever flare-ups in the eighteenth century, did nothing to enhance the art. It hardly helped, for instance, that Fellows of the College fled the capital during plague, or that the gaggle of royal physicians made such a botch of the final illness of Charles II, leading him regally to apologize to them for being such an 'unconscionable time a-dying'. Disease, in short, was rampant and the medical profession widely regarded as a double agent, sleeping with the enemy (illus. 5).

But if medicine did not dependably cure the sick, at least people did not seriously expect it to work wonders. Partly for this reason, it was not actually viewed at the time, and should not be adjudged by historians, solely in terms of technical proficiency, scientific breakthroughs and cure-rates. Rather, it offered itself, and was received by its public, whether supportive or suspicious, in a broader perspective, as a repository of texts and tenets, advice and apothegms, 'sick roles' and 'well roles', a corpus of identities, teachings and practices to be respected – or reviled – for their theatrical, spectacular and even magical aspects, procedures perhaps best interpreted in anthropological, dramaturgical, liturgical, spiritual and aesthetic terms.[24]

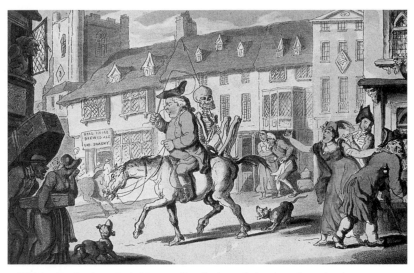

5 Thomas Rowlandson, *English Dance of Death*, pl. 23, 1816, coloured aquatint.

The prints in this sequence, issued monthly from April 1814 until March 1816, were accompanied by verses by William Combe. Drawing on medieval iconographic traditions, they show death present in the midst of life. Here the caption indicates the unholy alliance of the Undertaker and the Quack with the legend 'The Doctor's sick'ning toil to close, / "Recipe Coffin", is the Dose.' The undertaker in the window saw old Nostrum the practitioner riding upon his hack, with Death sitting behind him. As they reached his door, 'Death sneezed — and Nostrum was no more'. The undertaker lamented the loss of his good friend. Reproved by his wife, he replied: 'You foolish woman ... / Old Nostrum, there, stretched on the ground, / Was the best friend I ever found. / The good man lies upon his back; / And trade, will now, be very slack. / — How shall we Undertakers thrive / With Doctors who keep folks alive? / You talk of jobs. — I swear 'tis true, — / I'd sooner do the job for you. / We've cause to grieve — say what you will; — / For, when Quacks die, — they cease to kill.' For further discussion of the *English Dance of Death*, see Chapter 4.

Medicine thus ritualized made sense within a wider world view. Was not life itself, after all, played out on a sublunary stage bedecked with solemn pomp and pageantry? In the divine *theatrum mundi*, the playhouse, with all the roles, characters, make-up, rhetoric and gestures which marked the *tableaux vivants* of life throughout the seven ages of man, provided the organizing and explanatory categories for life's drama: all the world was a stage, whose players had their allotted lines, masks, props and cues, their entrances and exits.[25] Nor did such habits of thinking cease with Shakespeare. 'The word Person', commented the philosopher Thomas Hobbes:

> is Latin [and] signifies the *disguise*, or *outward appearance* of a man, counterfeited on the State; and sometimes more particularly that part of it, which disguiseth the face, as a Mask or visard ... So that a *Person* is the same that an *Actor* is, both on the Stage and in

23

common Conversations; and to *Personate*, is to Act, or Represent himself, or an other.[26]

'We are ... as in a Theatre', pronounced Joseph Addison in the significantly titled *The Spectator* magazine in 1711, 'where every one has a Part allotted to him. The great Duty which lies upon a Man is to act his Part in Perfection.'[27] 'My picture was my Stage', recalled William Hogarth, translating such views into the idiom of the visual arts, 'and men and women my actors, who were by Means of certain Actions and expressions to Exhibit a dumb shew.'[28]

In those stage-struck times, Parliament too nurtured the arts of oratory and performance, while street politics furnished a dazzling public theatre festooned with popular slogans and emotive props like the liberty tree, Magna Carta, the hustings, the sword of justice, the noose, Robin Hood, King Lud, St George and the dragon, and other folk heroes and bugbears.[29]

In such contexts, institutional and imaginary alike, small wonder that medicine too was not regarded as narrowly instrumental ('a pill for every ill') but was commended or condemned as performance and presentation, a theatre of healing (or cruelty) in which the doctor was a showman (or conman), and rhetoric and ritual were intrinsic to the art. In the medicine show, style, gesture and a studied bedside manner all counted – and even performed cures. Confidence was all – or maybe a confidence trick? – and a silver tongue possessed a wizardry which might work as a drug (or a turn-on): 'I can scarce express', marvelled George Baglivi, 'what Influence the Physician's Words have upon the Patient's Life, and how much they sway the Fancy.' In tune with his times, that Italian physician stressed the spell of imagination in creating trust: 'for a Physician that has his Tongue well hung, and is Master of the Art of persuading, fastens, by the mere Force of Words, such a Vertue upon his Remedies, and raises the Faith and Hopes of the Patient to that Pitch, that sometimes he masters difficult Diseases with the silliest Remedies.'[30] Medicine had always relied on the placebo effect, insisted John Haygarth in his *Of the Imagination as a Cause and as a Cure of Disorders of the Body* (1800), and the power of suggestion for good or ill was never lost on the early moderns, even if it provoked endless exasperation.[31]

Medicine was deputed, it was urged, to heal not just sores and chancres but minds diseased, indeed the maladies of the soul – to say nothing of wounds within the family, the social fabric and the body politic. These affinities between physic and ritual performance, clinched by the twinning of Apollo as the god of the arts and of healing alike, were reinforced by the notion that participation in spectacles, plays and demonstrations could itself prove cathartic and curative: the patient, observed Robert Burton, is 'sometimes an actor himself'.[32] The fact that quack doctors, mummers and buskers rubbed shoulders in the marketplace, competing for bystanders' attention with their hammy histrionics, confirmed their common functions as sources of diversion and distraction (illus. 39). In the upper ranks too, versatile individuals often doubled, Apollo-like, as doctors, artists and performers. Anatomists might teach art students at the Royal Academy, and many a poet, playwright and man of letters in the long eighteenth century had studied medicine – some even practised it; John Locke, John Arbuthnot, Richard Blackmore, Bernard de Mandeville, Samuel Garth, Mark Akenside, Oliver Goldsmith, George Crabbe and Erasmus Darwin, to name just the most illustrious.[33]

> For Physic and Farces,
> His equal there scarce is,
> His Farces are Physic,
> His Physic a Farce is.

Thus the herbalist, naturalist and playwright 'Sir' John Hill was deflated by a jingle: to endure his plays was, in other words, to swallow the proverbial bitter medicine.[34]

Medicine might be applauded for 'performing cures', but it was equally open to criticism for being a hollow sham, akin to bombastic speech, the seductive malarkey of popish priestcraft or the vacuous pomp of 'splendour at Court'.[35] Praised or disparaged, medicine's public presence was inextricably linked to recognition that it was a mode of theatre, be it a turn or a trick, cant, magic or mumbo-jumbo.[36]

Cast thus as rhetorical and performative, or, in its low and quackish mode, as festive and farcical, medicine will be explored in this book as an art (or 'mystery') transcending the narrow confines of a science or technique. It was a corpus of preachings and teachings, a vehicle of spiritual and psychological healing, a lancet of satire, a medium for moralizing, a social balm or caustic. As attested by such proverbial phrases as 'taking your medicine', it was 'a bitter pill' which purged, purified – or poisoned.[37] And by projection and transference, bodies were also invested as incarnations of moral judgments: beauty, harmony, health and goodness were fundamentally of a piece, as were the sick, the vicious and the ugly.[38]

Medicine was thus a quasi-religious morality play – 'Pain for Pain' it might have been called – addressing life and death and enacted in styles and idioms that far transcended criteria of the narrowly technical and functional. It was also contested territory, fought over by physicians, pastors and princes. Who possessed sovereignty over the body, quick or dead? Who had the right and responsibility to relieve? Until the Hanoverian succession (1714), monarchy had a stake of its own in healing, it being a vaunted privilege upheld by the Stuarts to 'touch for the king's evil' (that is, scrofula), the young Samuel Johnson being one of the last so to be 'touched', by Queen Anne in 1712.[39] Competing authorities staked claims to bodies of others: officers of the Crown in respect of military service and the execution of justice; the Church in regard to baptism, burial and resurrection (and the very occasional exorcism); to say nothing of fathers, masters and husbands, upholding the doctrine of patriarchal power.

The fact that medicine did not plainly and dependably 'work' bred controversy over its proper procedures and practitioners. Raising the tempo and temperature of such disputes was the post-Restoration print revolution – a veritable blizzard of pamphlets, poems, plays, journals, magazines, newspapers, *belles-lettres* and finally novels. About 6,000 titles appeared in England per decade in the early seventeenth century; by the 1710s this had leapt almost to 21,000, and it was over 56,000 by the 1790s. It was increasingly a world of paper, in which lives were becoming scripted by the printed word.[40]

Old genres flourished. Popular 'how-to' books and almanacs included scores of kitchen-physic and home medicine texts, offering *Physick for Families*, professing to make *Every Man his Own Physician*, or claiming to be *The Family Physician*. If many were authored by laymen – for instance John Wesley's *Primitive Physic* (1749) – a goodly proportion was penned by doctors, the most influential being Buchan's *Domestic Medicine*, just discussed.[41] Teaching readers a kind of home theatricals of healing, such writings purported to quell – though perhaps, as we have seen, they fanned – the anxieties stemming from living in plaguey times.

New genres materialized too. In 1700 the newspaper was still news. The annual total sale in 1713 was around the 2.5 million mark, but by 1801, when London alone was being served by thirteen daily and ten tri-weekly newspapers, that number had leapt to 16 million – how often in Hogarth's prints are people captured reading a paper (illus. 6)! 'Their cheapness brings them into universal use', enthused Samuel Johnson, 'their variety adapts them to everyone's taste.'[42]

Then as now, newspapers defined what counted ('news'), held up a mirror to events and opinion, moulded habits of thinking and made

26

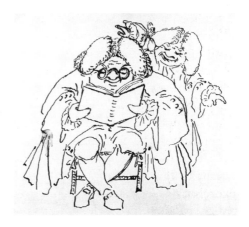

6 A pen-and-ink caricature of a fat man reading.

The vogue for reading in this period is indicated by the popularity of drawings and prints of people caught in the act. Note this man's engrossed satisfaction.

the news happen. 'A husband will warn the public not to lend or sell his wife anything on credit', wrote César de Saussure, in 1725. 'A quack will advertise that he will cure all ailments ... and by reading these papers you know of all the gossip and of everything that has been said and done in this big town.'[43] As that Swiss visitor noted, the papers were, not least, crammed with patent medicine advertisements, which, if only by relentless repetition, exercised a drug-like fascination.

Magazines were not far behind. Daniel Defoe's *Review* ran from 1704; Richard Steele founded *The Tatler* in 1709, and the first *Spectator* arrived on 1 March 1711, running to over 600 numbers. Hundreds more followed, particularly the *Gentleman's Magazine*, whose medical coverage was extensive, energetic and prestigious. Disease and doctors, hygiene and body management, medical ads, genuine and spoof – all featured in this barrage of light and improving reading.[44]

Between them, such ephemeral publications helped forge a national print culture, produced by metropolitan literati but consumed by the literate up and down the country, which gave the nation its daily diet of smart chat, anecdotes, amusement and instruction. Crucial to its appeal was the creation of stocks of cultural clichés and fictional types – notably Mr Spectator and the other members of his club, and John Bull and his double, Jean Maigre, the scarecrow, garlic-eating, barefoot French peasant, and other crude xenophobic stereotypes. Bit-players among such casts were the figures of the death-dealing doctor, the hypochondriac, the meddlesome lay know-all, the railer against the profession and, as we have seen with Buchan, the woebegone valetudinarian; some of these drawing upon pedigrees going back to antiquity, the *commedia dell'arte*, Ben Jonson and Molière (illus. 7).[45]

Familiarity with stock characters, moral messages, wisecracks,

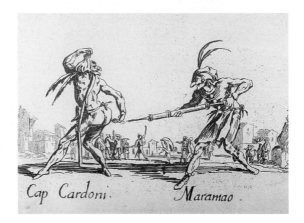

7 'Cap[tain] Cardoni [and] Maramao', etching after Jacques Callot.

How far this 17th-century print actually reproduces *commedia dell'arte* street theatre is hard to say; abundantly clear, however, is the conflation of medicine and theatre. The clyster or enema, squirting fluid up the anus, was associated with the violent sexual humour of 'up yours'.

Cap Cardoni.   *Maramao.*

backchat, catchphrases and 'sitcom' scenes counted in the 'culture of belonging' embraced by aspirant reading publics craving acceptance as insiders, would-be participants in the sophisticated, eligible circuits created and sustained by print.[46] In that narcissistic Spectatorial culture in which you were what you read, it was 'cool' to take from the media your cues for daily chat, your pet loves and hates and the right circles to join, and the roles of sufferer, patient and doctor became prescribed by reportage in the press.

During the Georgian century, fiction emerged as the medium for rethinking the self and trying out new identities.[47] Novels were just that – novel – and their 'humanitarian narratives' afforded ample opportunities for the scripting of sick roles.[48] Henry Mackenzie's best-selling tear-jerker *The Man of Feeling* (1771) was one relentless chronicle of misfortune, illness, suffering and weepy death; its human interest formula ran and ran.[49]

Anxieties were voiced that readers would so far lose themselves in their characters and plots that they would end up confusing romance with reality, trapped in the morbid fantasies peddled by pulp fiction. If empty heads thus filled up with idle thoughts, might not hypochondria and hysteria – rather than salutary home healing and self-improve-ment – prove the progeny of the print revolution? 'I cordially assent to the opinion of almost all men of reflection', thundered the radical Bristol physician, Thomas Beddoes, that of all popular prose 'NOVELS undoubtedly are the sort most injurious ... the imaginary world indis-posing those, who inhabit it in thought, to go abroad into the real.'[50] Fiction fed sick dreams: 'The common love-stories are justly regarded as abominable. They relax soul and body at once' – that is, it was implied, initiated teenagers into masturbation.[51]

Mirroring this came a vast expansion of image-making too. In 1700, Britain was quite overshadowed in that field by France, Italy and the Netherlands; by 1800, however, it led the world, with a rocketing output of prints on all manner of subjects: the kings and queens of England, celebrated actresses, racehorses, stately homes, townscapes, battlefield plans (as prized by Uncle Toby in *Tristram Shandy*), scenes from history and mythology, and, not least, reproductions of great art.[52]

In particular, the eighteenth century brought the rise of the political cartoon. Though distortion had been used for comic ends since time immemorial, its application to recognizable individuals did not become common till the Renaissance, and the work of specialist caricaturists reached Britain only in the 1740s, introduced by amateurs returning from the Grand Tour, who cultivated in-jokes as chic aristocratic divertissements.[53] It was mainly through William Hogarth, however, that a distinctive English tradition was established, his pungent satires on moral subjects transforming the craft from dilettante amusement into razor-sharp satire.

The scope of graphic satire broadened to include social targets, and political commentary fused with personal caricature. Early on, some three or four political prints appeared in the average week, but times of turmoil – Walpole's Excise Crisis, the Seven Years War, the Wilkite agitation, the American War, and later the French Revolution – boosted output and sales. While a few sold in very large numbers – Hogarth's malicious leering John Wilkes ran to 4,000 copies in a few weeks – limitations of both technology and market typically kept print runs short, and in general the circulation ceiling was quite low. Never cheap, the eighteenth-century black and white print cost three times more than a newspaper, a coloured one as much as a theatre ticket; it was not an item casually bought, chuckled over and chucked away, but an object occasionally invested in to be pinned up in the parlour (illus. 8).[54]

Matthew and Mary Darly, George Woodward and Robert Dighton, and other engravers and publishers paved the way for the genius of Thomas Rowlandson, James Gillray and George Cruikshank in what became the 'golden age' of British caricature. From the accession of Queen Victoria, however, British satirical art was to shed its savagery, and caricature was refined into less vicious forms of graphic humour, notably in *Punch*, founded in 1841, and *Vanity Fair* (1868).[55]

This book presents and analyses the medical side of a traditional Christian public culture which cast the human condition in terms of a repertoire of conventional acts and events upon a holy stage: God and

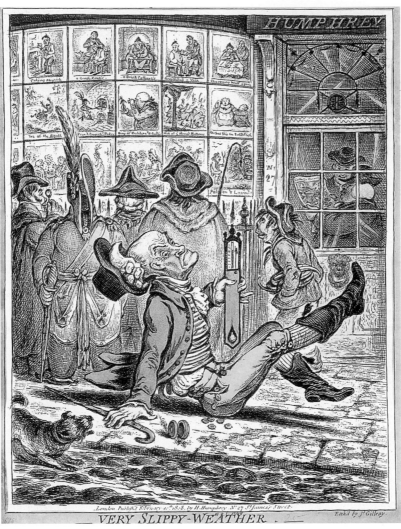

8 James Gillray, 'VERY SLIPPY WEATHER', 1808, etching. British Museum, London.
   This Gillray print shows the print shop of his employer, Mrs Humphrey, in St James's Street. On display in the window is Gillray's series of prints of patients undergoing foul medical treatments. Many who never bought prints (for instance, the yokel in front of the door) would have had the opportunity to see them in print-shop windows.

the Devil, the Fall, pilgrim's progress and other spiritual odysseys; birth and death, the *ars vivendi* and the *ars moriendi*, sin and redemption, death and resurrection. In such sacred dramas, medicine per se had always been a somewhat marginal player.

   Changes were afoot, however. The 'new science' of the seventeenth century, and then the Enlightenment, brought a shift from divine dramatics to more secular practices and naturalistic meanings, as part of that tendency through which, as noted by Mary Douglas, 'western medicine over its history has gradually separated itself from spiritual matters'.[56] In 1621, in his *Anatomy of Melancholy*, Robert Burton had entertained no doubt that Satan personally and directly visited sinful man with sickness.[57] By the end of the eighteenth century, however, such explanations no longer held water amongst the elite. When the physician Erasmus Darwin drew his Lunar Society friend James Watt's attention to the 'perpetual war carried on between the devil and all holy men', it was all badinage, a jesting black comedy:

> Now, you must know this said devil has played me a slippery trick, and, I fear, prevented me from coming to join the holy men at your house, by sending the measles with peripneumony amongst nine beautiful children of Lord Paget's. For I suppose it is a work of the devil! Surely the Lord could never think of amusing himself by setting nine innocent little animals to cough their hearts up. Pray ask your learned society if this partial evil contributes to universal good?[58]

Darwin the deist clearly found the old Christian theodicy (justifying the ways of God to man) exasperating fiddle-faddle. Fresh confidence in man's powers and dreams of human improvement were bringing a shift from gloomy to glowing readings of human nature and social prospects, even if the promise of progress invariably bred problems of its own.

Alongside the retreat of biblical myths, the age of Enlightenment also brought an embracing of modes of gentility, which raised the threshold of shame and prized politeness and the 'closed body' that went with it. The new stress on propriety in turn prefigured and pointed in the direction of the stricter codes of bodily control associated with Evangelicalism and Victorianism.[59] New disciplines and taboos were to govern the body – and breaking them could become more explosive.

With the accent shifting from the soul's salvation to temporal well-being, medicine took a move towards centre-stage, and medical men and health issues were to command heightened public attention and media space, if provoking decidedly mixed feelings. Of the 1,300 satirical prints produced by the prolific Rowlandson, quite a hefty proportion – around 50 – dealt directly with what might broadly be called medical subjects.[60]

Scholars dispute whether producers of the printed word and graphic prints had specific designs upon the viewer. In this book, what will be highlighted are deferred and indeterminate meanings, competing points of view (patient and doctor, male and female, elite and plebeian), and the polyvalency of representations. The satiric and ironic registers beloved of the Augustan temper ceaselessly destabilized signs, and it is arguably of the essence of visual images to carry no fixed point, no single ascertainable intention.[61] Whether or not pictures speak louder than words, they certainly have the power to communicate raw unconscious (Freudian) or subliminal significations,[62] and post-modernist criticism has rightly mocked facile authorial mind-reading and ventriloquism – simplistic notions of what pictures are saying.

Finally, a brief travellers' guide to what follows. The next two chapters amount to a scene-setting exploration of distinctive but complementary attitudes to 'thinking the body'.[63] Chapter 2 focuses upon the fallen flesh so fundamental to the Christian vision, probing various inflexions and implications of corporeal degradation. Chapter 3, by way of contrast, addresses the harmonious and healthy body prized by Classical and Renaissance thinkers and subsequently physiologized by Enlightenment philosophy. Involving preconceptions about class, race and gender, such modellings of ugliness and beauty, malady and health, the body bad and good, turn out to spawn surprising paradoxes: debasement, for instance, may invest the deformed body with a subversive energy, whereas the idealized body, though carrying high prestige, is shown to harbour pathologies of its own.[64]

Chapter 4 addresses representations of the body in suffering and sickness – and under the regime of medicine. Given that pain was regarded as, in large measure, unspeakable, how were diseases to be made visible? And did revealing them defuse their threat or render them all the more menacing? Exploration of the depiction of therapies bares a further puzzle: treatments were often represented as more agonizing than the disease. What does that tell us about attitudes towards the medical profession, or about the psychology of fear control and pain management?

Chapter 5 turns to the doctors themselves. Mirroring those authorized renderings, already explored, of bodies fair and flawed were public representations of healers good and bad. Before the Victorian era, the images of the noble doctor found in print and on canvas were essentially self-generated (above all, commissioned portraits or book title pages), whereas renderings of physicians by outsiders were overwhelmingly negative, underwriting the distrust expressed in popular proverbs: 'one doctor makes work for another.' Practitioners were pilloried in Georgian novels as 'Dr Slop' or 'Dr Smelfungus', and many a sufferer would have cried amen to Elizabeth Montagu's resigned sigh that she had 'swallowed the weight of an apothecary in

32

medicine, and what I am better for it, except more patient and less credulous, I know not'.[65] Why did an age which increasingly drew upon physicians nevertheless represent them so negatively? And why did doctors themselves seemingly collude in the production of such images?

The sixth chapter, by way of counterpart, turns to the patient as the hero, victim or butt of what might be styled a Hogarthian 'comic history'. Whether sketched sympathetically, or lampooned as foolish and fretful hypochondriacs, the sick as 'modern moral subject' became recruited in moral narratives which gave vent to the patient's dilemma, speaking to their needs, hopes and fears. But was the encounter with such representations of sufferers itself therapeutic, or quite the reverse?

Chapter 7 addresses the wider circles of the medical profession and those beyond the fringe. At a time of change within the occupation, how far were traditional representations of status hierarchies under-going attack? What new professional identities were taking their place? And what about quacks – the regulars' Waterloo or envy, those medical entrepreneurs who, albeit subject to non-stop vilification, nevertheless exerted enviable control over the mass-production of self-images? Should the quack be taken as the coming model of the medical man in an age of image-mongering?

The next chapter claps doctor and patient together, by addressing those conflict situations and professional crises which 'medical ethics' was eventually formulated to rectify.[66] Referring back to previous discussions, it emphasizes how the patient's body was represented as imperilled by the depredations of the doctors, in circumstances clinical, financial and sexual, and ultimately in matters of life and death. Was the formulation of codes of medical ethics truly a resolution of that problem, or just another mode of image-massage, but one more rhetoric?

Wider symbolic ramifications of the body/medicine couplet form the core of Chapter 9, which examines the transfer (and transvaluation) of the idioms of sickness and healing to the realm of politics. What made medicine at this time such an eloquent bearer of symbolic values? And if the politician was cast as the physician of society, what kind of connotations did that bear for the health of the state?[67]

The final chapter looks into the Victorian era, examining continuity and change in portrayals of patients and doctors in the light of earlier practices and values. Did new technologies of representation, notably photography, have much of an impact?[68] Or did innovations owe more to shifting cultural norms, as Victorianism succeeded Georgian and

Regency values? Did modifications in images map onto concrete developments in the practice and prospects of the medical profession? The wider implications of such matters are further considered in the Afterword.

This is a book, I wish to make clear, about the culture conveying the understanding of the body, the quest for health, and the practice of medicine. Alongside the tales and teachings embedded in texts, visual images form an important element. Prints and fictions together provided guides as to what was to be thought, said and done in painful, shameful and potentially life-threatening situations. The chapters that follow explore such images, verbal and visual, within the wider context of representations at large.

2 The Body Grotesque and Monstrous

I love the Pythagoreans ... for their ... getting out of the body, in order to think well. No man thinks right whilst he is in it.

LAURENCE STERNE, *Tristram Shandy*[1]

The body is not just a bag of bones; it is an expressive medium. We feel and experience through our bodies, they negotiate the boundaries and crossings of self and society, and furnish the models and metaphors (brow of a hill, head of state, footnotes, etc.) needed to name and navigate life and give it meaning. Language, especially perhaps the deadest of metaphors, attests our ceaseless need to envisage and engage with the world through the body and the body through the world: without a second thought we speak of bodies of knowledge, body politics, somebodies, nobodies and so forth.[2]

Proposing anthropocentric correspondences between microcosm and macrocosm, philosophers from Plato onwards elaborated analogies between the body human, the body social and the body cosmic, through which the little world of man was made to stand as the epitome of Creation ('man the measure of all things').[3] Christianity further contributed the idea of *corpus Christi*, the mystical body of the community of the faithful.[4] The iconoclasm of Protestantism and the 'new philosophy', it is true, denied the validity of such fanciful figures – such correlations were merely verbal! – but those strict metaphysical embargoes perhaps only heightened their popular aesthetic resonances and franchised the poet's pathetic fallacies (all those weeping skies and smiling daffodils). Invested as it remains with all such signs and associations, the flesh is thus eloquence itself, but it is also a contested semiotic site, and ours has ever been a culture embodying profoundly ambiguous – indeed, mainly negative – attitudes towards our incorporated selves.

As incarnations of prescribed order, body parts and sites pass judgments. Lofty and low, skinny and stout, front and back, straight and crooked, inner and outer, right and left, manly and effeminate, heads and tails and multitudes of other charged topographical referents – all flesh out social, ethical, gendered and political distinctions, as do 'Your Highness' and the 'handmaid' or 'footman' who attends him hand, foot and finger. Corporeality ceaselessly registers, underwrites or undercuts the socio-cultural status quo, supporting (or subverting) hierarchies of power and prestige. As a non-stop signwriter, the social body autographs all those activities of labelling and screening – vilification, marginalization, sublimation, stigmatization, repression, penalization and so forth – which put social actors in their places.

Bodywork mostly goes on surreptitiously: our obliviousness to it attests its omnipresence. But ours is a culture, it must be stressed, which traditionally enjoined a systematic occlusion and silencing of the body in the name of shame and modesty.[5] Whilst documenting in his autobiography the childhood infirmities he had experienced, Edward Gibbon, historian of the Roman Empire, assured readers that he would not 'imitate the naked frankness of Montaigne, who exposes all the symptoms of his malady, and the operation of each dose of physic on his nerves and bowels'.[6] As ever, the disclaimer doubles as an attention-seizing strategy, encapsulating thereby the inescapable ambiguities of abject corporeality: concealing is revealing, pride lurks in shame. It is this body, so mightily inglorious, which will be addressed below.

Christianity's master-narrative relates the tragedy of vile bodies; and key currents in Pauline, neo-Platonic and Puritan thinking, further rationalized by Cartesian dualism, have deemed the body inferior, indeed a threat, to the nobler endowments of the soul and spirit, reason and consciousness.[7] Christian theology pronounces the flesh fallen: gross, sordid, wormy, unruly – in short, so runs Hamlet's perfect pun, both too solid and too sullied. That has been a conclusion hard to escape: Freudian emancipationist attempts to counter psychic punitiveness towards the drives of the flesh, especially the libido, have arguably ended up restating and reinforcing such denigration and denial. The narcissism behind contemporary bodybuilding, cosmetic surgery and dieting has the same effect, ironically perpetuating dissatisfaction.

Broadly speaking, early Christianity, while lauding God's handiwork, mounted a defamation of the body, both theologically in the writings of Tertullian, Lactantius, St Augustine and fellow early Church fathers, and practically through the mortifications praised and performed by hermits and martyrs.[8] Such Christian asceticism was to draw upon, while disputing with, Stoicism and similar Graeco-Roman philosophies which set mind above body, and Eastern faiths, in the

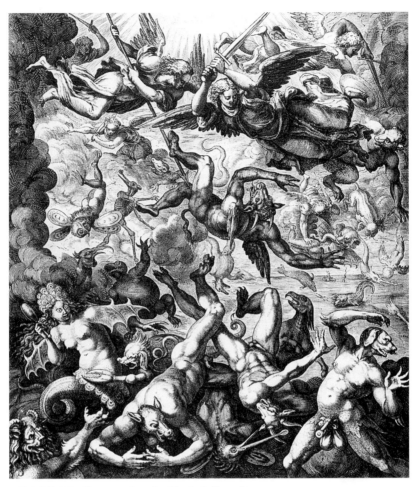

9 Ralph Sadeler, line engraving after Martin de Vos, 1583.
    A representation of the expulsion of the angels from heaven as related in the Book of Revelation. The angels' flesh has been literally bestialized. Note also the 'vanity' topos of the woman with featherless wings staring away from her mirror. (Dog-headed people figure later in this chapter.)

extreme case, Manicheism, which equated the flesh with wickedness and the Devil.[9]

Vest not your trust, taught the Church, in flesh which is base and ablaze with lust (illus. 9). Through original sin and the consequent expulsion from Paradise, Adam and Eve had brought disease and death upon their seed as vicarious punishment for disobedience; Genesis (3:16) warns women that 'in sorrow thou shalt bring forth children', while lapsarian man was condemned to labour by the sweat of his brow. Contemplating the Fall, John Milton explained how ugliness and illness were the fruits of the lusts of the flesh:

'Their Maker's image', answered Michael, 'then
Forsook them, when themselves they vilified
To serve ungoverned appetite, and took
His image whom they served, a brutish vice,
Inductive mainly to the sin of Eve,
Therefore so abject is their punishment,
Disfiguring not God's likeness, but their own,
Or of his likeness, by themselves defaced
While they pervert pure Nature's healthful rules
To loathsome sickness ...'[10]

Suffering was endemic, given fallen man's radical unworthiness, his self-inflicted afflictions. If God visited mankind with pestilence, what better reminder that His only Son had Himself been crucified to redeem wretched sinners? – and Christ the physician of souls was a dispenser of bitter medicines.[11] Early Christians had suffered martyrdom: must not latter-day miserable sinners bear their cross too?

The faithful were invited to contemplate a vile body which was, judged the early Stuart Puritan and 'painful preacher' Robert Bolton, 'an horrour to all that behold it; a most loathsome and abhorred spectacle'.[12] Guilty flesh deserved contempt. With the emblematic fig leaf covering its nakedness, its ignominy demanded due rectification through regimes of denial and mortification – fasting, for instance. Pride must be crushed. A Puritan streak censured the vain delights of the flesh. Philip Stubbes' *Anatomie of Abuses* (1585) was thus a sustained rebuke to the worldly for letting the concupiscent body off the hook; those who stooped to sensual pleasures would get their come-uppance for sure. Some conclude, he noted, that dancing 'is a wholesome exercise for the body, the contrary is most true, for I have known divers, that by the immoderate use thereof, have in short time become decrepit and lame, so remaining to their dying day'. Wretches, gloated that Calvinist, 'have broke their legs with skipping and vaulting'.[13]

A man so death-obsessed that he would rehearse for his quietus by swaddling himself in his own winding-sheet, John Donne, Dean of St Paul's, dubbed bodies 'boxes of poyson'. Falling gravely sick in 1623, he produced *Devotions upon Emergent Occasions*, reflections and prayers which opened with musings on the 'miserable condition of Man': 'this minute I was well, and am ill ... We study *Health*, and we deliberate upon our *meats*, and *drink*, and *Ayre*, and *exercises* ... But in a minute a Cannon batters all, overthrowes all, demolishes all'.[14] Pestilence insinuated itself into the ever-perfidious flesh: 'The *disease* hath established a *Kingdome*, an *Empire* in mee.'[15]

Mainstream Stuart divinity held that Creation was old and decaying,

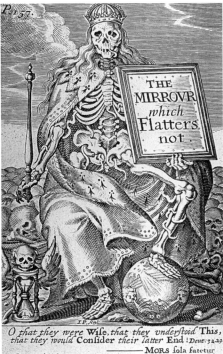

O that they were **Wise**, that they *underſtood* This,
that they *would* **Conſider** their *latter* End : *Deut: 32.29.*
———— Mors ſola fatetur
Quantula ſint hominum corpuſcula . ———— *Iuvenal:*

10 John Payne, engraved frontis-
piece for Jean Puget de la Serre,
The Mirrour which Flatters Not
(London, 1639).

The captioning includes 'O that
they were *Wise*, that they understood
This, that they would *Consider* their
latter End! *Deut*: 32.29.' Amidst the
paraphernalia of death (the hour-glass,
skulls and so forth), note Death's foot
upon the globe, an image which
recurs in Thomas Rowlandson's
English Dance of Death series,
discussed in Chapter 4. This print
involves a political thrust: kings
expect to be flattered.

as could be seen from its wrinkles (hills, valleys and cliffs) and baldness
(deforestation): 'tis all in peeces, all cohaerence gone':[16] the *mundus
senescens* (ageing world) and the *corpus senescens* (ageing body) matched
each other, and plagues, disasters, dearth, famine and wars all signalled
that the end, as prophesied by Revelation, was nigh. Disease should
thus serve as a perpetual *memento mori* (reminder of death), and death
would prove a blessed release (illus. 10).

The Lord, moreover, afflicted fallen mankind for His providential
purposes. As with the pestilences hurled against the Egyptians, plagues
smote the ungodly as bolts of divine wrath and warnings to the wicked. But
Providence worked in mysterious ways. When the pious Puritan Richard
Baxter fell sick and, by consequence, escaped involvement in bother-
some business, he praised the divine scourge for thus truly sparing him;
and for his older contemporary, the Revd Ralph Josselin, the fact that
the smart of a bee sting could be soothed by daubing with honey was
further proof of divine benevolence in supplying ready remedies for
doubtless well-deserved afflictions. Such barbs also alerted the Essex
clergyman to the incomparably more dangerous sting of sin.[17] Illness
was thus meant to teach Christians patience, endurance, love of God
and a loftier piety. 'Contempt' was in order, for the flesh was cursed.

39

Eighteenth-century Yorkshire: a woman goes into labour and the obstetrician is summoned. A servant, Obadiah, has tied the cords of Dr Slop's medicine-bag so tightly that the medical man cannot get at his surgical instruments. He draws his knife to cut the cords (a pre-echo of the umbilical) but cuts his thumb instead: 'May he ... be damn'd', explodes Dr Slop, 'for tying these knots':

> May he be cursed in eating and drinking, in being hungry, in being thirsty, in fasting, in sleeping, in slumbering, in walking, in standing, in sitting, in lying, in working, in resting, in pissing, in shitting, and in blood-letting.
> May he (*Obadiah*) be cursed in all the faculties of his body.
> May he be cursed inwardly and outwardly. – May he be cursed in the hair of his head. – May he be cursed in his brains, and in the vertex ... in his temples, in his forehead, in his ears, in his eye-brows, in his cheeks, in his lips, in his throat, in his shoulders, in his wrists, in his arms, in his hands, in his fingers.
> May he be damn'd in his mouth, in his breast, in his heart and purtenance down to the very stomach ... may there be no soundness in him.[18]

The action is, of course, fictitious – it forms a set piece in the Revd Laurence Sterne's *Tristram Shandy* (1759–65). That man of the cloth turned fashionable novelist was racked with the desires and defects of the body, maybe because he was dying a lingering death from tuberculosis and was acutely sexually frustrated to boot. Personal matters aside, however, the episode shows how the body stood as an object of official odium, from top to toe accursed. The malediction intoned by Dr Slop was authentic – it dates from Anglo-Saxon times – and far more brutal than the truncated extract just given suggests. And if the idea of literally performing a pious anathema upon the body had become a jokey anachronism by the age of reason, Sterne's novel itself was a sustained sermon upon the frailties and failings of the flesh.

Christianity posited a vale of tears, whose law was decay:

> Beauty is but a vain and doubtful good;
> A Shining gloss that fadeth suddenly;
> A flower that dies when first it gins to bud;
> A brittle glass that's broken presently:
> A doubtful good, a gloss, a glass, a flower,
> Lost, faded, broken, dead within an hour.[19]

All was vanity. 'The world's a bubble', elegized Francis Bacon,

> And the life of man
> Less than a span.[20]

'Alexander died', reflected Prince Hamlet,

Alexander was buried, Alexander returneth into dust; the dust is earth: of earth we make loam; and why of that loam whereto he was converted might they not stop a beer-barrel?

> Imperious Caesar, dead and turn'd to clay,
> Might stop a hole to keep the wind away.[21]

The eighteenth-century Dissenting doctor Richard Kay implored the Lord to remind him 'that I am dust'. He obliged: Kay was dead of a fever at 35.[22]

The pious trope of the vile body could be confirmed by the findings of medicine and science. Plague proved the infirmities of the flesh, and syphilis and other deadly and disfiguring afflictions clinched the ties between lust, sin and suffering.[23] Not least, that seventeenth-century wonder toy the microscope authenticated the Augustinian vision of man as a sack of shit, by revealing the teeming mass of repulsive bugs and grubs feeding off it. Nor was every parasite so microscopic. 'To *Lond: Royal Society*', wrote John Evelyn in his *Diary*:

> where Dr *Tyson* produced a *Lumbricus Latus*, which a Patient of his voided, of 24 foote in length, it had severall joynts, at lesse than one inch asunder, which on examination prov'd so many mouthes & stomaches in number *400* by which it adhered to & sucked the nutrition & juice of the Gutts, & by impairing health, fills it selfe with a white Chyle, which it spewed-out, upon diping the worme in spirit of Wine; nor was it otherwise possible a Creature of that prodigious length should be nourish'd, & so turgid, but with one mouth at that distance.[24]

If the tapeworm was wondrous in its own way, revealing the bounty of Creation, it also made the flesh creep.

The Platonic subjection of the body to Reason, and the Christian doctrine of its baseness bred ways of seeing which superimposed and conflated the sordid, the ugly and the brutish, the disorderly and the vulgar. The choleric Walter Shandy, so his son recounted, habitually disparaged his violent passions as his 'ass': 'It was not only a laconic way of expressing – but of libelling, at the same time, the desires and appetites of the lower part of us.'[25] In its anatomy and activities alike, the body thus epitomized all that was gross.

The correlations pervasive in early modern culture between the lower classes, the nether parts and base behaviour were spelt out with great acuity back in the early 1940s by the Russian critic Mikhail Bakhtin. 'To degrade also means to concern oneself with the lower stratum of the body, the life of the belly and the reproductive organs', he commented on this human 'underworld': 'it therefore relates to acts of defecation and copulation, conception, pregnancy and birth.'[26] Standing for vulgarity, the body is the hideous abode of unruly and irrational passions, nasty and disgusting urges (illus. 40). The identification, condemnation, control and punishment of this revolting flesh have been accorded high priority in Western philosophy and religion, art and ethics, law and order.[27] The remainder of this chapter will explore a few early modern expressions of this principled and thoroughgoing contempt.

Stigma, as defined by Irving Goffman, is 'the situation of the individual who is disqualified from full social acceptance'. The Greeks, noted that distinguished American sociologist, developed the term to refer to bodily signs designed to blazon something bad about the status of the signifier:

> The signs were cut or burnt into the body and advertised that the bearer was a slave, a criminal, or a traitor – a blemished person, ritually polluted, to be avoided, especially in public places. Later, in Christian times, two layers of metaphor were added to the term: the first referred to bodily signs of holy grace that took the form of eruptive blossoms on the skin; the second, a medical allusion to this religious allusion, referred to bodily signs of physical disorder.[28]

Goffman taught us to view stigma not, in the Greek way, as a natural, intrinsic badge of subservience but as a product of social labelling, involving projection of judgments about what is base, repugnant or disgraceful onto the body of a vulnerable individual or group, thereby translating disgust into the disgusting, fear into the fearsome. In the creation of such 'spoiled identity', the act of stigmatizing defines difference, dubs it inferiority, and blames those who are physically different for their otherness.

Psychologists and anthropologists have cast this demonizing process in terms of a gut need to order the world by way of demarcating selfhood and otherness: white and black, insiders and outsiders, natives and foreigners, straight and gay, pure and polluted. Through such polarizations our fragile sense of self-identity is shored up via the pathologization of pariahs. One stigma thereafter reinforces another: the blot of lunacy, for instance, has been intensified by the taints of blackness, homosexuality or femaleness, and vice versa.[29]

During the early modern centuries, the stigma-carrier par excellence was the witch, who bore on her body what were quite explicitly called the *stigmata diaboli* – birthmarks, warts, moles, and similar disfigurements. Often located in 'secret places', the armpit or the genitals for instance, and in the most heinous cases quite invisible to the common eye, these blemishes were to be flushed out by the expert gaze of priests, witch-finders and the courts. In *maleficium* accusations, the presence and purport of those stigmata could be a matter of life or death.[30]

The mad, those classic targets of more recent witch-hunts, were also seen to bear their stigma. Folk wisdom presumes that madness is as madness looks ('you know one when you see one'), and such popular assumptions have been backed by artistic and literary conventions.[31] In satires and on the stage, the insane figure is ferociously bestial, naked or clad only in rags, with locks dishevelled and matted with straw. Further tropes hammered such messages home. Just as the cuckold had his horns, the fool was portrayed with a stone bulging out from the forehead. This pre-phrenological 'stone of folly' thus stamped the character flaw into the very flesh. The court jester and the stage fool were additionally clad in motley, caps and bells, and sported bladder and pinwheel, the carnivalesque accoutrements of folly.

And in this stereotyping process art was assisted by psychiatry. From the Greeks onwards, medicine claimed to be able to identify madness alongside other conditions; for physical appearance, in particular the visage, told its tales within a medical humoralism whose holistic semiotics made humours, temperaments and complexions, the inner attributes and the outer, markers of a mind-body continuum. The choleric person who suffered from an excess of yellow bile became, in the extreme case, maniacal. A victim of surplus black bile (melancholy), the melancholic could for his part be identified by swarthiness of skin, dark hair and eyes or 'black looks' – note, as ever, the demonizing daub of blackness.

Such humoral identifications were supplemented by a further artistic and medical legacy derived from the Greeks: physiognomy, the art of using facial features to tell character and, by extension, (psycho-)pathology. Its rules taught the significance of both permanent, anatomical features: the size and shape of cheekbones, chin, nose, brow, etc. (we still talk of high-brow and low-brow), and also more labile aspects: dispositions to scowl, frown or smile, configurations of muscular tension and release. Artists made physiognomical studies of emotional transports – anguish, joy, anger, rage – while doctors, surveying asylum patients, would pay close attention to facial expression. Early in the nineteenth century, Charles Bell combined his anatomical training and artistic talents in exceptional physiognomical studies which included the mad (illus. 11). At a later stage, the anthropological criminology of degeneration associated with the

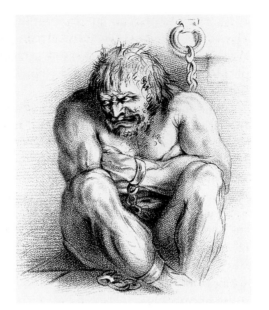

11 Illustration of 'Madness', from Sir Charles Bell, *Essays on the Anatomy of Expression in Painting* (London, 1806).

Reduced to a kind of animality, the maniac exemplifies the view that madness is all feeling, with knitted brows and swelling musculature. Bell writes about his 'deathlike gloom'. The maniac is fearsome but also an object of pity.

Italian criminal anthropologist Cesare Lombroso claimed to have elucidated the criminal, the lunatic and the defective types, seeing them as physically akin to the faces of the 'lower' races.[32]

Vileness taints all it touches, however. Stigma inexorably spreads from those studied to those who study it; medicine itself is liable to suffer from guilt by association, and the physician becomes tarred with the filthy waste products of the bodies he has to handle: blood, vomit and sweat, piss and shit. Administering clysters and enemas, abortifacients and poisons, sniffing turds and tasting urine, doctors have been represented – compare executioners, undertakers and butchers – as sullied accomplices to the degraded bodies of their patients, exposed to their contagion.[33] 'They are *shallow* Animals', declared Samuel Taylor Coleridge, 'having always employed their minds about Body and Gut, they imagine that in the whole system of things there is nothing but Gut and Body.'[34] Mad-doctors have been particularly stigmatized in this manner, endless 'world-turned-upside-down' jokes hinting that they are crazier than their charges.

The body being the signature of the soul, ridicule treats the ugly as bad and deems the bad hideous.[35] Revulsion against the flesh and exposure of its absurdities are deadly weapons in the satirist's scourging of evil and mockery of folly, and the grotesque is the art of fallen man in comic idiom.[36] Battening on those bodily parts or functions judged particularly impure, shameful or ugly, satire typically turns scatological, as in

Hogarth's elaboration upon an episode from *Gulliver's Travels*. Having quenched a fire in the royal palace by pissing it out, Gulliver is then, to his surprise, subjected to humiliating retaliation at the hands of the disgusted Lilliputians, who shove a huge clyster up his arse: the 'up yours' verdict is plain.[37]

Swift's own abhorrence for the flesh was misanthropic through and through and compulsively visceral, and savagery surfaces in his suggestions as to what was to be done with it – the solution to the Hibernian population problem proffered in the *Modest Proposal* (1729) intimated that home-reared babies would make delicious dinners, 'whether *Stewed*, *Roasted*, *Baked*, or *Boiled*; and I make no doubt, that it will equally serve in a *Fricasie*, or a Ragoust'.[38] Without exception, all the humanoids in *Gulliver's Travels* are grotesque – too big, too small, or, like the Yahoos, utterly foul: taking a swim, Gulliver is appalled when a nubile Yahoo makes up to him as a desirable member of her own species. Worst of all, perhaps, an end may be in store like that of the decrepit Struldbruggs, who having lost their teeth, sight and hearing, are reduced to the condition of wheezing cadavers: 'the most mortifying Sight I ever beheld; and the Women more horrible than the Men.'[39]

The Dean's most intense loathing, as this quotation attests, was reserved for women. Sanctioned by a creed that unabashedly identified womankind with sin, female flesh was singled out as particularly odious and treacherous.[40] Imagine an ageing trollop, preparing for bed after a night out:

> Now, picking out a crystal eye,
> She wipes it clean, and lays it by.
> Her eyebrows from a mouse's hide,
> Stuck on with art on either side,
> Pulls off with care, and first displays 'em,
> Then in a play-book smoothly lays 'em.
> Now dexterously her plumpers draws,
> That serve to fill her hollow jaws.
> Untwists a wire; and from her gums
> A set of teeth completely comes.
> Pulls out the rags contrived to prop
> Her flabby dugs, and down they drop.
> Proceeding on, the lovely goddess
> Unlaces next her steel-ribbed bodice;
> Which by the operator's skill,
> Press down the lumps, the hollows fill.
> Up goes her hand and off she slips
> The bolsters that supply her hips.
> With gentlest touch, she next explores
> Her shankers, issues, running sores.[41]

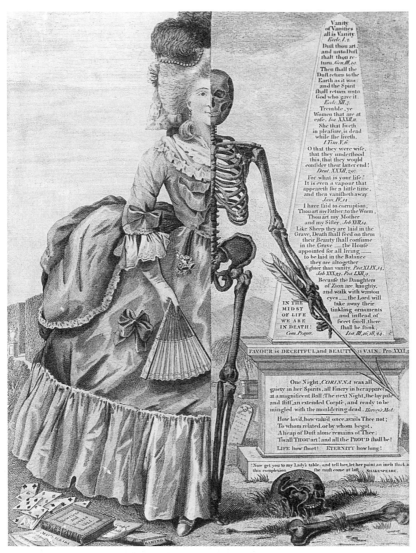

12 'LIFE and DEATH CONTRASTED – or, An ESSAY on WOMAN', 18th century, engraving.

A woman sectioned in two: half skeleton and half well-dressed lady, standing next to an obelisk inscribed with biblical quotations concerning vanity and pleasure. One further quotation is from James Hervey's *Meditations on the Tombs*, a favourite 18th-century work of moralizing sentimentality. It tells the tale of Corinna, partying one night, dead the next day. Anatomizing thus saw through the deception which was woman. On the ground to one side are playing-cards, a poster for a Masquerade, a volume of 'Romances and Novels' and a book on gaming. The idea of an 'Essay on Woman' echoes Alexander Pope's 'Essay on Man'.

Female sexuality was nauseatingly tricked out to conceal the sordid truth of decomposition and disease beneath. The deconstruction work undertaken just before bed revealed all, however (illus. 12).

Satire thus discharged volleys of violence against the body – its labels were libels; a further licensed weapon of anti-corporeal aggression was the law. With its judicial tortures (on the Continent) and other chastisements staged on the most official of public platforms, due legal process conducted a concerted punitive operation against unruly flesh, designed to produce not only pain but public shame, in line with a *lex talionis* which legitimized vengeance: 'eye for eye, tooth for tooth, hand for hand, foot for foot' (illus. 13).[42] For felons, capital punishment included the gallows, block or stake; for those guilty of lesser offences, there were the whip and branding iron, and the humiliating spectacle of the pillory or stocks – and, in traditional plebeian culture, the public shaming of 'rough-music' or the skimmington ride, in which a man might be bodily humiliated by being dressed in petticoats.[43] Conventionally all this was applauded as morally exemplary – the gallows formed the rostrum for the public triumph of Justice – though in actuality hangings tended to descend into mayhem, macabre farce or a ghoulishly voyeuristic theatre of horror.

Penal philosophy intended punishment to be of high public visibility and more cruel than the crimes it avenged.[44] At the Restoration, for instance, several of Charles I's regicides were tried and condemned to death, publicly suffering the horrifying fate of being hanged, hacked

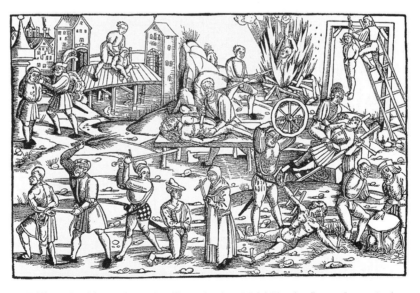

13 'Different Punishments', woodcut illustration from Ulrich Tengler, *Der neu Layenspiegel ...* (Augsburg, 1512).
    This print shows the multiplicity of punishments against the flesh, including beheading, scourging, drowning, quartering, burning at the stake, hanging, the cutting off of hands and ears, and breaking on the wheel.

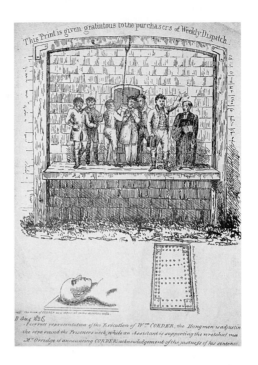

This Print is given gratuitous to the purchasers of Weekly Dispatch.

A correct representation of the Execution of W.ᵐ CORDER, the Hangmen is adjusting the rope round the Prisoners neck, while an Assistant is supporting the wretched ma. M.ʳ Orridge is announcing CORDER's acknowledgement of the justness of his sentence.

14 'A correct representation of the Execution of Wᵐ. CORDER ...', 11 August 1828, lithograph (by Bean and Mundays) given free to purchasers of the *Weekly Dispatch*.

The print also includes Corder's head 'as it appeared on the dissection table'. While executions themselves were gradually withdrawn from public view, images of them were circulated ever more widely in the media. Corder's murder of Maria Marten became the subject of popular Victorian melodrama.

down, and disembowelled while still conscious, after which their limbs and head were chopped off and their bloody members paraded. Not content with revenge against the living, public-spirited royalists later exhumed the bodies of Oliver Cromwell, Henry Ireton and John Bradshaw from their tombs in Westminster Abbey, and had the corpses dragged though the streets on hurdles before stringing them up, like common felons, at Tyburn.

Espousing the optimistic mentality of the Enlightenment, from the mid-eighteenth century penal reformers brought what they hailed as a mercy-mission for the body, the elimination of cruel and unnatural punishments, that system of pain and death theatrically meted out in the name of retribution – with the occasional melodramatic *deus ex machina* of regal mercy and (as in *The Beggar's Opera*) a happy ending. Tyburn hangings were abolished in 1783, and public executions ceased totally under Victoria (illus. 14).

Condemning corporal and capital punishment as no less futile than brutal, Jeremy Bentham, the founder of Utilitarianism, and other philosophical radicals touted new forms of correction designed to be at once more humane and effective. But if the body became spared spectacular public ferocity, it was still to be targeted in regimes of hard labour in the new rationalized penitentiary, under the gaze not of the public but of expert authority. In plans for his Panopticon prison,

Bentham prescribed a fourteen-hours-a-day work schedule, much on the treadwheel to the rousing accompaniment of martial music. The corrective discipline of toil (echoes of the Fall!) would inculcate the obedience and submission which would perfectly fit an ex-con for re-entry into society, not least into the factory labour definitive of industrialism. The traditional spectacle of bodily punishment thus yielded to more utilitarian approaches: the prison of the body sanctioned the body imprisoned as enlightened secularization brought an asceticism, indeed a Manicheism, of its own.

Judicial execution could pack a double punch, since hanging might be followed by the legalized posthumous violence of dissection. Starting in Renaissance Italy, public dissection of felons was staged as an official exhibition, held annually during carnival: ritualization within the upside-down world of that festival sanctioned the evident sacrilege of violating dead bodies.[45]

In England dissection was publicly authorized from 1564, when the Royal College of Physicians obtained a grant of four corpses yearly. The opening up of the body in the anatomy theatre – another theatre – provided a showcase for the progressive nature of the medical art, conspicuously laying bare the errors of hidebound Galenism. The anatomist's knife served as a blade of truth in a new and fashionable 'culture of dissection' expressed through poetry, plays, piety and (not least) the rituals of divine justice. Cutting up malefactors, however, indelibly tarred a medical procedure with the brush of violence and the violation of sacred taboos, kindling intense and enduring grass-roots distrust of dissection and providing fresh fuel for anti-medical moralizing.[46]

The final act of Hogarth's *Four Stages of Cruelty* series unfolds in an anatomy theatre (illus. 15). Tom Nero (*nomen est omen*: named after the cruel Roman emperor, evidently he is 'no hero') is undergoing dissection. The first print in the series had caught him red-handed, tormenting a dog. He then descended to seducing a maidservant, whom he subsequently slew. After his trial and execution, it is his own corpse's grisly fate to become a dissecting room exhibit, being ritually disembowelled and having his guts guzzled by a second dog, a truly canine *lex talionis*. A junior surgeon meanwhile gouges out one of Nero's eyes with a scalpel, and the rope and pulley attached to his skull mime the Tyburn hangman's noose.

The lesson is heightened by Hogarth's setting a surgeon, judge-like, in the President's chair beneath the royal coat of arms, replacing, but suggestive of, the skeleton of Death so conspicuous in the frontispiece

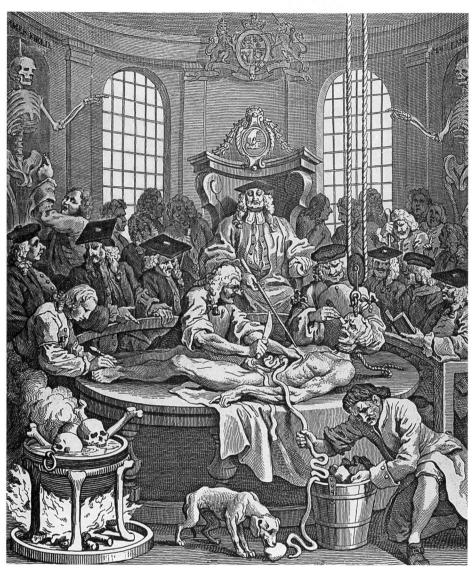

15 William Hogarth, 'THE REWARD OF CRUELTY' (The dissection of the body of Tom Nero), etching from *The Four Stages of Cruelty*, 1751.

to Vesalius' *De humani corporis fabrica* (1543). So upon what is the President – or Hogarth – sitting in judgment: the felon or the business of anatomy? And what precisely is there to choose, this moral twist invites us to ponder, between murderous malefactors and dissecting doctors?[47]

Dissection could also exact further humiliations upon the flesh, when its fruits were immortalized on paper. The eminent obstetrician

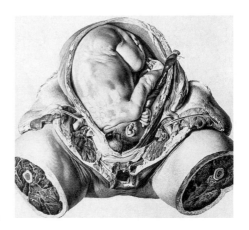

16 A foetus in presentation position, from William Hunter, *Anatomia Uteri Humani gravidi tabulis illustrata ... The Anatomy of the Human Gravid Uterus exhibited in figures* (Birmingham, 1774).

William Hunter, an eager dissector, published in 1774 his *Treatise on the Gravid Human Uterus*, which depicted the pregnant woman and her foetus in a stunning series of 34 folio-size engravings, by any standard an astonishing feat of medical knifework and artwork in the Vesalian manner. The troubling juxtaposition of limbs both whole and hacked was made all the more arresting by the female bodily zones in question and the hyper-reality of the graphic style. Plate VI (illus. 16), for example, displays the almost full-term child in the womb in its natural position; the full frontal view of a trunk with its legs apart guides the viewer's gaze towards the vagina, itself accentuated by the cropping off of the external genitals. While not unsympathetic, the image of mother and baby also exhibits carnage – the thighs eerily resemble joints of meat displayed in a shop (surgeons, of course, had a name for being 'butchers') – and gives off an air of sexual prurience.[48]

Dissection was not invariably depicted, as by Hogarth, as disgusting. For artists and anatomists worked together – after all, the object of both was the flesh – and the Royal Academy, founded in 1768, boasted a professor of anatomy to instruct its life-class students. Set in a skylit attic, Rowlandson's 'THE DISSECTING ROOM' (illus. 41) shows the first such professor, William Hunter, demonstrating to a cluster of students features on cadavers laid bare by the knife. No Hogarthian moralizing here, though there is always the tacit supposition in depictions of anatomy lessons that the 'stiffs' have been obtained unlawfully, through the stealthy nightwork of bodysnatchers or 'resurrection men' (see Chapter 8).

If also meant to nauseate, thrill or awe, all such takes on the body pointed to a moral: hideous flesh was the sign of evil deeds and base minds. Monstrosity at large was associated, for one thing, with

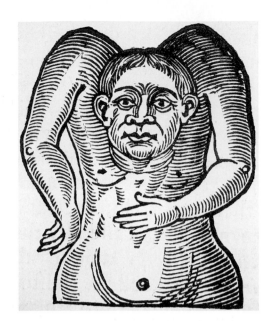

17 An engraved illustration of one of the 'Acephali, or headless Nation', from John Bulwer, *Anthropometamorphosis: Man Transform'd: or the Artificial Changeling Historically Presented* (London, 1653).

Such men, said Bulwer, 'have all the parts of their countenance in their Breast'.

'inferior' peoples and their depraved ways. In his *Anthropometamorphosis: Man Transform'd: or the Artificial Changeling Historically Presented* (1653), a vast compendium of false fashions and vitiated habits, John Bulwer addressed the gamut of bodily horrors, amongst them, the hideous deformations of the races of mankind, and advanced explanations for them (illus. 17). Take 'Cynoprosopi' or 'dog-headed men' – who, he insisted, were not mythic but real: '*Johannes de Plancarpio* and *Vincentius Burgundius* make relations of Nations lately discovered having such Dog-like-Heads.'[49] Bulwer hinted that such dog-headedness, amongst the Tartars for example, had arisen from unnatural sex: the practice of sexual intercourse *more canino* (doggy-style, from behind). In a comparable way, the fulfilment of the taste of the Macrones of *Pontus* for 'Macrocephali, that is, such Long Heads, as no other Nation had the like', had been artificially induced by mechanical manipulation of babies' soft crania, and all in pursuit of that tyrant, fashion.[50] These and other crazes for defacing the body earned Bulwer's censure, and over the generations similar anthropological judgments endlessly associated the woolly haired, low-browed, prognathous-jawed negroid type with mental and moral inferiority, and darkly hinted at their origination in bestial sexual practices – for example, miscegenation with monkeys.[51]

Monstrosities of all shapes and sizes were put on display nearer home, tricked out as wonders of creation teaching moral lessons. No less challenging to the mind than to the eye were 'Siamese twins'. 'At

Mr John Pratt's at the Angel in Cornhill', it was announced in the summer of 1708,

> are to be seen two Girls, who are one of the greatest Wonders in Nature that ever was seen, being Born with the Backs fasten'd to each other, and the Passages of their Bodies are both one way ... Those who see them, may very well say, they have seen a Miracle, which may pass for the 8th Wonder of the World.

'Siamese twins' from Hungary, Helena and Judith were joined at the buttocks; what was especially titillating about these girls was that they shared a single vagina, raising all sorts of questions about sexual pleasure and sexual property. What was the cause of their deformity? It was blamed by their mother on the fact that, early in pregnancy, she had been traumatized by the sight of a two-headed dog. While the credulous might believe that the dog was the Devil in disguise, for others the phenomenon confirmed the proclivity of the unruly and impressionable maternal imagination to visit monstrosity on its progeny – yet further proof of the frailty of the headpiece of the weaker vessel.[52]

Monstrosities of all stripes were exhibited at fairs and freak shows, if under the respectable cover of pious and didactic rhetorics. (*Monstrum*, the Latin term, means something put on show.) The Town gawped at a veritable Gulliver's parade of limbless midgets, giants, hunger-artists, hermaphrodites, stone-eaters – and, most bizarrely if briefly, Mary Toft, the Godalming peasant who claimed to give birth to litters of rabbits. Talked up first by a local doctor and then by leading London medical gentlemen, Toft went on display in 1726 in a Leicester Square bagnio, and inevitably became the subject of Hogarth's satirical eye (illus. 18).[53] 'Cunicularii' cast the doctors who promoted her as charlatans freakier than the freak. The ludicrous contrast between the full-bottomed wig of the obstetrician Sir Richard Manningham (labelled 'B') and his apron points to his meteoric rise from apothecary to physician and finally to knight. And the fiddle tucked beneath the arm of Dr St André, Mary Toft's original medical champion (exhibit 'A'), is Hogarth's reminder that the fellow had started out as a dancing-master, that incurably frivolous profession. So who are the true fools and knaves? The Toft family, who first cooked up the lucrative fraud? Or the doctors, who created the climate for such hoaxes, endorsed the reality of the rabbits, and got good publicity out of the affair, sustained in part by the vigorous public debate they kept up as to the causes of such monsters?[54]

The established belief that freaks were the fruit of the monstrous imagination of impressionable women was directly challenged by

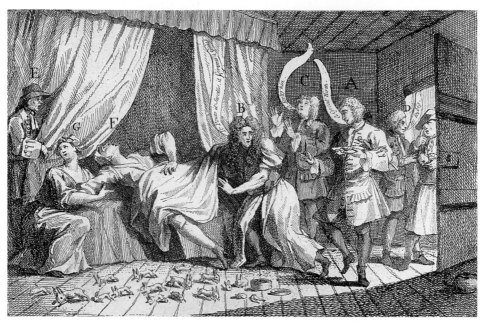

18 William Hogarth, 'Cunicularii or the Wise men of Godliman in Consultation', 1726, etching.
      The key runs as follows: 'A. The Danceing Master or Præternatural Anatomist; B. An
Occult Philosopher searching into the Depth of things; C. The Sooterkin Doctor Astonish'd;
D. The Guildford Rabbet Man Midwife; E. The Rabbet getter; F. The Lady in the stran; G. The
Nurse or Rabbet Dresser.' *Cunicularius*, Latin for 'rabbit' or 'coney', had obvious bawdy overtones.

James Augustus Blondel, a member of the College of Physicians. In
the thick of the 'rabbit breeder' hoo-hah, which had become the talk of
the town, that French-born physician brought out a treatise flatly
denying such a possibility: birth deformities were usually the result of
a botched delivery. The entrenched 'imaginationist' theory was thus a
self-serving medical excuse: monsters were not 'mind-forg'd', they
were down to the doctors.

Challenged by the surgeon Daniel Turner, who had reasserted the
'imaginationist' orthodoxy, Blondel blasted back with *The Power of the
Mother's Imagination Over the Foetus Examin'd* (1729), designed 'to
attack a vulgar Error ... I mean the common Opinion, that Marks and
Deformities, which Children are born with, are the sad Effect of the
Mother's irregular Fancy and Imagination'. Turner restated his
('vulgar') views in *The Force of the Mother's Imagination upon her Foetus*
(1730) which drew on 'the authority of Antiquity' and also Ambroise
Paré, Robert Boyle and Sir Kenelm Digby to establish that the disor-
dered female imagination was to blame. Particularly dangerous,
Turner affirmed, was the pregnant woman's craving for fruits – plums,
prunes and pineapples – while Mary Toft herself had been frightened

by rabbits while at work in the fields. For his pains, Turner was scurrilously satirized by his opponents, notably in burlesque verses in Hudibrastic octosyllables entitled *The Porter Turn'd Physician* (1731). In a further instance of guilt by association, those doctors who took up the question of the grotesque flesh thus ended up by becoming grotesques themselves. No less at stake was the question of female honour and female agency: in the age of modern gynaecological thinking, could women make *anything* distinctive of their own, even if it were only a freak? The power of the imagination equally lay in the balance, being challenged by the iconoclastic ('scientific') temper of the likes of Blondel.[55]

In such situations, it became a point of professional pride amongst men of science that they, unlike the crass herd, did not sensationalize monstrosities but viewed them coolly through eyes philosophical and detached. 'Since my coming to *Bruxelles*, I have seen a young *Friesland* Boy of about five years old, round the Pupil of whose Eye they pretend is naturally engraven *Deus Meus* and the same in *Hebrew*', reported a correspondent to the Royal Society, before going on to pooh-pooh the ignorant folly of the local Roman Catholics: 'This is looked upon as a prodigious Miracle in these parts; but upon nice surveying it, I could perceive it was only the *Iris* of the Eye, not circularly joyn'd.' Yet this stance was more rhetoric than reality. Seduced by public interest in marvels, doctors and natural philosophers did not, in the end, scant the role of the showman: after all, might not wonder prove the mother of wisdom? Coffee-house lecturers became the fashionable new spectacle-mongers.[56]

In the crescent curving from Covent Garden up through Soho, doctors' residences rubbed shoulders with anatomy schools, artists' studios, freak shows and exhibitions: the dwarf Robert Powell's puppet booth in the Little Piazza, Covent Garden; Mrs Salmon's waxworks in Fleet Street; the 'wonderful tall Essex woman' at the Rummer in Three King's Court, Fleet Street, who was 'seven feet high'; as well as the 'Ethiopian Savage'. 'This astonishing Animal', it was fanfared, 'is of a different species from any ever seen in Europe, and seems to be a link between the Rational and Brute Creation, as he is a striking resemblance of the Human Species, and is allowed to be the greatest Curiosity ever exhibited in England ... Also the Orang Outang, or real Wild Man of the Woods ... a Calf with eight legs, two tails, two heads, and only one body', on display 'opposite the New Inn, Surrey side of Westminster Bridge at 1s. each person.'[57]

Residing in the midst of all this in Leicester Square – precisely where Mary Toft had earlier sat and delivered – the surgeon and

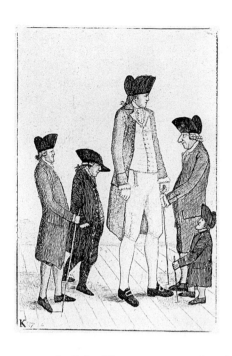

19 John Kay, 'Byrne, Cranstoun, & Others (Charles Byrne, a Giant; George Cranstoun, a Dwarf, and Three Other Normal Sized Men)', 1794, etching.

Scenes or prints like this might have put contemporaries in mind of *Gulliver's Travels*.

anatomist John Hunter, younger brother of William, netted the biggest freak of all. The Irish giant Charles Byrne had arrived in London in 1782 at the age of 21, to make a living by exhibiting himself as the 'tallest man in the world' – he allegedly stood over eight feet (illus. 19). Espying in him a prospective catch for his personal anatomical and pathological museum, Hunter made an advance offer for Byrne's bones – which provoked such terror that the Irishman, hating the idea of becoming a posthumous show, apparently made arrangements to be buried at sea in a lead coffin, fearful lest his body would be turned over to the anatomists.

The determined surgeon seized his chance in May 1783, however, when Byrne, in a drunken stupor, was dying in Cockspur Street, not 200 yards away from Hunter's home. Some deal was evidently struck with the attending 'corpse watcher' – £500 reportedly changed hands. The dead giant was whisked off to the surgeon's country house at Earl's Court, then a leafy village. He kept quiet for two years, before informing Sir Joseph Banks, 'I lately got a *tall man*, but at the time could make no particular observations. I hope next summer to be able to show him.' Byrne then made his debut as a skeleton, becoming one of the star showpieces at Leicester Square and subsequently, after Hunter's own death, at the Royal College of Surgeons, where his bones – unlike Hunter's – are still displayed alongside other freaks like Caroline Crachami, the 'Sicilian Fairy'.[58]

That eight–year old Sicilian dwarf hit the headlines in 1824, when she was exhibited in fashionable Bond Street – one shilling a look, another for a touch. Billed as the 'Sicilian Fairy', she was around twenty inches tall, with an enviable eleven-and-a-quarter inch waist. All dolled up, she had been, so one journalist reported, 'sat upon a small teacaddy with infinite grace', almost like a doll in a puppet-theatre.

Mademoiselle Crachami was a sensation, drawing fashionable crowds as 60 years later did Joseph Merrick (the 'Elephant Man'), another freak 'protected' by an eminent doctor (in that case, Sir Frederick Treves). She was, recounted the wife of the comic actor and freak-show fan, Charles Mathews, a 'most disgusting little withered creature', and the barker alluded to 'many particulars not mentionable to ears polite' – which surely explains her aversion to being touched. Alluring or not, some twenty years before Barnum brought Tom Thumb to London, the Sicilian dwarf was judged by *The Times* to be 'unquestionably the most curious of all the dwarfish candidates for public favour that have visited the metropolis'.

And why was she so stunted? Travelling while pregnant in the baggage-train of the Duke of Wellington, her mother (so the exhibition souvenir revealed) had been 'frightened into fits by an accident with a monkey' – in other words, Turner's old misogynistic line that 'maternal impressions' were to blame for birth defects was trotted out once more for public edification.[59]

Theologically discredited, morally condemned and shamefully exposed, the flesh has thus been pummelled, punished, exploited, and subjected to the prying, prurient gaze of science, medicine and the public. Yet, as already hinted in respect of the power of monsters, 'vile bodies' have had richer tales to tell. Christianity itself, after all, cast the mystery of incarnation in complex terms.

Of course, as already insisted, the faith disdained carnality: 'I know that nothing good dwells in me that is in my flesh', declared St Paul: 'who will deliver me from this *body of death*?'[60] Yet, exceptionally amongst world religions, Christianity holds that the Godhead becomes incarnate. In the flesh, Christ then performs miracles upon the ailing, failing flesh ('rise, take up thy bed and walk'); He raises the dead; He suffers and dies in the flesh ('My God, why hast Thou forsaken me?'); and, after the agony on the Cross, returns to His disciples in the flesh; and though, preceding the Passion, His command to Mary Magdalene is *noli me tangere*, Jesus thereafter invites doubting Thomas to finger His wounds, and, in the ultimate carnal gesture, breaks bread with His companions.

The Bible's unique promise for the faithful, typologically fore-shadowed by the drama of Easter, is that the saved will, in turn, be reborn in the flesh, arising from the grave at the last trump to enjoy an eternal happiness of a kind radically different from the bloodless, disembodied, aetherial perfection envisaged by other religions. And, at least as popularly interpreted, this Heaven would be an incorporated and sensuous bliss – if not quite the seraglio-like sensuality sometimes fantasized in disapproving Christian accounts of the Islamic afterlife. Meantime, by way of symbolic guarantee, the faithful were to partake of the body and blood of the Lord's only Son in the (cannibalistic) sacrament of the Eucharist.[61]

Albeit fallen, bodies were thus granted a central role in the divine drama – and even a voice of their own too, an opportunity to answer back. Written in the 1650s, Andrew Marvell's 'Dialogue Between the *Soul* and *Body*' dramatized the ceaseless civil war being waged within Everyman. In orthodox Christian-Platonic terms, Soul implores:

> O who shall from this Dungeon, raise
> A Soul inslav'd so many wayes?
> With bolts of Bones, that fetter'd stands
> In feet; and manacled in hands.[62]

Significantly, however, Soul does not have all the best shots. Body protests at how the Soul visits upon the flesh all manner of spiritual ailments that prove terrible torments:

> But Physick yet could never reach
> The Maladies Thou me dost teach;
> Whom first the Cramp of Hope does Tear:
> And then the Palsie Shakes of Fear.
> The Pestilence of Love does heat:
> Or Hatred's hidden Ulcer eat.

Body resents having to take the rap. If the flesh (it contends) is indeed a thicket of woes, who is to blame but the Soul for inflicting them in the first place?

> What but a Soul could have the wit
> To build me up for Sin so fit?[63]

Turning the tables on conventional tropes, and surely echoing the demotic struggles of the people against the monarch in the Civil War, as well as Marvell's own sympathies, it is the Body that craves release:

O who shall me deliver whole,
From bonds of this Tyrannic Soul?
Which, stretcht upright, impales me so,
That mine own Precipice I go ...
A Body that could never rest,
Since this ill Spirit it possest.[64]

After several sharp rallies, the contest proves an honourable draw, or
stalemate – himself an MP as well as a poet, Marvell was a political
trimmer – and his moral is the mutual interdependence, if inveterate
quarrelsomeness, of both participants in man's divided nature, rather
as in a stormy marriage.

In other circumstances, the very weakness of the flesh may inspire
not disgust but sympathy. Walter Shandy despised 'his ass', but readers of *Tristram Shandy* are invited to take pity upon the 'homunculus',
tiny Tristram, all marred and scarred, a manikin but nevertheless 'a
BEING guarded and circumscribed with rights ... created by the same
hand, – engender'd in the same course of nature, – endowed with the
same loco-motive powers and faculties with us'.[65] Our young hero –
'Unhappy *Tristram*! child of wrath! child of decrepitude!' – was a
victim not a villain, yet another whose bodily fate could be put down to
the fact that his parents did not have their minds on the job when they
(mis-)conceived him.[66]

Suffering, taught the Church, was the state and fate of fallen man:
we all, noted the medical moralist, Sir Thomas Browne, and after him
Tobias Smollett, surgeon and novelist, have our own hospital within.
The exemplary genre of the saint's life had traditionally showed,
however, how suffering was redemptive and mortification the *via crucis*
to holiness.[67] That precept was supplemented and superseded in
Protestant and enlightened Britain by medical narratives of the ailing
body being transcended either in release or in the restoration of health.
Take the autobiographical musings on his 'own crazy Carcase'
published by the pious physician, George Cheyne.[68]

Born in Aberdeen in 1673 and Edinburgh-trained in Newtonian
science and mechanistic medicine, Cheyne migrated to London to
make his fortune. 'A Scotchman with an immense broad back, taking
snuff incessantly out of a ponderous gold box', he hobnobbed in coffee-
houses and taverns with a free-living crowd, so as to get himself
known; the consequence, however, was that he grew 'excessively fat,
short-breath'd, lethargick and listless', blowing up by his mid 40s to
a vast 32 stone (448 pounds).[69] Though surviving an intermittent
fever, he remained in a 'jumbled and turbid' humour for a year, before
being struck by a 'vertiginous Paroxysm close to Apoplexy'. Deserted

by now by his boon companions, he withdrew to the countryside to try a simpler life. Despite therapeutic bitters, vomits, and chalybeate waters, he remained assailed by headaches and depression, however, and recourse to laudanum (opium) and mercurial medicines bred liver and gall bladder problems.

A life-and-death struggle ensued between 'that putrefied overgrown Body from Luxury and perpetual Laziness, scorbutical all over' and his spiritual hunger. Gross corpulence was not only aesthetically and physiologically disgusting; it was also morally and spiritually shameful to the devout Cheyne, who viewed his body as symptomatic of his failings, and as in need of purgation, medical and moral alike.[70]

His health still deteriorating, he travelled 'with great Difficulty' to the capital in December 1725, where he consulted professional friends who advised a light diet. He specifically took up vegetarianism, recommended as a spiritual remedy by the seventeenth-century mystic Jacob Boehme (animal flesh made one carnal). Warring against the spirit, the flesh then erupted in a final fulminating revolt: 'the whole Leg, Thigh, and Abdomen being tumified, incrusted, and burnt almost like the skin of a roasted Pig' – the hideousness of his flesh labouring under a paroxysm of erysipelas enacted the scaldings of his soul.[71] The contemptible flesh finally began to improve, however, and the bloated physician lost '16 or 18 Stone Weight of my rotten Flesh before I stopped wasting'.[72] Some ten years later, after further occasional bingeings, he made vegetarianism his choice. 'The thinner my diet is', he commented, 'the easier, more cheerful and lightsome I find myself' – 'lightsome' meaning not just being free from surplus fat but the carefree quality of a soul unoppressed.[73] This physician's tale reads as a somatization of the conversion experience familiar from spiritual autobiographies. Unlike such earlier Calvinist lives as John Bunyan's *Pilgrim's Progress* and *Grace Abounding*, Cheyne's transformation and deliverance were overtly grounded in the ailing, failing body, if also implicitly in spiritual transgression and remorse.

The spirit spoke through the flesh, and the medical advice Cheyne gave his patients fused faith and physic. 'It is true you are not a Physician, but you are I hope a Christian', he confided to one of them, the novelist and publisher Samuel Richardson:

> St. Paul kept his Body under. Our Saviour bids us fast and pray and deny ourselves without Exception, but for this there is no need of Revelation Advice. If you read but what I have written in this last in the Essay on Regimen in long Life and Health or Cornaro's and Lessius's little Treatise your own good Sense would readily assure you.[74]

In numerous other ways too, the Christian and Classical traditions alike taught that good could come out of fleshly ordeals. Pain, suffering and sickness might provide not merely the foundation for sanctified asceticism but the wellspring of literary and artistic creativity: 'the corruption of the senses', held Swift, rather enigmatically, 'is the creation of the spirit.'[75]

A tradition deriving from Aristotle and influential in the Renaissance associated genius with the psychophysical malady of melancholy. In his *Anatomy of Melancholy* (1621), Robert Burton portrayed the scholars' physical self-martyrdom: 'they live a sedentary, solitary life, *sibi & musis*, free from bodily exercise, and those ordinary disports which other men use', and their contemplative habit '*dries the brain and extinguisheth natural heat; for whilst the spirits are intent to meditation above in the head, the stomack and liver are left destitute, and thence come black blood and crudities by defect of concoction*'. Energizing the mind thus enervated the body.[76] Romanticism and, later, in the *fin de siècle*, the avant-garde, credited the body wasted by tuberculosis, addicted to drink and drugs, or beset by madness or epilepsy, with supercharging and releasing the imagination in the cause of art. Health was perhaps a small sacrifice for creativity and immortal fame.[77]

The grotesque flesh had powers of its own, not least the power to shock. Rather as with the freak show, the macabre mystery of death and the possibility of resuscitation drew crowds to executions, and folk wisdom proclaimed the miraculous healing properties of the hanged corpse, when touched.[78] As well as souring milk and turning butter rancid, menstrual blood supposedly possessed strange powers. The peasant woman's body – Mary Toft's, for instance – was magical indeed. Old crones repelled thunderstorms (folklore recorded) by baring their buttocks, while a virgin might send bad weather packing by mooning or flashing her vulva at the heavens. The pre-modern body had a repertoire of accompaniments like stigmata, levitations, ecstatic nosebleeds and visions, mystical lactations and pregnancies, all packing transgressive potential.[79]

Overall, faced by the tremendous if fearful energies of the vulgar body, it is worth returning to the contrast Bakhtin drew between the 'classical' body – the august, symmetrical figure endorsed by high culture, whose superiority depended upon keeping its cool and distance – and its subversive opposite, the 'grotesque' body, that mascot of the low and excluded. Irregular, uncoordinated, distended and undignified, and characterized by vulgarity (belly laughs), gut reactions and vital energies, the grotesque body irrepressibly violates boundaries and taboos in pursuit of excess and festivity. Dominated by its nether parts – legs, feet, buttocks, belly and genitals – it is an embodiment of sullied corporeality that is nevertheless expressive of joyous vitality. In literary and artistic depictions – classically in Rabelais and Brueghel, and later conspicuous too in Fielding, Hogarth, Rowlandson, Goya's *Caprichos* and all their ilk – low life was a succession of gormandizing, gorging, farting, belching, spewing, shitting and sex, punctuated by violence, pregnancies and dismemberments – traditions living on in slapstick and cartoon animations.[80]

No wonder, then, that the plebeian body, with its potent blood and its filthy but healing waste products, its smells and swagger, was widely condemned as a threat to the established order, in need of being disciplined. In what has been called the reformation of popular culture, the festive, drunken bodies associated with carnival, blood sports and fairs became targets of censure, and low behaviour was subjected to surveillance and repression, initially through witch trials and Church courts, and then through stricter sexual codes and the Poor Law.[81] A parallel *self*-disciplining amongst the better sort of the once raucous, boisterous social body has been styled by Norbert Elias 'the civilizing process'.[82]

These cultural contestations converge in a figure who achieved her fifteen minutes of fame in the Regency era, the millenarian prophetess Joanna Southcott. This Devon-born milkmaid who proclaimed the second coming attracted an enthusiastic plebeian following, first in the West Country and later in London. In her later years, this 64-year-old virgin claimed to be divinely impregnated, destined to give birth to 'Shiloh', the son of God, a marker of the imminent millennium. Convincing numerous doctors of her pregnancy – again compare Mary Toft – she died (of dropsy) in 1814, and her subsequent dissection brought the religious revival she led to a traumatic spiritual climax.

In 'MEDICAL INSPECTION, OR MIRACLES WILL NEVER CEASE' (illus. 43), Rowlandson captures the Devonshire prophetess defying 'the most Learned Doctors' while, with a revealing coarse gesture, baring 'the Naked Truth'. Simultaneously exposing and withholding her body, she spurs the surgeons into ogling her sex. 'Seeing is believing', runs her taunt, 'Behold the Naked Truth, most Learned Doctors', while the medical trio consult and chorus: 'I can't help suspecting.'[83] It is the time-honoured, if mythic, revenge of grotesque flesh over authorized knowledge, of female over male, peasant over professional.

3 The Body Healthy and Beautiful

In 1929 J. D. Bernal gazed into his crystal ball, and forecast in his *The World, the Flesh, and the Devil* an essentially cerebral future for the human race, a utopian tomorrow in which the brain would be surgically excised from the dross of the flesh and placed in an entirely artificial environment – a synthetic shell immersed in a constantly circulating fluid. 'Instead of the present body structure', he enthused, playfully,

> we should have the whole framework of some very rigid material, probably not metal but one of the new fibrous substances. In shape it might well be rather a short cylinder. Inside the cylinder, and supported very carefully to prevent shock, is the brain with its nerve connections, immersed in a liquid of the nature of cerebro-spinal fluid, kept circulating over it at a uniform temperature ... The brain thus guaranteed continuous awareness, is connected in the anterior of the case with its immediate sense organs, the eye and the ear.[1]

For that communist crystallographer, we'd be better off without the body, which he saw as 'parasitical', a drain upon the higher intellectual functions of the being rightly named *Homo sapiens*.

As highlighted in the previous chapter, Judaeo-Christian teachings expressed contradictory feelings about the flesh, but it was not, as it was for the atheist Bernal, an appendix of indifference, devoid of intrinsic meaning or value, a burden best jettisoned. Far from it: in that godly world we have lost, the body was not a mere mechanical receptacle or servant, but a replica of the divine, a noble piece of work – if also an eternal conundrum.

Though for Judaeo-Christianity the flesh was primarily and perennially a crisis point, corrupt in itself and prey to Satan's wiles, the Bible did present an alternative. Before the Fall, the human clay had been resplendently moulded by the Divine Potter in His own image.[2] And, however often disparaged as the dungeon of the soul (paralleling Plato's view, expressed in the *Phaedrus*, that 'we are imprisoned in the body, as in an oyster-shell'), it could also be regarded as its mirror or mansion. 'Know ye not', taught St Paul, 'that your Body is the Temple

63

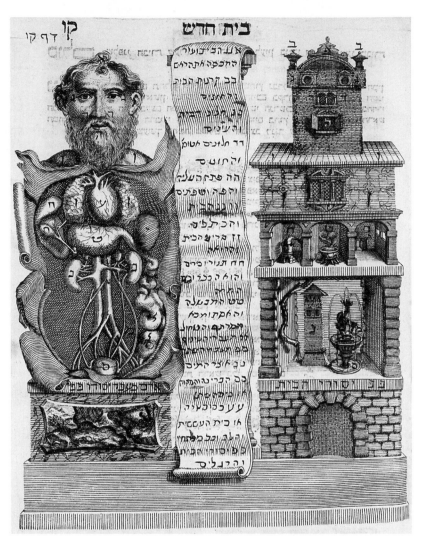

20 Illustration from Tobias Cohn, *Ma'aseh Tobiyah* (The Work of Tobias) (Venice, 1708).
    Cohn (1652–1729) was one of many artists who compared human anatomy to the construction of a house or temple, likening the hair to the roof, the roof's corners to the ears, the eyes to the windows, and the mouth to the door. The lungs are the upper, ventilated storey; the stomach, liver and spleen are the middle storey where the baker cooks and the cellar (spleen) are located. The kidneys are the water reservoirs, the lower intestines the lavatory, and the feet are the foundation. William Harvey (1578–1657) similarly referred to the thorax as a 'parlour' and the stomach as the 'kitchen' or 'shop', and spoke of 'furnaces to draw away the phlegm, rayse the spirit'.

of the Holy Ghost, which is in you, which you have of God?'[3] (illus. 20). It was thus as the Lord's tabernacle that George Herbert, Anglican minister and metaphysical poet, early in the seventeenth century imagined the architecture of the body harmonizing with Creation at large:

Man is all symmetrie,
Full of proportions, one limbe to another,
And all to all the world besides;
Each part may call the furthest, brother:
For head with foot hath private amitie,
And both with moons and tides.[4]

The Fall notwithstanding, the prototype of the human animal remained divine. 'The BODY OF MAN [is] a MACHINE of a most astonishing Workmanship and Contrivance!' exclaimed the Massachusetts minister Cotton Mather nearly a century later: 'My God, I will praise Thee, for I am strangely and wonderfully made!' In true natural theologian vein, Mather rejoiced in the anatomical marriage of beauty and utility: 'in the Body of Man there is nothing deficient, nothing superfluous, an End and Use for every thing ... There is no Part that we can well spare, nor many that can say to the rest, I have no need of you!'[5]

If even the lapsarian body still manifested God's stamp, once resurrected would it not shine in glory indeed? The precise shape of physiques to come in that Heavenly City was highly debatable – would we be like angels? and if so, what were angels like? But a blissful and beautiful reincarnation was widely anticipated. Elizabeth Singer Rowe's best-selling *Friendship in Death* – it raced through an impressive fifteen editions between its first appearance in 1728 and 1816 – presented a series of communiqués from the beyond. Altamont expired grieving for his deceased spouse Almeria. As he ascended to heaven, Rowe had him gushing,

> The first gentle Spirit that welcom'd me to these new Regions was the lovely Almeria; but how Dazling! how divinely Fair! Ecstasy was in her Eyes, and inexpressible Pleasure in every Smile! ... With an inimitable Grace she received me into her aetherial Chariot, which was sparkling Saphire studded with Gold: It roll'd with a spontaneous Motion along the Heavenly Plains, and stop'd at the Morning Star, our destin'd habitation. But how shall I describe this fair, this fragrant, this enchanting Land of Love![6]

In visualizing the body heavenly, a fine line had to be drawn between nebulous allegory and bathetic literalism. What, for instance, would be the fate at the last trump of those carcasses which had been mutilated, dissected or cannibalized (illus. 21)? And what about 'monstrosities' like the Siamese twins mentioned in the previous chapter? Lazarus Coloreda and his brother John Baptista, who grew from his navel, had been exhibited in freak shows during the reign of Charles I. The problem of their heavenly fate was later posed to *The Athenian Gazette*, the pioneering all-your-questions-answered magazine launched in 1691

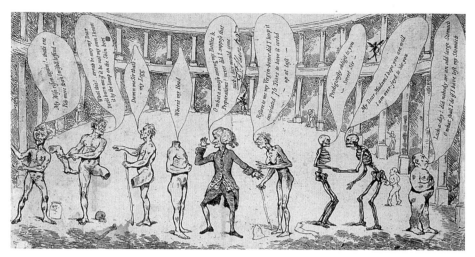

21 'The Resurrection or an Internal View of the Museum in Wind-mill Street, on the last Day', 1782, engraving.

    William Hunter was the most famous, or notorious, dissector of his day. The cartoon conjures up the confusion caused on Judgment Day by his anatomizing activities. The captioning runs: 'My Wife risen again! – that's one Rib more than I wish'd to find – ; / What this! arrah be easy my Dear Devil burn me if it be not my own / I know it by the lump on the Shin here; / Damn me Sir that's my Legg; / Where's my Head; / O what a smash among My Bottles and Preparations! never did I suppose that such a day could come [annotated in pen and ink: 'Dr. Hunter']; / Restore to me my Virgin-honor did I keep it inviolated 75 Years to have it corked up at last ; / Prodigiously oblig'd to you Sweet Sir; My Dear Madam I hope you are well I am over-joyd to see you; / Lack-a-day! did nobody see an odd large Stomach O what shall I do if I have lost my Stomach.' The rising of the dead is the reason for the shattering of the jars of preserved body parts, which Hunter, standing clothed and wigged at the centre of the print, is lamenting. Around him, figures demand the return of their missing parts. On the anatomist's right, a male and a female skeleton greet each other warmly, while the figure on the right is in search of his lost stomach. On the left, two one-legged men contest the ownership of a leg, while the man on the far left despairs at the prospect of his wife's resurrection. In the background, a hunchback rings a bell to call the souls back to life, and in the background, two figures hug each other. Two winged devils prance along the two-storied colonnade in anticipation of those souls who will be damned. One of the reasons for public distrust of dissectionists seems to have been religious fears of this kind.

by the enterprising Grub-Street journalist John Dunton. 'We find no lineaments of a Rational soul in *Baptista*, nor so much of the Animal as Brutes have', came the judicious reply:

> his brother shall rise without him at the Day of Judgment, for there will be no Monsters at the Resurrection ... but if he has a Rational Soul ... then he will be ranked among Children, Fools and Ideots at the last Day; but will rise separate with a perfect Body, not with another Body, but the same specifick Body, adapted and fitly organised for a future State.[7]

Despite such understandable anxieties as to what sorts of physiques had divine sanction, in its fetching images of baby Jesus, in the

Madonna or in beatific saints, Christianity had traditionally found little difficulty in imagining the beauty of holiness incarnate, as pious painters, of course, had recorded down the ages.

Quite independently, Classical aesthetics for their part endorsed the body harmonious and handsome, a testimony to the consonance of mind, society and cosmos, the celestial and the natural.[8] From archaic times – Olympic games date from at least 776 BC – the Ionians' passion for athletics had given rise to instructors in exercise, bathing, massage, gymnastics and diet (illus. 22). Greek ideals of manliness required that the physique should be kept in peak condition – admiration for the lithe, fit, athletic warrior shines through ancient myths and the visual and plastic arts. Dancing, gymnastic and martial arts and working out with a trainer – predominantly men-only practices, women being excluded from public life – were regarded as essential for the virile and virtuous.

The warrior as celebrated by Homer was gradually transformed into the ideal of the beauty-loving citizen, pursuing in the *polis* the goal of a cultivated mind in a disciplined body. Athenian sculpture and painting delighted in the human form, proudly displaying its naked graces and those geometrical ratios, governing the limbs, which encoded the fundamental harmonies of nature. The Delphic oracle's

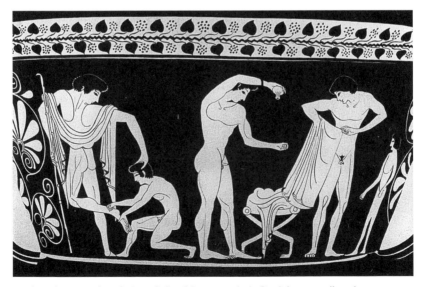

22 A modern gouache painting of a late 6th-century Attic Greek *krater*, attributed to Euphronios, in the Berlin Museum.
    On the left, an attendant massages an athlete's ankle; in the middle, an athlete pours oil for anointing himself; towards the right, another athlete scrapes himself with a strigil.

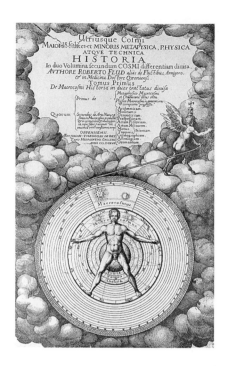

23 Theodore de Bry, line engraving from
the title page of the first volume of Robert
Fludd, *Utriusque Cosmi majoris scilicet et
minoris … historia* (Frankfurt, 1617).
  Fludd was a hermetic or Rosicrucian
thinker who developed elaborate ideas
about human harmony with the cosmos.

'know yourself' included knowing your body. A tradition was thus
inaugurated – man as the measure of all things – which would climax in
the Renaissance conceit of 'Vitruvian man' (illus. 23), the nude male
figure inscribed at the core of the cosmos, which was to exercise such a
hold over artistic imaginations and practices beyond the Renaissance.[9]

In a chapter of his *De Architectura*, dealing with temple design, the
Roman architect Vitruvius (first century AD) proposed the use of
certain archetypal shapes and natural proportions to demarcate
ground plans, elevations and other dimensions in building. Declaring
it the measure of perfection, he inscribed the body of a male with limbs
outstretched within the primary geometrical shapes of the square and
circle. This perfectly circumscribed figure in turn generated various
further sets of proportions. It provided, for example, a guide for
column design – the column being the closest architectural analogue to
the body. There are, Vitruvius gauged, nine head-heights in the total
height of the well-proportioned figure; the height of a column should
therefore be the equivalent of its capital (Latin *caput* = head) multiplied by nine. Different columnar types (Doric, Corinthian, etc.) were,
moreover, to be read as expressive of human diversity, male and female,
young and old, plain and fancy. Such ideas were in due course elaborated in the Renaissance: Filarete, for example, treated doors and
windows as a building's 'orifices'. As man was patterned on the heavens,

so the city and its buildings should be reflections of the human.[10]

It was this body classical which bore the imprimatur of art and the rules of beauty, defining the golden and the ideal world as proposed by Michelangelo and enshrined in the academic tradition in later centuries.[11] Countering the Augustinian tradition of the humiliated naked body, so poignantly captured in late medieval Gothic representations of the Fall, the classical nude, reincorporated in the Renaissance, vaunted the human form in all its idealized anthropocentric glory.[12] (It was, as one might expect, the Puritan Oliver Cromwell who insisted on being painted warts and all.)

If Vitruvianism highlighted the affinities of the body with architecture, the eighteenth century brought to fruition a comparable tradition melding art and anatomy. The body, it was claimed, could not be adequately depicted artistically without an exact knowledge of the fundamental architectonics of its bone structure; anatomists for their part needed to be able to draw correctly in order to see well. To celebrate that happy marriage of craft skills, brought together by the new institution where Sir Joshua Reynolds delivered his celebrated 'Discourses' on the principles of art, Johann Zoffany produced two

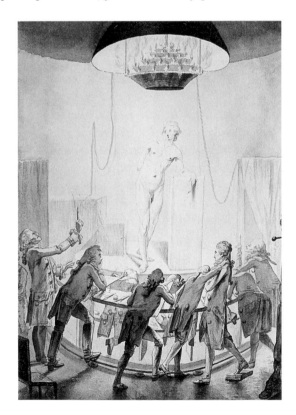

24 Elias Martin (attrib.), 'The Life School at the Royal Academy of Arts, with William Hunter Teaching Anatomy', *c.* 1770, black chalk and pen and ink with grey wash.

Like Johann Zoffany, Martin depicted Hunter at the RA.

group portraits, *The Life School at the Royal Academy of Arts* and *Dr William Hunter Lecturing at the Royal Academy of Arts*, Hunter being the first Professor of Anatomy there, appointed in 1768 (illus. 24).[13] Tall muscular males (London's carters, coachmen and draymen were often used) served as the Vitruvian models in the life class; muscular bodies might be flayed after death, as *écorchés*, to reveal the secrets beneath the skin.

Physical beauty, symmetry and harmony were not only for the greater glory of the Heavenly Artist, they were also meant to be morally inspiring and instructive, outer manifestations of inner excellence. In particular, according to a genre of sacred anatomy, the body, as investigated by science, would further reveal God's design; anatomy and physiology progressively laying bare the divinely exquisite proportions and contrivances of the human machine (*machina carnis*).

In *De Praxi Medica* (1699), a work popular in English translation, the Italian physician Giorgio Baglivi asserted that the key to the scientific understanding of the human body lay in the fact that it 'operates by number, weight, and measure ... by the wish of God, the highest Creator of all things, who ... seems to have sketched the most ordered series of proportions in the human body by the pen of Mathematics alone'.[14] With anatomy's foundations already laid, the perfecting of 'animal economy' (today's physiology) seemed just a matter of time, even if the natural philosopher Walter Charleton had thrown up his hands at the labour involved in the exploration of this internal New Found Land. 'There are yet alas!', he sighed, 'Terrae incognitae in the lesser world, as well as the greater, the Island of the Brain, the Isthmus of the Spleen, the streights of the Renes.'[15] Was it not shameful that Galileo had discovered Saturn's rings before Harvey demonstrated the circulation of the blood! 'It was highly dishonourable', reflected the great experimenter Robert Boyle, 'for a Reasonable Soul to live in so Divinely built a Mansion, as the Body she resides in, altogether unacquainted with the exquisite Structure of it.'[16] Potent taboos against the 'desecration' of the sacrosanct body, and the old bugbear of 'forbidden knowledge', may go some way towards explaining that paradoxical predicament.

Science was, however, making rapid strides towards disclosing the new found lands of the great body systems, and popularizers trumpeted knowledge of what had recently been Charleton's *terrae incognitae*. The versified anatomical descriptions in Sir Richard Blackmore's *The Creation* (1712) represent the most august example of Augustan veneration of the divine handiwork:

> The salient point, so first is called the heart,
> Shap'd and suspended with amazing art,
> By turns dilated, and by turns comprest,
> Expels, and entertains the purple guest.
> It sends from out its left contracted side
> Into th' arterial tube its vital pride:
> Which tube, prolong'd but little from its source,
> Parts its wide trunk, and takes a double course;
> One channel to the head its path directs,
> One to th' inferior limbs its path inflects.[17]

The heart and the vascular system may not have made for palatable poetry but they were prized as the finest proofs of a wise and benevolent God.[18]

The religious, scientific, moral and other traditions just reviewed combined to underwrite the ideal of the proper body, and a magazine of body images demarcated the normal and noble from the defective, offensive and unseemly. The exemplary body, as spelt out for instance in artists' manuals, was to be upright rather than crooked; its face was to be symmetrical and display a high forehead – or, as we meaningfully say, 'temples'; it was to have an aquiline, rather than a flat or snub nose. A becoming appearance was debonair not ferocious; and, most important of all perhaps, the ideal body was to be light-skinned rather than dark (swarthiness betrayed animality and melancholy). Fair means light, pale-skinned, but also exalted of feelings, or simply beautiful, as with Shakespeare's Sylvia in *The Two Gentlemen of Verona*, 'lovely fair', or the 'fair sex'. In all such matters, as will be obvious, we are in the realm not of mere human biology or chemical pigments – no human is snow white or jet black – but of metaphorical tints, the hues of imagination.[19]

Mikhail Bakhtin styled the forms endorsed by official high culture the 'classical body', in contrast to the 'grotesque body' discussed in the previous chapter.[20] Well-proportioned and symmetrical by design, the classical body and face had their own prescriptive geometry upheld and rationalized by such traditions as physiognomy (the art of reading the face), and, later, phrenology (illus. 42), whose key doctrine that the contours of the skull revealed character presumed the homology between a good head and a good temperament.[21] The distinguishing characteristics of the approved body and its bearing were further classified in terms of rank and station. 'Every class of society has its own glory', noted Mary Anne Schimmelpenninck: 'The poor, his physical strength; the middle, the power of mental research; the elevated, the charm of manner, the amalgam which fits them as keystones to solidify the arch of society.'[22] The body beautiful (or as that prim Midlands Quaker put it, 'charming') was, unsurprisingly, indexed onto the 'higher', or ornamental, ranks. Indeed the 'upper' class body was, in actuality, more elevated – anthropometric studies have shown that, a couple of centuries ago, the elite were perhaps four or five inches taller than the poor.[23] And not only were the high-born taller, they were credited with superior tone and bloom. 'The skin, pores, muscles and nerves of a day-labourer', remarked the philosopher David Hume, 'are different from those of a man of quality.'[24]

Elaborate social parade, courtly protocols, gesture and dress codes vaunted and flaunted the superior ('classical') body upon the social stage. Yet, with more than a touch of conspicuous paradox, in a tradition ultimately owing much to Baldassare Castiglione's *Book of the Courtier* (1528), its effortless superiority was held to reside in disciplined understatement and in such perfect self-control (*retenu*) that it would never attract attention to itself – indeed, might almost vanish. Grace or elegance was the essence, for instance, of the dance, but such footwork and bodywork as the minuet required impeccable control of timing, balance and gesture. Fashionable carriage was a strictly regulated ballet.[25] While Junior Keeper of the Robes at George III's court, Fanny Burney, soon to be a celebrated novelist, drew up '*Directions for Coughing, Sneezing or Moving*, Before the King and Queen', a mock-serious list of commandments for courtly comportment designed to perfect the body by making it utterly immobile, invisible and inaudible. 'In the first place you must not cough', she instructed,

> If you find a cough tickling in your throat, you must arrest it from making any sound; if you find yourself choking with the forbearance, you must choke – but not cough. In the second place you must not sneeze. If you have a vehement cold, you must take no notice of it; if your nose-membranes feel a great irritation, you must hold your breath; if a sneeze still insists upon making its way, you must oppose it, by keeping your teeth grinding together; if the violence of the repulse breaks some blood-vessel you must break the blood vessel – but not sneeze. In the third place, you must not, upon any account, stir either hand or foot. If, by chance, a black pin runs into your head, you must not take it out. If the pain is very great, you must be sure to bear it without wincing; if it brings the tears into your eyes, you must not wipe them off; if they give you a tingling by running down your cheeks, you must look as if nothing was the matter. If the blood should gush from your head by means of the black pin, you must let it gush; if you are uneasy to think of making such a blurred appearance, you must be uneasy, but you must say nothing about it.[26]

Enlightened England was, however, a realm which prided itself upon its liberty, even at Windsor. Hence, noted Burney, the theatre of cruelty respected civilized limits:

> If, however, the agony is very great, you may, privately, bite the inside of your cheek, or of your lips, for a little relief, taking care, meanwhile, to do it so cautiously with that precaution, if you even gnaw a piece out, it will not be minded, only be sure either to swallow it, or commit it to a corner of the inside of your mouth till they are gone – for you must not spit.[27]

Flawless self-mastery marked the execution of the superior presentation of the social self, rather as what made the dandy the best-dressed man was that the exquisite austerity of his get-up betrayed not a whiff of excess or accident.[28]

Exhibition of the body in all its glory ranged from the meticulously choreographed grand opera (or *opera buffa*) of court down to the perfectly eccentric. On her demise in 1775, the surgeon and dentist Martin Van Butchell opted to have his wife's corpse embalmed, dolled up and displayed to view. With the assistance of William Hunter, her blood vessels were injected with camphorated spirit of wine and carmine dye, so that the lips retained their colour; and, packed with camphor, the body remained uncorrupted as if in a state of sleep. Van Butchell, further discussed in Chapter 8, long took pleasure in displaying her preserved and beautified corpse to friends and visitors.[29]

What Mrs Van Butchell would have made of all this we do not know. Some other singular souls were keen, however, to have their own remains put to public profit. One was the fashionable Georgian physician, Messenger Monsey, who, as an unbeliever, stipulated that on his death his corpse should be dissected, before being tossed into the Thames.[30] The pioneer Utilitarian, Jeremy Bentham – also, significantly, no Christian – set a public-spirited example by bequeathing his carcass to posterity, professing that 'how little service soever it may have been in my power to render to mankind during my lifetime, I shall at least be not altogether useless after my death'. He should be dissected, Bentham directed, and thereafter displayed, preserved and fully clothed, in a glass case as an 'auto-icon'. He is still thus on show, or on guard, near the entrance of University College, London (illus. 25).[31]

Published just before his death, Bentham's *Auto-icon; or, Farther Uses of the Dead to the Living* (1831) commended such exhibition of the preserved bodies of the good and the great: having 'every man [as] his own statue' would not only be more edifying but also cheaper than investing in marble or bronze. His atheistic and materialist philosophy

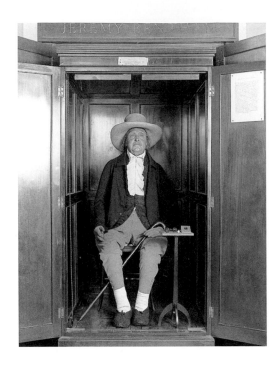

25 'Auto-icon' of Jeremy
Bentham (1748–1832) in
University College, London.

thus envisaged a double use for corpses, one 'anatomical, or dissec-
tional', the other 'conservative, or statuary'.[32]

Overriding the Church's condemnation of pride, vanity and lubricity, parade of the eroticized female form was sanctioned in the names of
beauty, charm and aesthetics, and all the more so after the Restoration
as public morals relaxed and the media and fashion industries were
fuelled by sex appeal. As well as being Charles II's 'Protestant whore',
Nell Gwyn performed as an actress and artist's model. Born in Soho in
1738, Kitty Fisher's charms came to the attention of London's leading
gallants; she enjoyed a succession of prominent lovers, and, as a belle
turned celebrity, was twice painted by Sir Joshua Reynolds. Then
suddenly she fell sick, due, perhaps as malicious gossip had it, to over-
use of the highly poisonous lead-based cosmetics ('paints') of the day,
and within five months, at the age of 29, she was dead. Attractiveness,
said the moralizers, was a treacherous gift, and painted ladies would
pay dearly for their vanity.

Starting out in the capital in domestic service, the buxom country
girl Emma Hart (also known as Lyon) similarly attracted attention
through her 'exquisite beauty', moving on to become George
Romney's favourite sitter. Gaining entrée into fashionable society, she
became, successively, mistress to Sir Harry Fetherstonehaugh and to
the Hon. Charles Greville, who, in return for the discharge of his

debts, passed her on to his uncle, Sir William Hamilton, British Minister Plenipotentiary in Naples. Rather eccentrically, that ageing gentleman went on to marry her before she finally became Nelson's lover (on his death, Nelson famously left her 'to the nation').

Emma won notoriety for her 'postures' (illus. 26), gauze-draped poses representing renowned scenes from classical mythology, the tasteful eighteenth-century equivalent of striptease enjoyed by ex-pats in Naples (excavations in nearby Pompeii and Herculanaeum had been revealing the eroticism of Ancient Rome). If initially disposed to be amused and titillated, in due course the fickle public back home took revenge on her for her meteoric rise to renown by spitefully rejoicing in revelations of her middle-aged descent into blowsy corpulence.

In a man's world, the accent inevitably fell upon the display of female bodily assets as an erotic commodity, appreciated by the discerning male, be he painter, beau, rake or connoisseur. The mutilated Nelson was a hero, Emma just a body. What it was precisely which differentiated male and female and thus constituted the 'looks' of the 'sex' which the male gaze could appropriate stirred heated debate: was

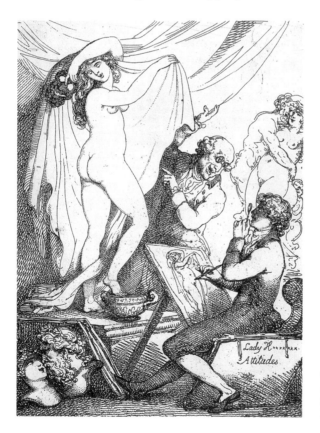

26 'Lady H*******
Attitudes', undated
engraving. British
Museum, London.

the female physique a version of the male? – albeit smaller and weaker, and so evidently imperfect and inferior; or did it constitute a distinct prototype?[33] 'The habite [flesh] of a woman is fatter, looser and softer', wrote the physician Helkiah Crooke, in one seventeenth-century attempt to resolve that riddle of riddles:

> The flesh of men is more solide ... and beside, [women] liue an idle and sedentarie life ... The woman was ordayned to receiue and conceiue the seede of the man, to beare and nourish the Infant, to gouerne and moderate the house at home, to delight and refresh her husband forswunke with labour and well-nigh exhausted and spent with care and travell; and therefore her body is soft, smooth and delicate, made especially for pleasure.[34]

Crooke thus read the female build as ordaining the 'helpmeet' part. Backed by what seemed scientific and medical testimony, eighteenth-century opinion elaborated the notion that hers was a constitution designed to be nurturing, James Thomson lecturing the 'British Fair' on their consequent 'natural' duties:

> Well-order'd Home Man's best Delight to make;
> And by submissive Wisdom, modest skill,
> With every gentle Care-eluding Art,
> To raise the Virtues, animate the bliss,
> Even charm the Pains to something more than Joy
> And sweeten all the Toils of human Life:
> This be the female Dignity and Praise.[35]

Nature, it was claimed, had formed a woman principally for motherhood, proof of which lay not just in her curvaceous softness at large but specifically in the breasts, whose snowy, swelling amplitude was endlessly celebrated alike in erotic art, bawdy tales, medico-scientific writing on motherhood, and the sartorial shapes of the day.[36]

Commended as essential to physical well-being, sexuality acquired a new stamp of approval in the eighteenth century. Waving aside age-old Christian reproofs against the seductiveness of the flesh, enlightened and scientific discourses held that the youthful, nubile body was entitled to due hedonic gratifications – denied which, it would shrivel and breed psychophysical complaints. Properly channelled, sexual desire promoted matrimony and populated the nation. Rather than condemning carnality, as with Augustinian theology, or regarding coitus as legitimate only with offspring in mind, Georgian sexual advice literature maintained that the erotic constituted a pleasure in its own right and a contribution to physical health and conjugal bliss.[37] The leading physician Erasmus Darwin, who sired fourteen children,

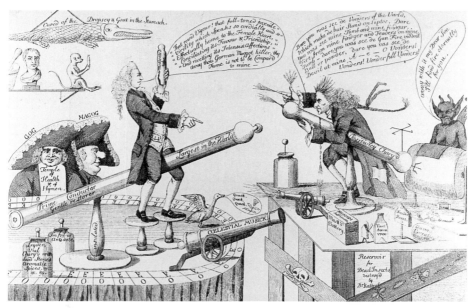

27 'The Quacks', 1783, engraving.
　　It was James Graham's claim that medical electricity could cure impotence; hence the giant phallic electrical conductor which he bestrides. Gustavus Katterfelto, by contrast, claimed that influenza had to do with plagues of insects, a view found preposterous in his day; he is shown standing on a 'Reservoir for Dead Insects'.

twelve of them in wedlock, panegyrized sex as 'the purest source of human felicity, the cordial drop in the otherwise vapid cup of life'.[38] For his part, the master-quack of the 1780s James Graham (illus. 27) insisted that erotic activity made you hale and hearty: 'The genitals are the true pulse, and infallible barometer of health.'[39] Promotion of the joy of sex was the message of the 'Lecture on the Generation, Increase and Improvement of the Human Species' which he would deliver with the assistance of a bevy of lightly-draped nymphs – one of them apparently Emma Lyon herself, got up as 'Hebe Vestina', the goddess of health.[40] Gratification of sexual instincts, Graham insisted, was not merely a male privilege, for he regarded the fair as no less libidinous: 'Were we to be made acquainted with the real sentiments of the sex', he ventured,

> even the chastest, coldest, most reserved, and least amorously complexioned woman in the world, we would find her to be precisely of the same taste, with the bishop's lady, who very frankly declared that, for her part, she liked to have a GOOD THING in the house, or in the bed by her, whether she made use of it or not.[41]

Debate over the erotic raised the sensitive question as to whether the body possessed supreme sex appeal and attractiveness naked or when adorned by clothes and art. Conventional wisdom deemed that, as well as protecting modesty, finery enhanced natural attributes. An article 'On Taste in Female Dress', published in 1817 in the *Chester Chronicle*, thus declared that clothing was 'the natural finish to beauty'; without it, 'a handsome woman is a gem, but a gem that is not set'. 'The love of dress is natural to women', insisted the writer:

> This has been seen and attested in all ages and in all countries of the world, in the most savage as well as in the most polished states. It is a laudable, a useful, and interesting propensity; but it requires to be chastened and regulated by the hand of taste, by a sense of the beautiful in nature, of the correct and harmonious in art.[42]

Womanliness was indeed being judged in terms of modish new criteria of 'femininity'; an eligible lady was expected to glamourize her looks by recourse to art. A fading, ageing complexion could be salvaged by cosmetics – a term with a wider application than today, including hygiene and grooming;[43] while patches, powder, wigs, lace, gauze, perfumes, etc., as well as face paint sometimes so coarse it was compared to 'rough cast' or Plaster of Paris, could be used to repair or hide the ravages of time.[44] A beauty industry arose to meet such needs, one Piccadilly shopkeeper commending her own preparations to women, in hopes that their husbands 'might not be offended at their deformities and turn into other Women's chambers'.[45] Vendors specialized in washes that removed unwelcome suntan (darkened skin bespoke rusticity), and lotions to hide scars or raise or lower the hairline. She could 'make the hair fall out, where it is too much, and make it grow, where it is too little',[46] boasted a certain Sarah Cornelius de Heusde, while another shopkeeper claimed her unique pomatum 'makes the Aged appear youthful to a wonder'.[47] As with patches, such preparations were commonly meant to mask venereal infections: 'if *Venus* should misfortunately be Wounded ... by tampering with *Mars*', claimed 'Agnodice', she could cure it 'without fluxing'.[48]

Beauty aids proliferated. *Mundus Muliebris: or The Lady's Dressing Room Unlock'd*, a poem of 1690, enumerated various devices in its 'Fop-Dictionary'. *Plumpers* ('light Balls') would 'fill up Cavities of the Cheeks'. Improvements to the coiffure included *Crushes* – 'certain smaller Curls, placed on the Forehead'; *Confidants* – 'smaller Curles near the Ears'; the *Choux* – 'the great round Boss or Bundle'; and *Meurtriers* – 'murderers, a certain Knot in the Hair, which ties and unites the Curls'. Further aesthetic aids were down to the dressmaker. The whaleboned stay, hoop and padded rump were all designed to

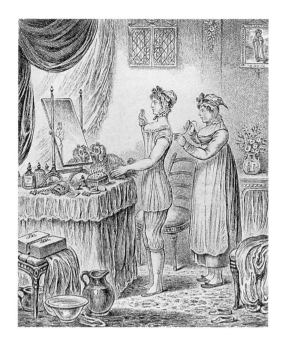

28 James Gillray, 'Progress of the Toilet. THE STAYS', 1810, engraving after himself.

Gillray depicts a woman standing at a dressing table while a maidservant laces her stays. Art was meant to perfect nature, and a genteel 18th-century woman would have been expected to wear hefty under-garments to create a sound foundation for her clothes. Gillray's satire subverts that message.

impart to women the desirable ample, curvaceous shape dictated by fashion (illus. 28).

All told, wigs, powdered hair, false curls and knots, paint and beauty spots, masks, fans, feathers, elaborate head-dresses and a multitude of other flights of costume effectively embellished, or concealed, nature's endowments.[49] But was this a good thing?

That was a question which assumed some urgency when European males encountered indigenous peoples and were forced to confront the looks of the 'noble savage'. Exploring Tahiti on Captain Cook's first expedition in 1769, Joseph Banks, later eminent as President of the Royal Society but then a young blade, was bowled over by the native women. 'It is reckond no shame', he observed, 'for any part of the body to be exposed to view except those which all mankind hide; The women at sun set always bard their bodys down to the navel, which seemd to be a kind of easy undress to them.'[50] In a letter written after his return, Banks delivered his aesthetic judgment of Paris as to relative beauty: did the West outdo the rest?[51] Native African or American women, it went without saying, were hardly in the running at all – they were physically hideous, and that was precisely because they were not treated as dishes by their men: 'the regard and attention paid by us Europeans to the fair sex is certainly one of the chief reasons why our women so far exceed those of Climates most favourable to the produce of the human species in beauty.'[52] African and American women could not possibly have any feel for 'the refinements of Love', because in those regions men were so brutish as to covet women not as charmers but as 'Servants'.[53] Such strictures obviously could not apply to Tahiti, however, for on that paradise island 'Love is the Chief Occupation, the favourite, nay almost the Sole Luxury of the inhabitants'.[54]

The true beauty contest was thus between Polynesian and European eroticism, which meant, Banks explained, the choice between nature and art, in itself an expression of the contrast between indolence and industry;

> Idleness the father of Love reigns here [i.e., in Polynesia] in almost unmolested ease, while we inhabitants of a changeable climate are Obligd to Plow, Sow, Harrow, reap, Thrash, Grind Knead and bake our daily bread.[55]

The time thereby saved was so much 'Leisure given up to Love'.[56] As befitted isles of love so blessed by nature, the fair sex dazzled: 'I have no where seen such Elegant women', insisted Banks, 'as those of Otaheite such the Greecians were from whose model the venus of Medicis was copied.'[57]

What explained that surpassing loveliness? It was, above all, natural – 'undistorted by bandages nature has full liberty'.[58] Thus, without any need for stays and other synthetic foundation aids, fecund nature produced 'such forms as exist here [Europe] only in marble or Canvas nay such as might even defy the imitation of the Chizzel of a Phidias or the Pencil of an Apelles'. And it was all natural: 'Nor are these forms a little aided by their dress nor squezed as our women are by a cincture.'[59] Natural shapes were preferable to Europe's 'exaggerated smallness of waist, an artificial beauty not founded at all on the principles of nature'. Britain boasted the hoop, but what did that do but conceal the buttock, 'natures favourite ornament'? Not least, Banks continued, Tahitian women sported a wonderful 'Luxury' of appearance which was 'also not a little aided by a freedom which their differing from us in their opinion of what Constitutes modesty'.[60]

What, after all, was this so-called 'decency' prized so highly by the civilized? Was it not rather a species of hypocrisy? 'A European thinks nothing of Laying bare her breast to a certain point but a hairs breadth Lower no mortal eye must Pierce.' With the Polynesian no such 'modesty' – or was it, in truth, coquetry? – applied:

> An Otaheitean on the other hand will by a motion of her dress in a moment lay open an arm and half her breast the next maybe the whole and in another cover herself as close as prudery could contrive and all this with as much innocence and genuine modesty as an

English woman can shew her arm or as women of the spanish west Indies her breast.[61]

Tormented by decorum or scruples over decency, the English woman 'can not shew her breast nor the [Spanish] her foot without commiting the highest indelicacy'; the Tahitian, by contrast, had no such inhibitions.[62]

When it came to looks, Europeans were thus on the horns of a dilemma: appearances should be perfected yet appearances deceived – and disappointed. Clothes maketh the man, and wonderful sartorial displays were put on.[63] But what allegedly enhanced bodily dignity readily, in the judgment of severe moralists, no less than the 'back to nature' brigade, betrayed it. With its splendid subtitle – *Historically Presented, In the mad and cruel Gallantry, Foolish Bravery, ridiculous Beauty, filthy Finesse, and loathsome Lovelinesse of most Nations, Fashioning & altering their Bodies from the Mould intended by Nature. With a Vindication of the Regular Beauty and Honesty of Nature* – John Bulwer's mid-seventeenth century *Anthropometamorphosis: Man Transform'd; or, the Artificial Changeling*, as we have already seen, was the classic iconoclastic condemnation of the vainglory of artifice. 'Our Ladies here', ranted the author, 'have lately entertained a vaine Custome of spotting their Faces, out of an affectation of a Mole to set of their beauty, such as Venus had, and it is well if one black patch will serve to make their Faces remarkable ... This is as odious, and as sense-less an affectation as ever was used by any barbarous Nation in the World.'[64] The craze for beauty spots proved enduring – as did such denunciations of artful deception. 'Cloaths', pronounced Bernard Mandeville, reiterating this complaint a couple of generations later,

> were originally made for two Ends, to hide our Nakedness, and to fence our Bodies against the Weather, and other outward Injuries: To these our boundless Pride has added a third, which is Ornament; for what else but an excess of stupid Vanity, could have prevail'd upon our Reason to fancy that Ornamental, which must continually put us in mind of our Wants and Misery, beyond all other Animals that are ready cloathed by Nature herself?[65]

Applying a different spin, however, Mandeville, no Puritan but a cynic, then held that such personal vanity was in truth a social desideratum, for private vices were public benefits: take fashion away, and the economy would grind to a halt.

With fashion growing ever more imperious, a civilization seemed to be emerging, so critics complained, not of honest faces but facades, undermining the old faith that bearing and presence were escutcheons of birth and worth. A grande dame like Lady Stucco in *School for Scandal* (1777) was an object of censure and ridicule for hiding nature's face behind a visor, using powder, paint, patches and puffs, masks, fans, lace and gauze to fabricate a make-believe (and more youthful) self. Nor was it only women who found themselves in a sartorial dilemma: in the wake of the Restoration, male beauty was problematized as the molly (homosexual) emerged. The Restoration comedy *Love's Last Shift* (1696) has Sir Novelty Fashion strutting his stuff as the upstart fop, consumed with chic ostentation: 'the Cravatstring, the Garter, the Sword-knot, the Centurine, the Bardash, the Steinkirk, the large Button, the long Sleeve, the Plume, and full Peruque, were all created, cry'd down, or revived by me.' This fop of fops made a point of conspicuously leaving the theatre before the performance ended, so as to give 'the whole Audience an Opportunity of turning upon me at once'. The tubby Prince Regent's slavish pursuit of fashion was endlessly ridiculed, while the macaroni was pilloried as the embodiment of the dangers of narcissistic display.[66]

By the eighteenth century, the weakening of hard-line Calvinism was permitting the body beautiful its place in the sun. But female attractiveness did not cease to arouse suspicion, especially when it owed much to artifice, while male display drew new reproof.

If looks were therefore equivocal indicators of the proper body, would not a truer proof of the pudding lie in good health? 'Banish money – Banish sofas – Banish wine – Banish music – But right Jack Health, – Honest Jack Health, true Jack Health – banish Health and banish all the world,' sang the consumptive John Keats, probably aware even then his days were numbered.[67] 'Health is the basis of all happiness this world gives', ruled Samuel Johnson in 1782, then sinking into the grave.[68] 'O blessed health', declared that arch-dogmatist Walter Shandy, 'thou art above all gold and treasure.'[69] Such sentiments were ten-a-penny, as were health plans designed to keep the body fit. But whose bodies were really healthy? And what brought sickness on?

One line, spun by laity and doctors alike, was that the pursuit of refinement ironically compromised the constitution. Our ancestors, it was widely held in a narrative paralleling Banks' views on native erotic appeal, had been strong and sturdy; needs were few, exercise plentiful, food plain and wholesome.[70] Necessity had made men hardy, and hardiness had inured them to pain. 'True health and vigour of body', asserted the late eighteenth-century Scottish physician, Thomas Trotter, 'are the inheritance of the untutored savage'; disease, by contrast, was the child of 'excess' or 'debauch'. 'The encouragement of manufactures', remarked Thomas Beddoes, 'is the creation of a miserable and sickly population.'[71] How had this 'fall' come about?

> By Chase our long-liv'd Fathers earned their Food;
> Toil strung the Nerves, and purifi'd the Blood:
> But we, their Sons, a pamper'd Race of Men,
> Are dwindl'd down to threescore Years and ten.
> Better to hunt in Fields, for Health unbought,
> Than fee the Doctor for a nauseous Draught.[72]

Far from producing fitness and vitality, civilization, in other words, according to a golden-age myth peddled by poets, bred disease:

> The first Physicians by Debauch were made:
> Excess began, and Sloth sustains the Trade.[73]

Nostalgic doctors rued the demise of old frugality, and told luxury-lubbers to learn from the robust life of the virtuous rustic. The fashionable physician William Cadogan, a passionate advocate of maternal breastfeeding, held up 'the Poor, I mean the laborious' as an example, for they – unlike the luxurious and the licentious – had 'Health and Posterity'.[74] Whereas the simple life was the healthy one, the affluent and aristocratic had brought sickness upon themselves through fast and hard living, notably the gluttony endemic in a nation of 'gullet-fanciers'.[75]

Notorious for heavy eating, the English, so the proverb ran, were digging their graves with their teeth. Hearty appetites admittedly had sanction from the traditional model of the constitution as a throughput system, designed energetically to digest food into strength and expel waste products. The active body needed regular fuel to supply warmth and vigour ('vital heat'). Hence the stress on a healthy stomach, dubbed by Edward Jenner the 'grand Monarque of the Constitution'.[76] For that reason, John Bull was meant to be stout, the converse of France's scrawny Johnny Crappo.[77] 'Man is an eating animal, a drinking animal, and a sleeping animal', Mary Anne Schimmelpenninck reported the corpulent Erasmus Darwin as declaring, 'and one placed in a material world, which alone furnishes all the human animal can desire.'[78] Perhaps such nutritional logic encouraged overindulgence; certainly many Georgian doctors felt obliged to counter-argue that excessive eating, or the fad for over-sophisticated food, must give way to restraint and moderation. Here some drew upon a tradition of prolongevist writings stemming from the celebrated Luigi Cornaro.

By the age of 35, that sixteenth-century Paduan nobleman found his constitution utterly ruined by overindulgence in sensual gratifications. In these desperate circumstances he embraced a temperate life and rapidly recovered. It proved a quasi-religious conversion, and he became a health freak. Eventually, at the age of 83, he composed his *Discourse on the Temperate Life* (1550), and propounded his regimen of health; a second was added at the age of 86, a third at 91 and a fourth at 95.[79]

Despite his advanced years, insisted Cornaro, his senses were in tiptop condition, his teeth remained well preserved, he could easily climb stairs and even mount his horse unaided. He waxed lyrical over the joys of life, his love of reading and writing, his discussions with scholars and artists, and, dearest to his heart, the company of his grandchildren.

The secret of his regimen lay in temperance. As one grew older, food intake had to be reduced, because 'natural heat' decreased in the elderly. In time, his diet came to consist of tiny portions of meat, bread and egg broth. 'I always eat with relish', he claimed, and 'I feel, when I leave the table, that I must sing.' The nobleman confidently predicted the extension of the lifespan beyond the biblical 'three score and ten' (Psalms 90:10). All could live to 100, while those blessed with a robust constitution could aspire to 120. This paragon of health passed away prematurely in 1565, at the disappointing age of 98.[80] Praised by Joseph Addison in *The Spectator*, Cornaro's *Discourse* went through at least 50 editions in English translation in the eighteenth and nineteenth centuries. Much like us, the Georgians binged on diet books.[81]

The best-selling English-language writings in the temperance tradition were those of George Cheyne, already discussed, whose *Essay on Health and Long Life* (1724) enjoyed some twenty editions in fifteen years. This British Cornaro became a somebody: when Lady Pembroke wanted to give some health advice to her son – it concerned that irresistible and evergreen subject, flannel underwear – she transcribed a page from Cheyne, and rounded off her letter: 'So says Doctor Cheyne, from whose Book the above is copied (*so you see what a wise woman I am*).'[82] Cheyne owed his popularity in part to the fact that, as documented in the previous chapter, his was a high-profile case of self-cure, having practically eaten himself into the grave and then written up his own 'case'.[83]

While also addressing air, sleep, exercise, evacuations and the passions, Cheyne's *Essay on Health and Long Life* concentrated on the rules for a healthy diet. Poultry, hares and rabbits, and other young and tender white flesh were better than the traditional English beef, but healthiest of all was a greens-and-grains diet.[84]

Before it could be preserved, however, the good constitution had first to be created. In *Some Thoughts Concerning Education* (1693), easily the most influential educational treatise of the Enlightenment, John Locke stressed the positive value, nay, the very necessity, of early physical hardening – nothing could be worse than to pamper the young. An overheated birth-room was harmful; swaddling was counterproductive – it would enfeeble rather than strengthen; and the ritualistic dosing of infants with medicines and alcoholic cordials would equally weaken by inducing dependency. Overall, 'cockering and tenderness' first created and then confirmed constitutional delicacy, thereby spawning spindly hothouse valetudinarians dependent on stimulants, tonics and medicines.[85]

Diet should be simple, meals irregular – youthful stomachs should not be pandered to – but excretion regular. Costiveness 'being an indisposition I had a particular reason to inquire into', Locke had found infants could be trained to go to stool directly after breakfast.[86] Indulgence was a mistake, 'for if the child must have grapes or sugarplums when he has a mind to them ... why, if he is grown up, must he not be satisfied too, if his desires carry him to wine or women?'[87]

Once created, the healthy constitution must then be sustained by moderation in lifestyle. 'The temperate', declared Erasmus Darwin in his youth, before he ran to fat, 'enjoy an ever-blooming Health free from all Infections and disorders luxurious mortals are subject to.' Were moderation to triumph, he fantasized, 'the whimsical Tribe of Phisicians' would go without their fees – another enigmatic consequence for the aspirant doctor.[88]

In time critics feared that the temperance message was being taken too much to heart, moderation was being immoderately pursued. As is evident from fashion plates, society portraits and satirical cartoons, partly with a view to health though more in response to fashion, a cult of elegant etiolation became dominant in the late Georgian era, carrying as it did strong connotations of youthful sexual attractiveness (illus. 44).

Once thin was in, trendy girls in the process of being 'manufactured into a lady' were allowed by their parents, complained the Clifton physician, Thomas Beddoes, ever fashion's scourge, to get away with finicky eating. Hoodwinked by pseudo-medical faddery – perhaps by reading Cheyne! – parents were even going in for vegetarianism: 'There are ... among the higher classes, some who keep their children to the fifth, or even the seventh year, upon a strict [Cheynian] vegetable and milk diet,' fumed the appalled physician, seduced by the 'false hope of rendering the blood of their children pure, and their humours mild'.[89] All this, he feared, was the slippery slope to tuberculosis ('consumption' – being consumed rather than consuming).

The right balance was obviously hard to achieve, and letters, diaries and journals reveal anxious searches for the royal road to health. The mid-eighteenth-century Sussex grocer Thomas Turner constantly pondered his see-saw condition – indeed, was a bit of a hypochondriac, though this did not stop him from getting blotto when on parochial binges that resulted in positively Boswellian hangovers. In principle, at least, a model of petty-bourgeois prudence, Turner set about safeguarding his constitution, boning up on medical books and culling advice from magazines. Not least, he dictated to himself 'rules of proper regimen':

> First, be it either in the summer or winter, to rise as early as I possibly can; that is, always to allow myself between 7 and 8 hours' sleep, or full 8, unless prevented on any particular or emergent occasion. 2ndly, to go to breakfast between the hours of 7 and 8 from Lady Day to St. Michael, and from St. Michael to Lady Day between the hours of 8 and 9. 3rdly, my breakfast to be always tea or coffee and never to exceed 4 dishes. If neither of those, half a pint of water or water gruel; and for eatables, bread and cheese, bread and butter, light biscuit, buttered toast, or dry bread, and one morn in every week, dry bread only. 4thly, nothing more before dinner, and always to dine between the hours of 12 and 1 o'clock if at home. 5thly, my dinner to be meat, pudding, or any other thing of the like nature, but always to have regard, if there is nothing but salt provision, to eat sparingly; and to eat plenty of any sort of garden stuff there is at table, together with plenty of bread and acids, if any, at table; and always to have the greatest regard to give white or fresh meats and pudding the preference before any sort of highly seasoned, salt, or very strong meat; and always one day in every respective week to eat no meat.[90]

And so on and so on. Health maintenance was evidently in danger of becoming a Sisyphean struggle and a source of high anxiety; a new physical puritanism was being born.

Cornaro and his devotees were concerned with long life; certain champions of Enlightenment went one stage further, dreaming of earthly immortality. In a future rational society, predicted the anarchist William Godwin in his *Enquiry Concerning Political Justice* (1793), there would not only be no government; there would also 'be no disease, no anguish, no melancholy and no resentment'.[91] Once humans comported themselves rationally, ill health and ageing would end. Nor would this occasion overpopulation, since sexual appetites, being themselves irrational, would equally wither away. The consequence? 'The whole will be a people of men, and not of children. Generation will not succeed generation, nor truth have ... to recommence her career every thirty years.'[92] This crankily confident rationalism sounds curiously like Bernal over a hundred years *avant la lettre*.

Citing Benjamin Franklin's supposition that 'mind will one day become omnipotent over matter', Godwin reflected: 'if the power of intellect can be established over all other matter, are we not inevitably led to ask, why not over the matter of our own bodies?'[93] In support of his claim he adduced psychosomatic evidence: did not sorrow produce a 'broken heart' and bring about organic disease, while good news set physical complaints to rights? The active had the power to resist setbacks sufficient to reduce the idle to illness. 'I walk twenty miles, full of ardour', he declared,

> and with a motive that engrosses my soul, and I arrive as fresh and alert as when I began my journey. Emotion, excited by some unexpected word, by a letter that is delivered to us, occasions the most extraordinary revolutions in our frame ... There is nothing of which the physician is more frequently aware, than of the power of the mind in assisting or retarding convalescence.[94]

Whereas post-Freudians regard such forces as unconscious, Godwin considered them open to rational control. Right thinking prompted longevity; the prescription for immortality was 'chearfulness, clearness of conception and benevolence'; and through such a moral medicine man would 'attain as nearly as possible, to the perfectly voluntary state'. Death would thus at last be conquered, and reason would resolve the problem of the unruly body – in an unexpected stroke of Cartesian revenge, it would virtually disappear.

This chapter has explored models of the 'good body' in the early modern era and how to manage it. Its ideals, visual and personal, were articulated in religious, scientific and aesthetic idioms and pursued in terms of decorum, beauty, sexual attractiveness and health. Within limits, the early modern body was meant to serve as an uplifting moral spectacle, teaching the triumph of civilization over savagery, the lofty over the low.

The outcome, however, was anxiety as much as achievement. The deliberate and determined pursuit of health arguably led to the hypochondriacism to be touched on in later chapters. The quest for sexiness sparked moralistic counter-discourses, which condemned artifice and voiced misogynistic fears of deceptive appearances; nature and art were seen to conflict. Finally, the search for long life produced not only what was seen as the inordinate, absurd, and indeed impious, Godwinian faith in immortality but the new puritanism evident in the demand for the perfect bodily subjugation. The rational discourse of better, more enduring, more satisfied bodies ironically thus tended towards their further problematization, indeed their very denial.[95] It is against the backdrop of the body painted in this and the previous chapter that the following essays will explore cultures of sickness and their medical representations.

4 Imagining Disease

High amongst medicine's priorities lies identifying the trouble.[1] The traditional way of getting a disorder's name involved the doctor prompting the sick person to tell him what was wrong: pains and symptoms, when and how they began, what had apparently precipitated them, their comings and goings. The patient would also recount relevant lifestyle details: eating and drinking habits, sleeplessness, bowel motions, recent emotional upsets and so forth, not to mention the perhaps embarrassing matter of indulgence in home or quack medicines.[2]

In fulfilment of his side in this diagnostic rite, called 'taking the history', the practitioner would further conduct some physical scrutiny, mainly by the unaided eye, paying attention to skin colour, inflammation, rashes, spots, signs of swelling, and so forth. He would also take the pulse, making a qualitative assessment (was it languid or racing, regular or erratic?) rather than timing its beats against a watch (illus. 29). He would also listen to coughs, wheezings and eructations, and sniff for any odour of putrefaction. Physical examination was, generally, however, rather perfunctory – merely ritualistic, some might say; what truly counted were the patient's words and how the physician decoded them. Hopefully blessed with a fine memory, the clinician had thus, rather like a Freudian psychoanalyst, to be proficient at listening and cross-questioning, using skills best called humanistic and hermeneutic.[3]

It is only in consequence of the new disciplines of pathology, pioneered by Giovanni Morgagni in the 1760s and then systematized in early nineteenth-century Parisian hospital medicine by René Laennec and others, that this style of diagnosis gave way to one in which the living body itself was rendered transparent and forced to display and yield up its diseases.[4] The new pathological thinking (disease is localized not holistic) made thorough physical examination essential, signally with the introduction of Laennec's invention, the stethoscope, and the technique of auscultation that paralleled it.

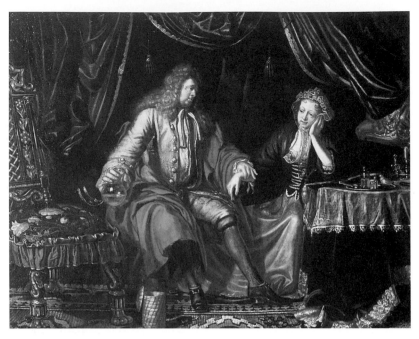

29 This oil painting on wood by Matthijs Naiveu (1647–1726) depicts a theme common in 17th-century Dutch domestic art: the love-sick woman, betrayed by her melancholy and her erratic pulse. The doctor's touch doubles as an erotic gesture: is the doctor the source of his patient's complaint?

Auscultation still required the doctor to be a good listener, but now he was listening primarily to body functions, not to the patient. In Britain, perhaps for reasons of propriety, 'physicals' did not become standard practice till the Victorian age, and the Queen herself held out, her personal physician Sir James Reid noting her 'great aversion' to the stethoscope. In all the twenty years he attended her, 'the first time I had ever seen the Queen ... in bed', he reported, was when she was dying, and it was only post mortem that he discovered she had a prolapsed uterus – proof that he had never once given her a thorough 'physical'.[5] Other skills and devices were introduced in the nineteenth century to bypass the patient and get direct access to organic function, notably the thermometer, for measuring body temperature, and the sphygmo-manometer, which read blood pressure.

The technical history of diagnostics thus tells of a steady if dilatory, progress in getting the body, initially a 'black box', to reveal its interior; later developments along the same lines included X-rays (illus. 30), ultrasound, MRI, CAT, PETT and many other scanning technologies familiar today.[6] Nevertheless, if disease was long clinically hidden, in the wider sense, as proposed in Chapter 1, disorders have always been on parade. In the ancestral *theatrum medicinae*, illness was acted out in a grand opera of gestures of suffering, and symptoms, as already discussed, were read as divine and highly public verdicts, encoded in blemishes and buboes, boils and blisters. The 'Chosen People' knew that pestilence was a judgment:

> But it shall come to pass, if thou wilt not harken to the voice of the Lord thy God, to observe to do all his commandments and his statutes which I command thee this day; that all these curses shall come upon thee, and overtake thee; ...
>
> The Lord shall smite thee with a consumption, and with a fever, and with an inflammation, and with an extreme burning, and with the sword, and with blasting, and with mildew; and they shall pursue thee until thou perish ...
>
> The Lord will smite thee with the botch of Egypt, and with the emerods, and with the scab, and with the itch, whereof thou canst not be healed.[7]

Medical philosophies and popular wisdom alike held that outer symptoms spoke eloquently of inner states: like the label on a bottle, bodily appearance advertised contents, and a divine Trades Descriptions Act hopefully guaranteed the tag's veracity. Implicitly or explicitly, doctors themselves depended on this correlation – it formed a basic diagnostic decoder: redness meant inflammation, yellow spelt jaundice, and death was heralded by the *facies Hippocratica*, the pinched, drawn, hollowed visage. Folk wisdom too traded on such beliefs. As we saw in Chapter 2, birthmarks like a club foot or a port wine stain were telltales of something sinister in the baby's conception – a syphilitic father or steamy adulterous sheets. Disease was

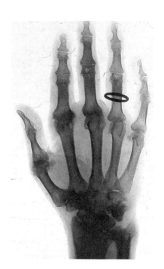

30 An early (1896) X-ray made under the direction of Sir Arthur Schuster; a note on the back of the print reads 'rheumatoid arthritis'.

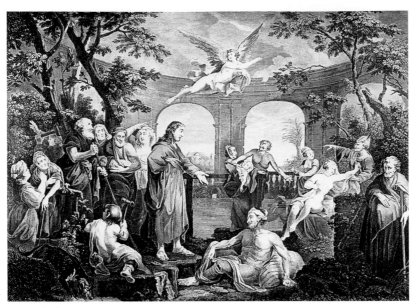

31 Ravenel and Picot, *The Pool of Bethesda*, 1772, engraving after a painting by William
Hogarth in St Bartholomew's Hospital, London.

standardly the signature of wrong, and could create or reinforce
stigma.[8]

Yet the very conspicuousness of a disorder might paradoxically serve
the patient. The visibility of external symptoms – a rash, for instance –
guaranteed that a malady (here perhaps a fever) was authentic and
would not be judged imaginary or fraudulent. The somatic (the 'truth
of the body') may be the crucial voucher of the real – or it may, through
an ironic twist, lead to the labelling of a condition 'psychosomatic', and
hence 'merely' hysterical. Not taking the 'truth of the body' at face
value but putting it to the test became a further diagnostic refinement.[9]

As the lame and the halt always hoped, the spectacle of disease
might in itself also command sympathy. Donated to St Bartholomew's
Hospital, of which the Smithfield-born artist was a Governor,
Hogarth's *The Pool of Bethesda* (illus. 31) displayed the sick with a
view to arousing the visitor's pity: a woman suffering from jaundice, a
blind man carrying his long stick, a cretinous girl, a lame man with a
bandaged arm, a woman with inflammation of the breast and a mother
with a child suffering from rickets (or perhaps from hereditary
syphilis). Such paintings, hung in hospitals, were intended to stir the
charitable impulse and to sanctify the institution itself.[10]

Hospitals themselves were designed to be quasi-public spaces
which put the sick on show for moral and philanthropic purposes –

92

once healed, they might be expected to perform conspicuous gratitude, before donors and the public, in parades or church services.[11] Set
up in 1741, London's Foundling Hospital staged concerts and art exhibitions; the quality was meant to attend these, admire the healthiness
and discipline of the infants in the charity's care, and place their grateful guineas on the plate. Similar protocols applied to 'lock' hospitals for
venereal diseases and 'Magdalene' foundations for prostitutes.[12] And
all such institutions would also stage an annual thanksgiving service
with a charity sermon in a fashionable church.

Showing sickness for pious, fund-raising and moralizing ends was
most systematically practised at London's Bethlem Hospital, which
was for centuries a public spectacle, the model visitor to this madness
show being the 'person of quality', attending with the intention of
'releiving ... the poore Lunatiques'.[13] The insane were displayed as
part of an appeal to godliness and compassion, an inscription on the
poor box entreating visitors to 'remember the poore Lunaticks'.
Alongside the fund-raising function, insanity was exhibited as a didactic spectacle. Satisfying that 'desire for instruction' supposed to draw
the 'enlightened visitor', patients were meant to serve as object lessons,
living exemplars of the penalties consequent upon vice and disorder.
There was no 'better lesson [to] be taught us in any part of the globe
than in this school of misery', judged *The World* magazine in 1753:

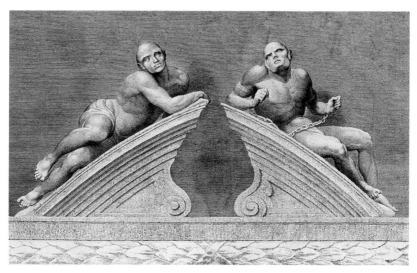

32 William Sharp, 'Bethlemii ad portiis ...', 1783, engraving after Thomas Stothard of Caius
Cibber's Bethlem ('Bedlam') Hospital pediment.
     Cibber's statues (1680) reclined on a broken segmental pediment crowning the gates of
Bethlem Hospital in London. 'Melancholy' is listless and, characteristically, has the hidden
hands of idleness. 'Raving Madness' is muscle-bound and needs to be restrained.

> Here we may see the mighty reasoners of the earth, below even the
> insects that crawl upon it; and from so humbling a sight we may learn
> to moderate our pride, and to keep those passions within bounds,
> which if too much indulged, would drive reason from her seat, and
> level us with the wretches of this unhappy mansion.[14]

The utter degradation of the mad, their pathos, their mockery of
normality, were meant to impress sincere hearts and minds. In *The
Guardian* in 1713, 'PHILANTROPUS' thus wrote of having 'rambled about
the galleries at Bedlam ... for an hour' and 'thoroughly reflected' on
what he 'beheld'; and the statues of 'Melancholy and Raving Madness'
(illus. 32), displayed above the gateway of the new Bethlem building
at Moorfields, opened in 1677, were displayed as warnings of the
madness lurking within – within Bethlem, within every breast. 'Seeing
the insane' was thus meant to be instructive, and the miseries of
Bethlem, like Tyburn tree, were hammered home as object lessons to
impressionable youngsters. In 1709, Sir Richard Steele took three
young brothers, to whom he was (significantly) guardian, 'to show
'em ... *Bedlam*' and other sights.[15]

The reality of public visiting may have been the reverse – an air not
of edification but of the funfair for, especially at holiday times,
Bethlem notoriously attracted hordes of tipsy voyeuristic gawpers, out
for raucous sport, and the Bedlamites would themselves put on performances, singing, capering and telling riddles in return for pennies.
And was not going to stare at the mad itself a crazy thing to do? Richard
Newton's cartoon (illus. 33) poses the question: who are the truly
insane – the inmates or the visitors? The physiognomies of the man
and his wife betray the stereotypical features of the deranged, with
their gross gestures and mouths agape, eyebrows raised and goggle-
eyed. But they must be the sightseers, since the bizarre headgear of
chamberpot and crown announce that certified insanity lies on the far
side of the door, with the handle drawn to suggest the crescent moon,
symbol of lunacy. Under such circumstances – the mirror held up to
madness further confusing the issue – no wonder critics deplored the
madness circus; and around 1770 the curtain was run down on the
Bethlem show, shortly before the ending of the public theatre of
executions at Tyburn in 1783.

Till then, however, Bethlem served as so much more than a therapeutic centre pure and simple for the insane. Moralists, journalists and
cartoonists had relished embroidering the theme of Bedlam as the
mirror and microcosm of Britain, with patients transformed into such
archetypes as the demented politician, the warmongering general, the
compulsive stock-exchange speculator, the vainglorious emperor, the

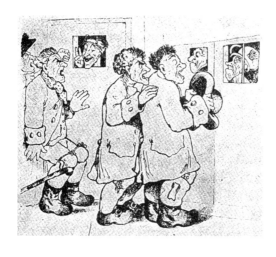

33 Richard Newton, 'A Visit
to Bedlam', 1794, etching.
Newton's print was made
after the end of general public
viewing at Bethlem Hospital.
Evidently the place continued
to loom large in the public
imagination.

religious enthusiast and the lovesick maid. It is a theme to which we
shall return in Chapter 9.

Madness was, in the main, a 'bad' disease, melodramatized in its
representations (nakedness, wildness, animality) by way of a warning;[16] and a similar negativity applies to most other disorders. But
occasionally a malady was worn, like a battle-wound or a duelling-scar,
as a badge of pride. Gout, for example, conferred dignity because, as
the lord of diseases and the disease of lords, it bespoke pedigree and
fine breeding, and was reckoned the price to be paid for a superior
lifestyle: being wheeled round in their bath chairs with their feet heav-
ily bandaged, sufferers would flaunt, in a phallic way, the magnitude of
the swelling. Lord Gout was one of the few illnesses conducive to the
comic muse: numerous prints depicted rubicund, corpulent gour-
mands (illus. 45) guzzling away and swilling their port, their feet
reclining on gout stools, swathed in shock-absorbing bandages.[17]

Though there have been certain other droll or desirable disease
representations – for example, elegant thinness in Rowlandson's
Dropsy Courting Consumption (1810), reproduced in the previous chapter, far more common has been the casting of illness in the tragic,
horrific or disgusting mode, rendered, as with syphilis, as the wages of
sin.[18] Published in 1683, Robert Gould's 'Love Given O'er' maligned
an actress for her lust:

> When she found that she could do no more,
> When all her Body was one putrid Sore,
> Studded with Pox, and Ulcers quite all o're;
> (Which show'd most specious when they most beguil'd)
> Sh'enrolled more Females in the List of Whore,
> Than all the Arts of Man e're did before,

95

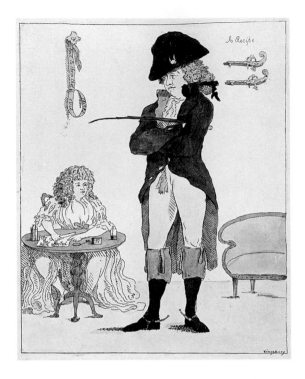

34 Henry Kingsbury, 'THE KING'S EVIL', 1786, engraving (coloured impression). British Museum, London.

The garter on the wall bears the motto of the Order of the Garter, 'evil to him that evil thinks'. The female doctor (Mrs Fitzherbert) has written a prescription addressed 'to the man affected' (her clandestine husband, the Prince of Wales).

> Prest with the pond'rous guilt, at length she fell,
> And through the solid Centre sunk to Hell.[19]

Venereal disease was ever shocking as a moral marker, especially when it was the quality who were touched. 'THE KING'S EVIL' (illus. 34) trades on the affinity between the pox and politics. The Prince of Wales straddles the foreground as Mrs Fitzherbert his mistress – nay, clandestine wife – sits encircled by medicines with a knife in her hand meaningfully pointing, and as lettering reads, 'to the part affected'. Her outspread legs and state of undress further emphasize the need for the cure – if the Order of the Garter hanging above her head tenders an ironic reminder: 'evil to them that evil thinks.' No coincidence, surely, that its outline intimates a noose or that the pair of pistols is pointing at the Prince's head.[20]

Diseases themselves were commonly personified. Samuel Garth's *The Dispensary* (1699), to be discussed in the next chapter, made a cavalcade of them before the reader – fever, dropsy, and so forth:

> Febris is first: the hagg relentless hears
> The Virgin's Sighs, and sees the Infant's Tears ...
> In her parch'd Eye-balls fiery Meteors reign;
> And restless Ferments revel in each Vein.

96

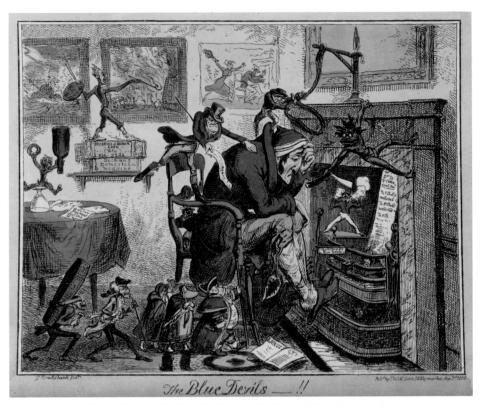

35 George Cruikshank, 'The Blue Devils—!!', 1835, etching with watercolour.
The 'poor debtor' faces bills from a doctor and 'J. Coke, coal merchant'; his fire-grate
is empty.

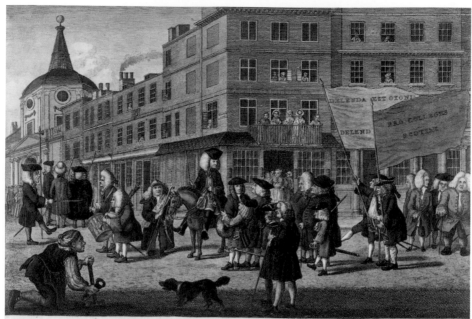

THE MARCH of the MEDICAL MILITANTS to the SIEGE of WARWICK-LANE-CASTLE in the Year 1767.

36 John June, 'THE MARCH of the MEDICAL MILITANTS to the SIEGE of WARWICK-LANE-CASTLE in the Year 1767', 1768, coloured etching.

   The premises of the Royal College of Physicians (the domed building) were in the City of London. The banners read: 'DELENDA EST OXONIA' (Down with Oxford) and, presumably, 'Down with Cambridge' and 'Up with the Scottish Colleges'. The print attests to public interest in the spectacle of intra-professional rivalry amongst the doctors spilling onto the streets.

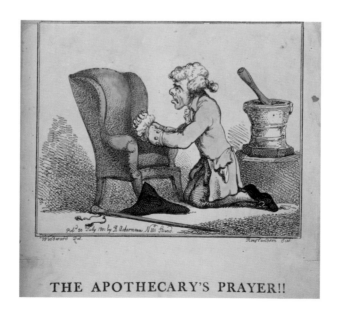

THE APOTHECARY'S PRAYER!!

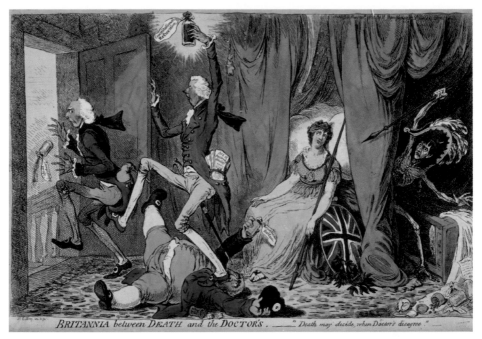

BRITANNIA between DEATH and the DOCTOR'S . ___ " Death may decide, when Doctor's disagree "

38 James Gillray, 'BRITANNIA Between DEATH and the DOCTOR'S', 1804, coloured etching.

The captioning below trots out the old saying 'Death may decide, when Doctor's disagree'.

37 Thomas Rowlandson, 'THE APOTHECARY'S PRAYER!!', 1801, coloured etching after George Moutard Woodward.

An apothecary prays for a host of illnesses to descend so that he can make more money: 'O mighty Esculapius! hear a poor little man overwhelm'd with misfortunes, grant I beseech thee to send a few smart fevers and some obstinate catarrahs amongst us, or thy humble supplicant must up shop — and if it should please thee to throw in a few cramps and agues it would greatly help thy miserable servant, for on the word of an apothecary I have scarcely heard the music of mortar these two months. Take notice also, I beseech thee, of the mournful situation of my neighbour Crape the undertaker, who suffers considerably by want of practice, and loses many a job of my cutting out; enable him to bear his misfortunes with philosophy, and to look forward with new hope for the tolling of the bell. Physic those, I beseech thee, that will not encourage our profession, and blister their evil intentions, viz. Such as their cursed new-invented waterproof; and may all the coats be eaten by the rats that are so made: but pour down the Balm of Gilead on the overseers of the village, and all the friends of Galen. May it please thee to look over my book of bad debts with an eye of compassion, and increase my neighbours' infirmities; give additional twinges to the rector's gout, and our worthy curate's rheumatism; but above all, I beseech thee to take under thy especial care the lady of Squire Handy, for should the child prove an heir, and thy humble servant so fortunate as to bring the young gentleman handsomely into the world, it may be the means of raising me to the highest pinnacle of fortune.' The print suggests the unholy alliance between doctor and disease and mocks the puritanical strand of faith which welcomes miseries. Aesculapius was the Greek god of medicine.

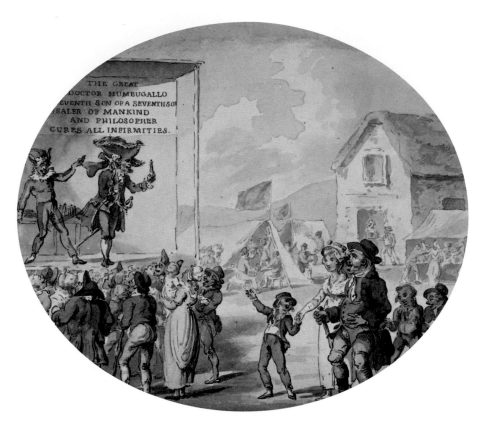

39 Thomas Rowlandson, 'The Great Doctor Humbugallo Seventh Son of a Seventh Son Healer of Mankind and Philosopher Cures all Infirmities', watercolour.

Rowlandson brings out the essential theatricality of quack medicine, with its stage, fancy dress and captivated audience. Seventh sons of seventh sons, as Humbugallo claimed to be, were traditionally believed to possess inherited healing powers.

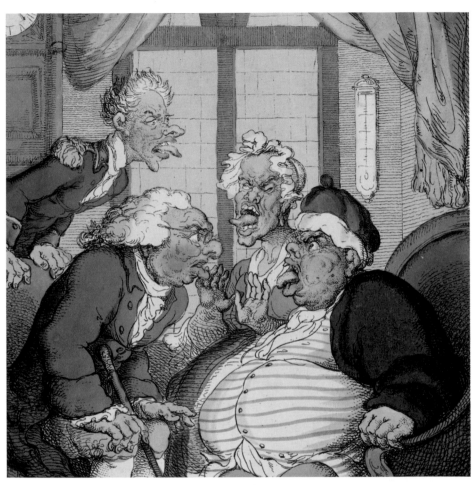

40 Thomas Rowlandson, coloured etching, 1813.

    A doctor examines an obese man and his wife and servant for suspected food poisoning from toadstools. As over-eating produces sickness, obesity and ugliness, the doctor is, by association, as hideous as his patients.

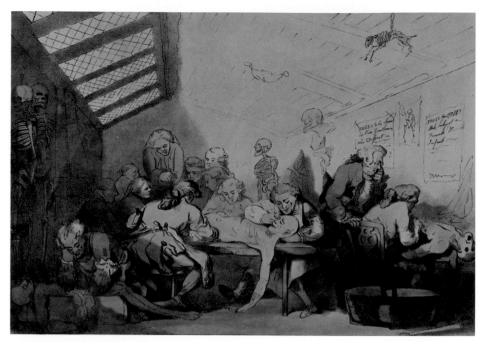

41 T. C. Wilson, 'THE DISSECTING ROOM', lithograph after a pen and wash drawing by Thomas
Rowlandson in the collection of the Royal College of Surgeons of England.

Identifiable amongst the gathering are famous medical men associated with William Hunter –
his younger brother John, Cruikshank, Hewson, Pitcairn, Baillie, Howe, Sheldon and Camper –
all brought together retrospectively to form a composite portrait of some of Hunter's pupils and
colleagues. One of the notices on the wall advertises 'Prices for Bodys' (presumably to be
charged by Hunter to the students, rather than the costs exacted by the body-snatchers).
Rowlandson had probably sketched in such dissecting rooms; however, this scene may be
fanciful, since the dissecting rooms at Hunter's Great Windmill Street premises were in the
basement, not the attic.

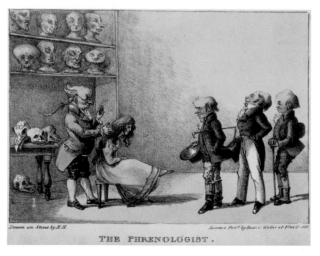

THE PHRENOLOGIST.

42 'E. H.', 'THE PHRENOLOGIST',
1825, coloured lithograph.

Franz Joseph Gall, the co-
founder of phrenology, is shown
examining the head of a pretty
young girl, while three gentlemen
wait in line. Conventionally the
subject is an attractive female; the
men in line are grotesques, as is
Gall himself. Note the skulls and
phrenological busts in the
background. Phrenology was
controversial since its basic
premises were materialistic (mind
is a function of the brain); hence it
was widely recruited as a subject of
satire.

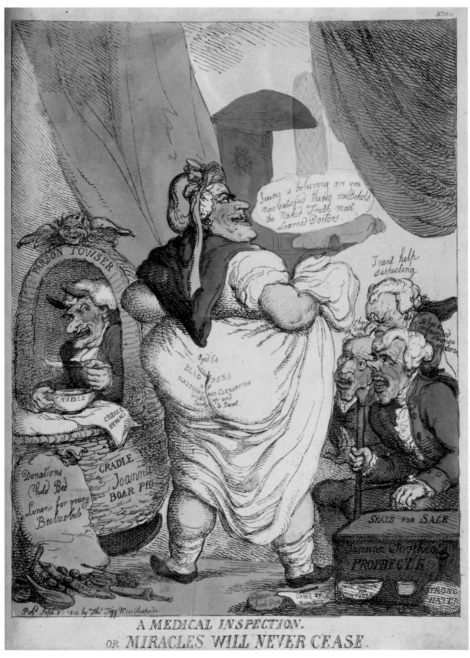

43 Thomas Rowlandson, 'A MEDICAL INSPECTION. or MIRACLES WILL NEVER CEASE', 1814, coloured etching.

Joanna Southcott the prophetess exposes herself to three physicians in order to validate her pregnancy. The print includes medical paraphernalia and lewd captions suggestive of the doctors' lubricity. Sex, medicine and fringe religion are all tarred with the same brush.

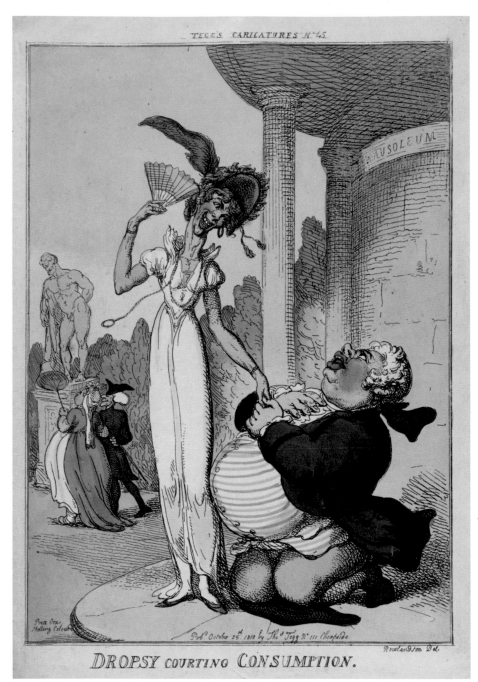

MAUSOLEUM

Price One
Shilling Coloured

Pub.d October 25.th 1810 by Tho.s Tegg N° 111 Cheapside

Rowlandson Del.

DROPSY COURTING CONSUMPTION.

44 Thomas Rowlandson, DROPSY COURTING CONSUMPTION', 1810, coloured etching.
   Rowlandson satirizes the fat/thin obsessions of the time by depicting an obese man wooing a
tall, cadaverous female, skinny, simpering and very bony, outside a mausoleum, hinting that both
are close to death. In the background, an obese lady and her thin escort gaze with envy at a statue
of Hercules.

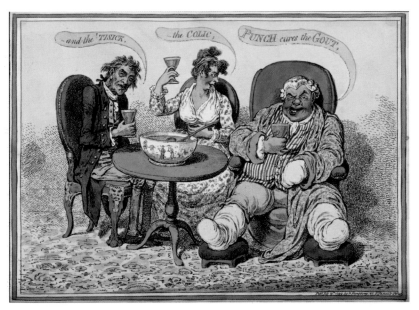

45 James Gillray, 'PUNCH cures the GOUT, — the COLIC, — and the 'TISICK', 1799, soft-ground etching with watercolour.

    Gillray depicts gout accompanied by a man with the 'physick', or tuberculosis, and a woman with colic. All drink to drown their sorrows.

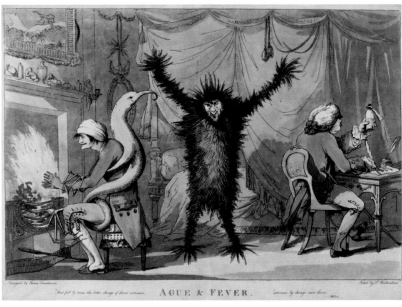

46 Thomas Rowlandson after James Dunthorne, 'AGUE & FEVER', 1788, coloured etching.

    The captioning runs: 'And feel by turns the bitter change of fierce extremes, Extremes by change more fierce (Milton).'

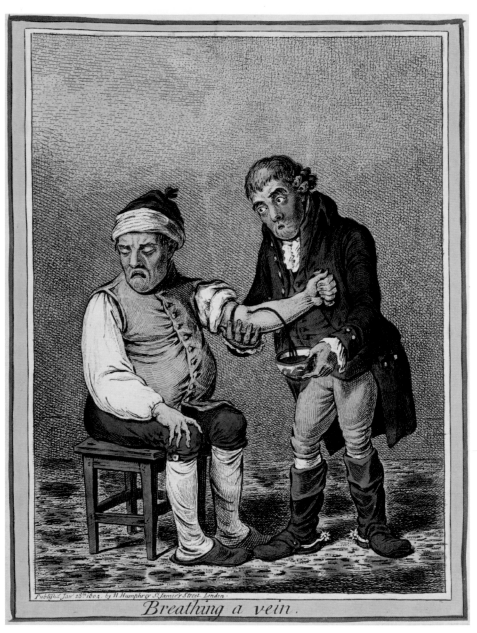

Breathing a vein.

47 J. Sneyd, 'Breathing a vein', 1804, coloured etching after James Gillray.

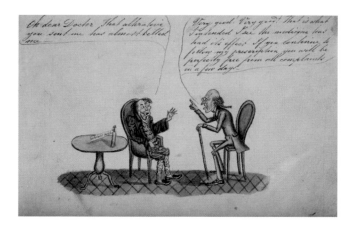

48 In this undated watercolour, the patient says: 'Oh dear doctor that alterative you sent me has almost killed me.' Replies the doctor: 'Very good! Very good! That is what I intended I see the medicine has had its effect if you continue to follow my prescription you will be perfectly free from all complaints in a few days.' A bottle labelled 'Vitriolic Acid' lies on the table by the patient.

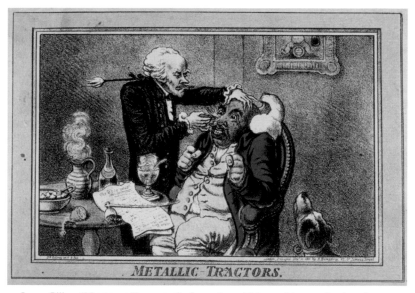

METALLIC-TRACTORS.

49 James Gillray, 'METALLIC TRACTORS', 1801, coloured lithographic reproduction of an aquatint after himself.

Gillray shows an operator (Benjamin Perkins, an American quack) treating the carbuncled nose of an obese patient with 'Perkin's tractors'. A radical newspaper ('The True Briton') announces: 'Theatre Dead Alive ... / Grand Exhibition in Leicester Square / just arrived from America the Rod of Esculapius / Perkinism in all its Glory being a certain cure for all Disorders Red Noses Gouty Toes Windy Bowls Broken Legs HumpBacks / just Discover'd the Grand Secret of the Philosp[hical] Stone with the true way of turning all metal into Gold pro bono publico.'

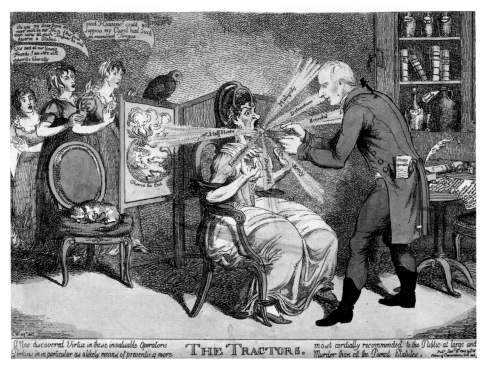

50 Charles Williams, 'THE TRACTORS', 1802, etching with watercolour.

The captioning runs: 'A New discovered Virtue in these invaluable Operators most cordially recommended to the Public at large and to Dr Perkins in particular as a likely means of preventing more Murder than all the Pœnal Statutes.' The rays from the open mouth – 'Half-Hints', 'Malignity', 'Destruction', 'Scandal', 'Envy', 'Hypocrisy' and 'Innuendoes' – have set fire to a screen. Amongst the other specifics on the shelf is a large jar labelled 'Cherry Brandy'. The notion of medical treatment being prescribed for women who were themselves a pain is an archaic joke. Tractors will make her tractable.

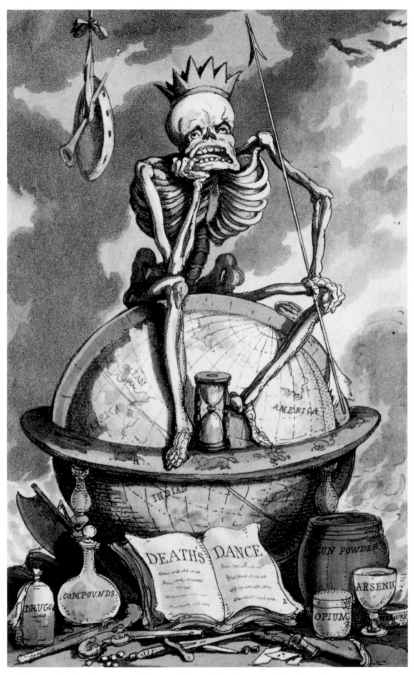

51 Thomas Rowlandson, *English Dance of Death*, frontispiece, 1816, coloured aquatint.

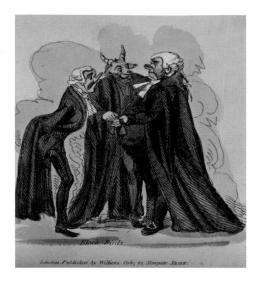

52 'Black birds': a physician, a lawyer and a vicar, represented as outlandish figures in an anonymous coloured etching, *c.* 1820.

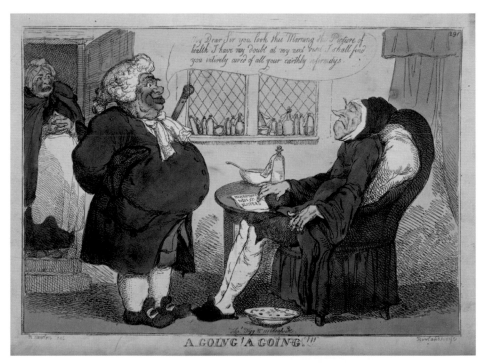

53 Thomas Rowlandson, 'A GOING! A GOING.!!!', 1813(?), coloured etching after Richard Newton.

The Doctor says: 'My Dear Sir you look this Morning the Picture of health I have nay doubt at my next visit I shall find you intirely cured of all your earthly infirmitys.' The patient holds a sheet with the words 'Prescriptions bolus &c. blisters'.

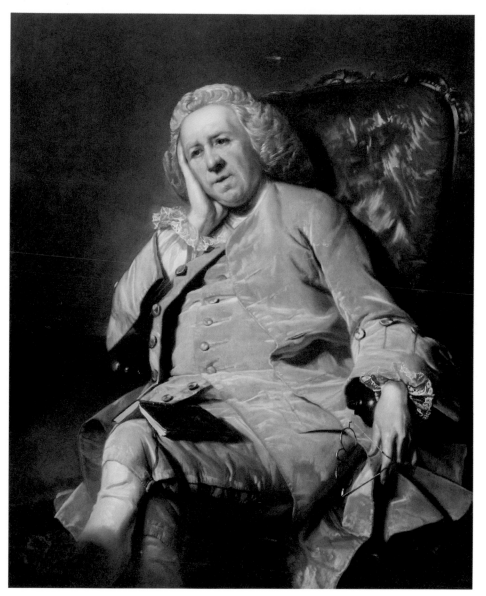

54 Mary & Thomas(?) Black, *Messenger Monsey*, 1764, oil on canvas. The Royal College of Surgeons of England.

On qualifying, Monsey set up in practice in Bury St Edmunds and had a stroke of luck. Lord Godolphin, the son of Queen Anne's Lord Treasurer and grandson of Sarah, Duchess of Marlborough, fell sick while on the road to Newmarket. The nearest medical man happened to be Monsey. Called in, he so pleased his noble patient by both his skill as a doctor and his personality that Godolphin persuaded him to come to London. To ensure a steady income for his *protégé*, Monsey's patron presented him with the post of physician to Chelsea Hospital, though he lived in fashionable St James's. Monsey soon numbered many of the leading Whig politicians among his patients, including Sir Robert Walpole, who became a friend. Georgian medicine worked less by professional rules than by patronage.

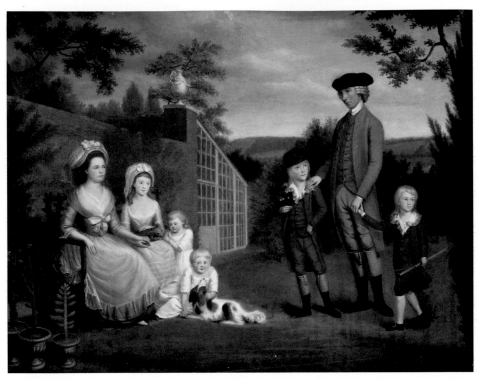

55 John Coakley Lettsom with his family, in his garden at Grove Hill, Camberwell, *c.* 1786, oil on canvas.

This painting was designed to depict a Georgian ideal of domestic virtue and conjugal informality.

> The Hydrops next appears amongst the Throng;
> Bloated, and big, she slowly sails along.[21]

Thus anthropomorphized, disease was a device later exploited by William Thompson:

> Of SICKNESS, and its family of woes,
> The fellest enemies of life, I sing …

The maladies Thompson personified included

> … The knotted Gout;
> The bloated Dropsy; and the racking Stone
> Rolling her eyes in anguish; Lepra foul;
> Strangling Angina …[22]

In his Lucretian philosophical epic, *The Temple of Nature* (1803), Erasmus Darwin similarly demonized disease as a foul fiend visiting evil and destruction upon innocents:

> Behind in twilight gloom with scowling mien
> The demon Pain, convokes his court unseen;
> Whips, fetters, flames, pourtray'd on sculptur'd stone,
> In dread festoons, adorn his ebon throne;
> Each side a cohort of diseases stands,
> And shudd'ring fever leads the ghastly bands …[23]

If enlightened men like Darwin no longer believed in the Devil and the other demons of darkness, disease had by no means been divested of its malign and moralistic associations – a victim-blaming situation which, to the American critic Susan Sontag's exasperation, has continued to this day.[24]

Arresting literary and artistic devices wrung comment and comedy out of the interchangeability of people and diseases. A correspondent to the *Chelmsford Chronicle* in January 1765 felt 'induced to look on the town I live in as an hospital, and everyone in it, by close or remote analogy, to be qualified for that admission they have obtained', proceeding to conduct a facetious local population survey of the diseases there resident. In a bantering account, he found diseased with

Vertigo	100 youths of both sexes
Blindness on one side	20 husbands
Deafness in one ear	40 wives
Short sightedness	200 inexperienced
Plica polonica	4 sluts

Lethargy in the morning	Half the town
Vigilia Nimiae at Night	12 rakes
Facies Hippocratica	The physicians sets
A vitiated taste	6 connoisseurs
Asthma	2 Scolds
Foul tongue	2 Scolds
An irregular tumour of the abdomen	1 virgin
Diarrhoea of words	16 women, 8 men
Continuity of sense	16 women, 8 men
Vapours	1 bully
Gravel–in conversation	4 formalists
Lameness of argument	4 formalists
Comibus	one cuckold
Fluor Albis	2 milkmaids
Urinae incontenentia	499 children
Relaxation of the reins – of government	17 parents
Excessive transpiration	6 gossips
Ruptures incurable	2 married pairs
Ruptures curable	16 friends
Eruptions	10 schoolboys
Fistula in ore	30 smokers, 2 musicians
Piles – of wealth	1 miser
Breeding	500 children
Labour	Their fathers
An unnatural delivery	1 parson
False conceptions	2 pretenders to wit
Miscarriages	12 projectors
Eructations	2 clowns
Tympany	The bellman, 12 ringers
Concussio capitus	30 parents
Contusio ejusdem	70 children
Adura mater	70 children
Miserere mei	500 poor
Tinea	10 shopkeepers
Worms	1 distiller
Cramp	1 in prison

and so forth.[25]

Displacement and substitution could work in various ways. Anthropomorphism, the caricaturist's favourite trick, drew comically disturbing effects out of the incongruous look of dumb animals, manikins or, in the present case, diseases, when made to assume human attire, airs and expressions. Anthropomorphization rendered diseases threatening – indeed, they could be all the more insidious precisely because thus envisaged as such diminutive invaders – but simultaneously it might help to draw their sting through ludicrousness.

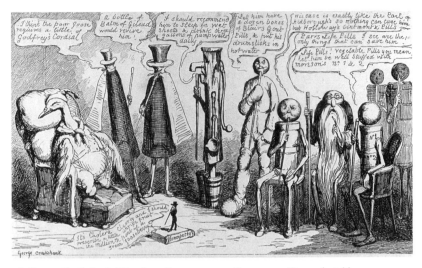

56 George Cruikshank, 'THE SICK GOOSE AND THE COUNCIL OF HEALTH', etching.
    A large group of doctors, deliberating around a patient, are mimed by figures characteristic of the cures they are prescribing. A bottle says: 'I think the poor Goose requires a little of Godfrey's cordial'; another bottle says: 'a bottle of balm of Gilead would revive him!' A hydropath water pump suggests: 'I should recommend him to sleep in wet sheets & drink three gallons of pump water daily'; a pill says: 'let him have a dozen boxes of Blairs Gout Pills, & put his drumsticks in hot water.' A bottle of ointment says: 'His case is exactly like the Earl of Aldborough's so nothing can cure him but Holloway's Ointment & Pills'; an old man says: 'Parrs Life Pills I see are the only things that can save him!' Another bottle of pills (labelled 'n°.1 and n°.2') replies: 'Life pills! Vegetable Pills you mean, let him be well stuffed with Morison's n°.1 & 2.' A minute man on top of a book entitled 'homœopathy' says: 'It's cholera clearly and I should prescribe a little unripe fruit – the millionth part of a green gooseberry.'

Rowlandson excelled in caricature personification of maladies. 'AGUE & FEVER' (illus. 46) shows a sick man, teeth chattering, warming his hands before a blazing fire. A sinuous, snaky monster, Ague – that is, malaria, still then common in low-lying areas like Romney Marshes and the Fens – clings to him, while Fever, a bear-like furry fiend, dominates the chamber.[26] In various Cruikshank prints likewise, maladies are transmogrified into goblins, demons and imps, kin to the mythical beasts, fairies, nymphs and nereids comprising the supernatural squadrons of Pope's *The Rape of the Lock* and other mock-heroic epics.

The agents of Illness were rendered into graphic foes. A series by Cruikshank, issued between 1819 and 1825, depicts cholic, headache, indigestion and (as seen in Chapter 1) the *Blue Devils* (depression), all as miniature puppet diseases helplessly contemplated by doctors. He also conjured up a 'sick goose' (illus. 56) attended by a grotesque 'Council of Health', whose physicians, clad in prescriptions by way of overcoats, are pillboxes who raise their mandatory canes to their medicine-bottle heads. A waterpump, its spout a nose and its handle an arm, is doubtless intended as a charade hydropath.

In 1803 an influenza epidemic raged through Europe. In a print, 'Mr Influenzy' is shown attired in the *bonnet rouge* (cap of liberty) of revolutionary France, implying that the epidemic was (like syphilis) yet another French disease, which had smuggled itself across the Channel during the brief Peace of Amiens (1802). The nine practitioners paying their respects to the Continental caller are those illustrious medics suspected to have done well out of the visitation. Paying homage on his knees is the recently elevated Sir Walter Farquhar, physician to Prime Minister William Pitt and Physician-in-Ordinary to the Prince of Wales, while behind him, bowing low, is Sir George Baker, a former President of the College of Physicians who had earlier published a paper on 'Influenza or Epidemic Catarrhal Fever'. Thomas Beddoes, included presumably because he was a supporter of the French Revolution, is at the back on the left.[27]

In the medical theatre of cruelty, not only maladies but treatments too are standardly represented as a pain, creating an ironic symmetry of suffering: 'The disease torments us on one side', Montaigne had lamented, 'and the remedy on the other',[28] while Lady Holland was to complain, with an epigrammatic turn, 'my plague is physic'.[29] At first sight perversely, the ferocious painfulness of a treatment might even serve as a positive recommendation in its favour – the earnest of its efficacy lay in its bite or sting ('if it's not hurting, it's not working'). Disapproving of 'popgun remedies', Samuel Johnson frequently requested, nay, demanded, to be bled by his surgeon, and sometimes he did it himself. In January 1777 night-time breathing difficulties led the ageing and ailing lexicographer to consult his friend Thomas Lawrence, who ordered the removal of twelve ounces of blood. Finding he still could not sleep lying down, he 'therefore did what the Doctor permitted in a case of distress. I rose and opening the orifice let out about ten ounces more.' After a third bleeding in four days he was 'much better, at the expense of about thirty-six ounces of blood'.[30] Psychologically at least, heroic remedies often seemed to work and hence appealed to hardy souls (illus. 47). The nineteenth-century Yorkshire naturalist squire Charles Waterton recorded, near the close of his life, that he had bled himself 136 times.[31]

Even so, treatment might still seem like futile torture. 'I took physic today', moaned Elizabeth Wynne, 'it gave me the Belly ake all day and made hardly no effect.'[32] Ever the cynic, Byron shrugged his shoulders at the bizarre palaver: 'I have been most painfully ill', he told a friend in

1812, 'cupped on the loins, glystered, purged & vomited, *secundum artem*': he made it sound as though the physic was the illness. As Lady Holland suggested, medicine partnered malady in a masked ball in which identities were reversed.[33]

Jonathan Swift, for his part, took mulish glee in the paradoxical nauseousness of treatments of the *Drekapotheke* (shit medicine) kind. Finding that the chief affliction amongst the Yahoos was called the 'Yahoo's Evil' – obviously a mocking reference to the 'King's Evil', that is, scrofula – and that its remedy was 'a Mixture of *their own Dung* and *Urine* forcibly put down the *Yahoo's* Throat', how gratified was Gulliver the surgeon to discover the resemblance to the business of undergoing medication back home. For European physicians, we are told,

> from Herbs, Minerals, Gums, Oyls, Shells, Slats, Juices, Seaweed, Excrements, Barks of Trees, Serpents, Toads, Frogs, Spiders, dead Mens Flesh and Bones, Beasts and Fishes, form a composition for Smell and Taste the most abominable, nauseous, and detestable, they can possibly contrive, which the Stomach immediately rejects with loathing; and this they call a Vomit.[34]

On medicine's battlefield, practitioners are represented in prints and stories endlessly performing procedures which invade, wound and hurt their patients – and, the implication is, sometimes despatch them fast (illus. 48). They wield the lancet and let blood; Gillray's *Taking Physic* – a common image – expresses through the patient's anguished grimace the medicine's dreadful taste; and they perform surgery, always, in the pre-Victorian era, without anaesthetic. The effect is usually depicted as excruciatingly painful, though sometimes an amputee may be portrayed as superhumanly and unimaginably stoical.

To the patient, such medical apparatus as the enema (or clyster) might appear as an offensive weapon, an engine of sexual assault. Other illustrations of therapies wring wry laughter out of pain, often so as to discredit the unscrupulous practitioner and deride the credulous patient. The painfulness of physic is basic to anti-doctor satire: doctors do not only make you sick, but pile on the agony with their agonizing ('heroic') cures for those conditions. Let us return to gout. Dismissing 'the Prescriptions of the Faculty' which, he said, 'consist generally of Flannels, Patience and sleeping Draughts', the quackish 'gout doctor' Abraham Buzaglo instead implausibly touted 'exercise and means of restoring Limbs and joints to their usual state'. As described in his *A Treatise on the Gout* (1778), his treatment involved the sufferer in exhausting balletic routines of muscular activities

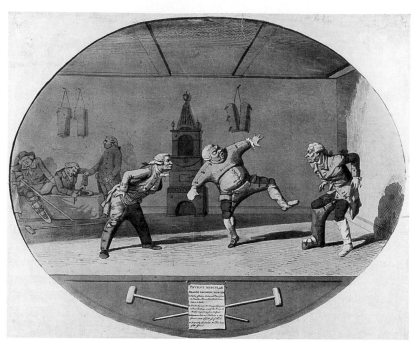

57 Paul Sandby, 'LES CAPRICES DE LA GOUTE, BALLET ARTHRITIQUE', 1783, lithograph.
  The captioning ('PATENT MUSCULAR HEALTH-RESTORING EXERCISE') touts Buzaglo's treatment: 'I. It takes off within the hour all Pains from the Shoulders, Elbows, Sides, Back, Knees, Calves and Ancles. II. It radically cures the Cramp, dissipates callous Swellings round the Knees & Ancles originating from the Gout. III. It restores wasted Calves to their former state of fullness of Flesh. IV. It greatly facilitates the Discharge of the Gravel.'

drawing on the aid of 'wedges and pegs'.[35] In an ironic representation of that medical entrepreneur's gout-cure establishment (illus. 57), Paul Sandby showed him fitting up a sufferer with wooden 'bootikins', whilst other martyrs to the gout are caught whirling and twirling around, encased in assorted bizarre contraptions, an enactment of pure farce.

Another quackish remedy inviting humorous representation was Perkins' tractors. Patented in 1798 by the American Elisha Perkins, who perished of yellow fever in New York the following year while demonstrating his cure, the tractors had only to be drawn across the affected part – so their inventor claimed – for relief to be achieved at a stroke through the magic of electricity. The marvel was brought to Britain by his son, and a 'Perkinean Institution' was founded for the free treatment of the poor who could not afford the regular five guinea charge for the wonder gadget. The patients' metal was evidently turned to gold in that theatre of healing: Perkins Junior returned to America supposedly £10,000 in pocket.

His powdered hair tied back in a queue, a thin but resolute operator is shown by Gillray (illus. 49) clenching one tractor between his teeth while applying the other to the carbuncled nose of a seated John Bull-figure. Electrical sparks issue, the startled patient's wig falls off, and his dog is surprised. The device put to more sinister ends is shown in another print, in which an operator is treating Mrs Philip Thicknesse to stop her venomous tongue (illus. 50). The Thicknesses notoriously quarrelled in public, and there was nothing new in the notion that medicine might serve as a means of silencing shrewish women.

Confirming the old jest, or suspicion, that psychiatrists are crazier than their patients, treatments for insanity have frequently seemed indistinguishable from torture engines. Take the cold-water-jet therapy outlined by the Lincolnshire physician Patrick Blair in 1725 in 'Some Observations on the Cure of Mad Persons by the Fall of Water'. Referring back to earlier shock treatments like ducking, the 'Cataractick Way of Cold Bathing' had various advantages, claimed that Fellow of the Royal Society, notably 'the Surprize upon being blindfolded [which] is a great means to the recovery of Reason [and] the Terror of the former creates such a dread & horrour of it [as] much contributes to produce the desir'd effect.' Cold water had many symbolic properties and madness was supposedly susceptible to shocks.

The dose was to be determined according to the tenacity with which the mad person clung to his – or, one imagines, more often her – delusional feelings and beliefs. Treating a married woman who, showing 'dislike to her husband', had become mildly distracted, Blair went in for an appallingly punitive mode of treatment which makes the barbaric, knockabout, farcical handlings of the mad on the Jacobean stage seem mild indeed:

> I ordered her to be blindfolded. Her nurse and other women stript her. She was lifted up by force, plac'd in and fixt to the Chair in the bathing Tub. All this put her in an unexpressable terrour especially when the water was let down. I kept her under the fall 30 minutes, stopping the pipe now and then and enquiring whether she would take to her husband.

Still the lady was not for turning:

> She still obstinately deny'd till at last being much fatigu'd with the pressure of the water she promised she would do what I desired on which I desisted, let her go to bed, gave her a Sudorifick as usual. She slept well that night but was still obstinate. I repeated the Tryal by adding a small pipe so that when the one let the water fall on top of her head the other squirted it in her face or any other part of her head

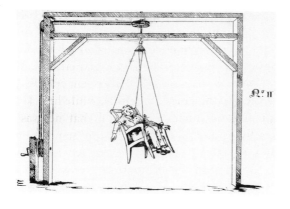

58 Rotatory-motion machine, or 'swing chair', for the treatment of the insane, from Alexander Morison, *Cases of Mental Disease* (London and Edinburgh, 1828).

neck or breast I thought proper. Being still very strong I gave her 60 minutes at this time when she still kept so obstinate that she was laid a bed as formerly but next day she was still obstinate.

At last she broke under the physical and mental torture.

> Evacuations being endeavoured for 90 minutes under it, promised obedience as before but she was as sullen and obstinate as ever the next day. Being upon resentment why I should treat her so, after 2 or 3 dayes I threatned her with the fourth Tryal, took her out of bed, had her stript, blindfolded and ready to be put in the Chair, when being terrify'd with what she was to undergo she kneeld submissively that I would spare her and she would become a Loving obedient and dutiful Wife for ever thereafter. I granted her request provided she would go to bed with her husband that night, which she did with great chearfullness.[36]

Therapy, torture and sexual bullying dissolve into each other, and make bad worse; madness taints all it touches.

The various swing chairs (illus. 58) touted by asylum-keepers around 1800 and resembling items out of a fairground merry-go-round, likewise blended physical and psychological torture in awesome spectacle, as, strapped into the contraption, the patient was revolved at up to a hundred gyrations a minute. At his Fishponds Asylum just outside Bristol, Joseph Mason Cox noted the varied effects produced by different velocities: slow speeds proved soothing, while faster ones induced violent and disorienting giddiness, a traumatization anticipated to break the hold of a delusory system or a vicious stubbornness of will. Extreme 'vertigo' would 'often contribute to correct the morbid state of the intellect', for, Cox argued, the 'valuable properties of this remedy are not confined to the body', but 'its powers extend to the mind', especially by inducing terror.[37]

A respected asylum-keeper, Cox was far from a conventional 'sadist' but a practitioner enthusiastic as to the therapeutic potential of spectacle, calling for an absolute environmental control designed to outwit the devious delusions of his patients, a stage upon which he could orchestrate that gothic anti-carnival which he termed, using an old Roman Catholic idiom, 'pious frauds'.[38] Such enactments might involve dramatizing the patient's hallucinations, while hijacking or rewriting the script. Take a lunatic convinced that he was doomed to perish because a living animal had become lodged in his belly and was devouring him. It was useless to attempt to reason him out of this error; one had rather to 'humour the insane idea', but then outsmart him, for instance by introducing a frog into his chamber pot, thereby persuading him that he had voided it himself, and so was cured.[39]

More broadly, Cox believed in orchestrating the total environment to create a theatre of terror. One patient was shaken out of his conviction of being the Holy Ghost by the introduction of a bit-part player who insisted *he* was.[40] Or, affirming great stage-managerial talent, Cox would use scenic devices 'contrived to make strong impressions upon the senses, by means of unexpected, unusual, striking or apparently supernatural agents'. Thus he would awaken patients 'by imitated thunder or soft music, according to the peculiarity of the case'; or, in a more sinister manner, he would deploy 'signs executed in phosphorus upon the wall of the bed chamber', or 'make strong impressions on the senses' by 'some tale, assertion, or reasoning'.[41]

Sometimes dramatic use might be made of a helper 'in the character of an angel, prophet, or devil' – though, he added, 'the actor in this drama must possess much skill, and be very perfect in his part'. Such pyrotechnics, Cox confessed, might seem 'ludicrous' pantomimes, but they were 'sometimes indispensably necessary'.[42]

Cox was quite fetched by the management of sound – the strains of distant, hidden music were beneficially soothing. Particularly valuable, however, was the art of 'producing unpleasant impressions' through other senses, as when yells and screeches were made in an apartment painted glaring white or black and red, through all of which 'every man must be painfully affected' and 'the maniacal patient, however torpid, must be roused'.[43] Or a raging patient might be set 'in an airy room, surrounded with flowers breathing odours, the walls and furniture coloured green, and the air agitated by undulations of the softest harmony'. All such synaesthetic stage-managerial stunts were designed to batter and disorientate the senses, grab the attention, break resistance and the grip of delusions, and wrest the maniac out of his raving.[44] The theatre of illusion would outwit delusion in the battle as to who – doctor or patient – was to define reason and reality, who was to serve as *Schauspieldirektor*.

The perennial doubling of therapy as torture – yet also perhaps as the agent provocateur of therapeutic shock or laughter – shows itself uncommonly frequently in representations of toothache and its treatments, the mortifying pain of that affliction being an inspiration for Robert Burns's muse:

> My curse upon thy venomed stang
> That shoots my tortured gums alang;
> And through my lugs gaes many a twang
> Wi gawing vengeance;
> Tearing my nerves wi bitter pang
> Like wracking engines.[45]

Because it was not life-threatening, the agonies of toothache, especially when redoubled by the dentist, became comic material – and also exemplary tests of fortitude. 'My father and mother constantly desired me to bear pain like a Philosopher or a Stoic,' the Quaker Mary Anne Schimmelpenninck recalled of her childhood. One day the Friends' dentist arrived to examine her teeth:

> I agreed to have my front teeth drawn before my mother came in from her walk, that I might puzzle her as to my classification, as I should want the four teeth in the upper jaw, the distinctive mark of the Primates. I sat still and had them all out, that it might be over when she arrived. George Bolt said I was 'the best little girl he had ever seen;' and took from his pocket a paper of comfits as my reward. But I drew up, and said, 'Do you think Regulus, and Epictetus, and Seneca, would take a reward for bearing pain; or the little Spartan boys?'[46]

Little Miss Schimmelpenninck had certainly learned how to put on a Stoic disposition.

One of the Whig physician Messenger Monsey's many eccentricities, according at least to the caricature of him which circulated in gossip and anecdotes, was his unorthodox approach to extraction:

> Round the tooth sentenced to be drawn he fastened securely a strong piece of catgut, to the opposite end of which he affixed a bullet. With this bullet and a full measure of powder a pistol was charged. On the trigger being pulled, the operation was performed effectually and speedily. The doctor could only rarely prevail on his friends to permit him to remove their teeth by this original process.[47]

The incongruous juxtaposition of tiny tooth and mighty weapon is not unique: a favourite image of French quack 'dentistry' depicts extraction apparently being carried out by the application of a sword point. In such cases, however, it is hard to tell tooth-pulling from leg-pulling, and probably foolish to try. Certainly, bizarre and grotesque treatments proved the source of unerring titillation.[48] Under the pseudonym of 'Tim Bobbin', John Collier published in 1773 *The Human Passions Delineated in about 120 Figures, Droll, Satirical and Humorous*, a series of prints accompanied by a verse text. Four of them depicted tooth-pulling, in each case extraction being accomplished, in true Monseyan manner, by means of a thread affixed to the tooth. Within that basic scenario, different devices, all equally terrifying, are depicted expediting the operation.

In Collier's first print, laughing scornfully, the dentist draws the offending tooth with a thread wound about his hand. His head pulled forward, the patient unwittingly reinforces the tug of the thread by making a grab at it:

> A Doctor once much puzzl'd was
> To find out ways and means,
> How teeth to draw of ev'ry class,
> Without such wracking pains,
>
> A packthread strong he ty'd in haste
> On tooth which sore did wring:
> He pull'd, the patient follow'd fast,
> Like Towzer in a string.

In the second (illus. 59) the callous toothdrawer immobilizes his

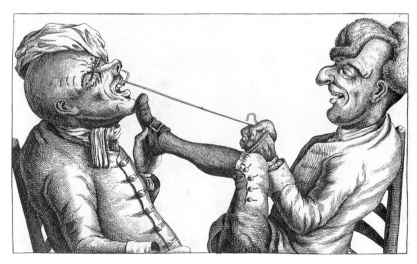

59 'Tim Bobbin' [John Collier], etching for his *The Human Passions Delineated in about 120 Figures, Droll, Satirical and Humorous* (Manchester, 1773).

123

victim's head by wedging his foot against his chin. Eyes squeezed tight in pain, the latter tries in vain to push it away:

> He miss'd at first, but try'd again,
> Then clap'd his foot o'the chin;
> He pull'd – the patient roar'd with pain,
> And hideously did grin.
>
> But lo! – capricious fortune frown'd,
> And broke the clewkin string,
> And threw him backwards on the ground,
> His head made floor to ring.

In the third the dentist jerks on the thread wound round the doomed tooth with one hand, while with the other approaching the sufferer's face with a glowing lump of coal, gripped in a pair of tongs. Yanking back his head in terror, the patient accomplishes a self-extraction. The fourth picture deals with a perennially fascinating topic, forceps extraction, a gadget dear to artists' hearts not only because of its look but because it suggested the low humour of the blacksmith. Laughing cruelly, the doctor grips the handles in his fists and nips the one tooth remaining in the old hag's mouth. While she clenches her eyes shut in dread, her husband leans forward in outright detachment so as to observe the progress of the extraction.[49]

As with all violent slapstick, the psychology underpinning such black humour is evidently complex: is it, as Thomas Hobbes might have said – following his definition of laughter as 'nothing else but sudden glory, arising from some sudden conception or eminency in ourselves, by comparison with the infirmity of others' – an expression of gloating glory and aggressive superiority, a cruel laugh shared between artist and onlooker? Or does it soften the blow to a potential sufferer? – surely actual extractions can't be so bad! Or does the artist-audience relationship mirror that of dentist and sufferer? – does the draughtsman have us on a string? The full meaning may be difficult to extract.

Finally the Grim Reaper. 'DEATH himself knocked on my door,' Tristram Shandy tells us, conveying its terrifying personal immediacy.[50] People of all ages, ranks and stations wended their pilgrim's progress in Death's shadow; Christianity hinged upon that grave mystery; funerals were celebrated with far more pomp than marriages; and new secular media forms, notably newspaper obituary columns, emerged to pay death due homage. What else was certain, asked Ben Franklin, 'except death and taxes'?[51]

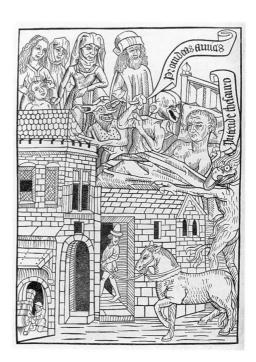

60 Woodcut from the medieval
*Ars Moriendi, or De Tentationibus
Morientium: l'art de bien mourir,
or les tentations des moribonds.*

Christianity had portrayed dying not as a finale but as the threshold
to eternity. To the Catholic the last dispensation of grace was para-
mount: a good person who perished suddenly without the sacraments
might be committed to hell, the sinner who received them, saved. The
Protestant, by contrast, was instructed to meet his Maker with
conscious fortitude. Either way, the pious deathbed staged a high
drama of its own, and the *ars moriendi* scripted the conquest of Death,
to prove one's exit held no terrors. Expiring on a public platform, the
dying person was meant to put on a good show (illus. 60).

Death did, of course, have its terrors; and deathbed scenes
record the intractable fears entertained by Christians of what the
beyond might have in store – Samuel Johnson for one feared eternal
damnation.

Combating such 'morbidity', enlightened deists and sceptics like
David Hume, Edward Gibbon and Erasmus Darwin sought to demys-
tify death, replacing the old 'art of dying' with a new one promoting
frankness towards physical decomposition and annihilation.[52] Central
to this was an onslaught upon the orthodox theology of eternal punishment, now exposed as one of priestcraft's perverted devices devised to
cow the credulous and thereby maximize ecclesiastical power and
profit. The enlightened also strove for dignity in the final scene of life.
Overcoming the remonstrances of his friends, the ailing anatomist

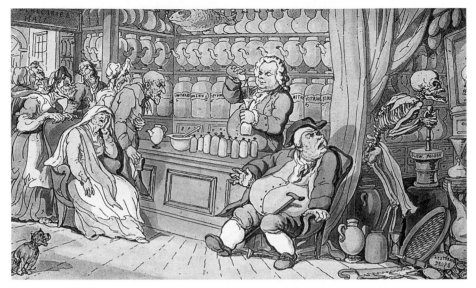

61 Thomas Rowlandson, 'Death and the Apothecary or the Quack Doctor', pl. 11 from his
English Dance of Death, 1816, coloured aquatint.
    The accompanying text by William Combe reads: 'Of this grand shop behold the Master, /
Who deals in Bolus, Pills and Plaister. / See how his visage he disposes, / As his hands measure
out the doses; / While his round paunch most truly tells, / He never takes the Drugs he sells.'
Meanwhile, the patient in the foreground, who is complaining of loss of appetite, observes
Death pounding slow poison and decides, 'I'll take no Drugs that fellow pounds. / I'd better far,
to save my bacon, / Go back to those I have forsaken, / And look once more for healing knowl-
edge, / To the grave Sages of the College.' Beneath is the legend 'I have a secret Art, to cure /
Each Malady, which men endure.'

William Hunter rose from his sickbed to deliver a lecture. Exhausted,
however, he fainted away, and he was finally returned to his bed. 'If I
had strength enough to hold a pen', he observed, 'I would write how
easy and pleasant a thing it is to die.'[53] A noble exit line, indeed.

So how was death visually represented once medicine had become a
presence? If medical humour was in general the child of desperation in
the face of disease, Death became, in the eighteenth century, the hellish
jester par excellence, the prince of darkness, the grave enemy. The
Grim Reaper as a personal foe, dogging mankind, was magnificently
embroidered in all his guises in Rowlandson's *English Dance of Death*
sequence.[54] In the frontispiece (illus. 51), Rowlandson depicts Death
bestriding a globe surrounded by sundry engines of destruction, many
of them medical – drugs, compounds, opium, arsenic – alongside
gunpowder, blades and pistols in an image which perhaps alludes to
the Last Judgement in Holbein's *Dance of Death*, where Christ rides a
rainbow, his feet planted on the universe.[55]

Several prints in Rowlandson's series probe the collusion between death and the doctors. 'Death and the Apothecary or the Quack Doctor' (illus. 61) shows a sleek apothecary in his shop (which slyly contains the dried fish emblematic of the quack, and assorted tools of the trade) making up medicines from one of his recipes, whilst languishing clients await his attention. Peering over his shoulder, a gouty gent on the right is horrified to see an aproned skeleton, leering at him and grinding a pestle in a mortar labelled 'SLOW POISON'. 'I have a secret Art, to cure/ Each Malady, which men endure', darkly pronounces the apothecary, while he gives this sinister advice to the ladies,

> These Pills within your chamber keep,
> They are decided friends to sleep,
> And, at your meals, instead of wine,
> Take this digestive Anodyne.
> Should you invigoration want,
> Employ this fine Corroborant.
> These curious Panaceas will
> If well applied, cure every ill.
> So take them home; and read the bill,
> Which with my signature at top,
> Explains the medicines of my shop.
> On these you may have firm reliance;
> So set the college at defiance.
> And should they not your health restore,
> You now know where to send for more.[56]

Just as in the apothecary print, in other images of Death stalking the living Rowlandson has the doctor playing a menacing role as Death's deputy, adjutant or double. Death shadows the anatomist in the mortuary and rides with the undertaker. And in the dark and doubtful pact forged with Death, the doctor may end up as his master's dupe. Plate No. 15 of the sequence presents the *Good Man, Death, and the Doctor* with the legend:

> No scene so blest in Virtue's Eyes,
> As when the Man of Virtue dies.

The setting is a bedchamber. At the foot of the bed on which the newly deceased honest man lies are grieving members of his family, with the minister standing at the side in prayer. Disturbing the serenity, the ugly, corpulent physician (odious doctors are ever fat) is disgustedly turning his back upon the dead; sniffing the head of his cane in haughty disdain, he thrusts out his hand for his fee, but Death, with his dart, seizes him by the hair:

Thus, as the pious Churchman prayed,
The Doctor in a whisper said,
'My skill in vain its power applies'
'Tis Fate commands; the patient dies.
'No call requires me now to say:
'I've something else to do than pray.
'I feel my Fee'. – 'Then hold it fast',
said grinning Death, – 'for tis your last'.
The Doctor heard the dreadful sound;
The Doctor felt the fatal wound,
And hast'ning through the chamber door,
Sunk down, all breathless on the floor,
Ah, never more to rise again. –
Thus Doctors die like other men.

Dramatic revenge is thus enacted, by Death, but on behalf of humanity.

5 Prototypes of Practitioners

Though in recent times the medical profession has energetically massaged its own public image, identity-management is not unique to the modern era of spin doctors and public-relations consultants – indeed it dates back to the very first medical professionals. The provenance and early history of the Hippocratic Oath (illus. 62) remain highly contested, but what is beyond doubt is the oath-writer's desire to reassure: 'Whenever I go into a house', swears the physician, 'I will go to help the sick and never with the intention of doing harm or injury. I will not abuse my position to indulge in sexual contacts with the bodies of women or of men, whether they be freemen or slaves.'[1] What does this tell us of popular expectations as to the conduct of the medics of the time?

Zoom forward to Tudor and Stuart days, and we see medical men and their friends championing the physician's honour with equal solicitude: he is a man, we are told, whose protracted university education has rendered him a master in the liberal arts and sciences; he is upright, trustworthy and God-fearing, grave and sober, experienced and devoted to the love not of lucre but of learning.[2] Quoting the Oath, the Tudor physician John Securis reiterated Hippocrates' advice as to professional comportment:

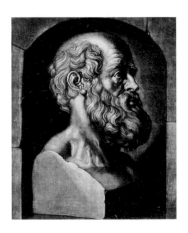

62 J. Faber, 'Hippocrates', undated mezzotint after Peter Paul Rubens.

There is no authenticated original representation of Hippocrates. This image conveys the features classically attributed to Greek sages: maturity, high forehead, baldness and beard.

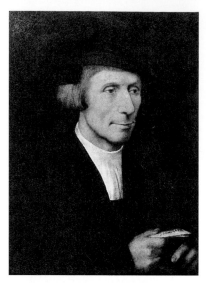 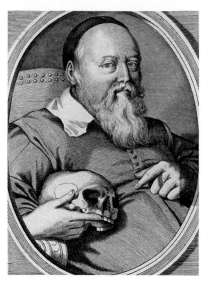

63 Quentin Metsys, undated photogravure engraving (perhaps from life) of Thomas Linacre (*c.* 1460–1524).

64 William Elder, line engraving of Theodore Turquet de Mayerne (1573–1655), *c.* 1680, after an anonymous etching derived from a portrait by Rubens.

Note the common features in these portraits from the Tudor and early Stuart periods: the gravity of countenance; the simple, sombre academic dress; the skull as a reminder of mortality.

> The phisitian must be of a good disposition of the body: he muste also be had in estimation among the common people, by comely apparel and by swete savours ... for by such meanes the pacientes are wont to be delited ... Hys countenance must be like one that is geven to studye and sadde.[3]

Above all, perhaps, the doctor was typecast, first and foremost, as a lofty scholar: '*Hippocrates*', proclaimed James Primrose in 1651, 'saies that a physician which is a Philosopher, is God-like.'[4]

This job specification for the good physician – one who gives wise counsel and inspires trust – was reinforced through the demonization of his antithesis in a rogues' gallery of the inept, ignorant and immoral: the money-grubbing pretender, the swindling foreign charlatan – that 'turdy-facy, nasty-paty, lousy-fartical rogue';[5] the greasy nurse, the gossiping midwife, and the threadbare druggist selling under-the-counter love philtres and poisons – recall the apothecary in *Romeo and Juliet*. Such blackening of one's co-workers may not have been awfully comradely, but the stigmatizing act was carried off with aplomb. Boosted by the pomp and circumstance following Henry VIII's chartering of the College of Physicians in 1518 – it gained its 'royal' tag in 1551 – the medical profes-

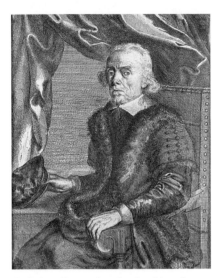 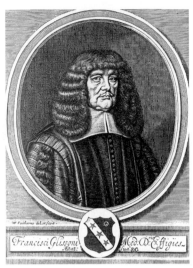

65 Robert Gaywood, undated etching of
William Harvey (1578–1657), possibly after
Wenceslaus Hollar.

66 William Faithorne, line engraving of
Francis Glisson (1598–1677), 1677, perhaps
after himself.

sion showed dexterity in promoting a high-minded image of itself.[6]

There was, it goes without saying, no shortage of disparaging
caricatures in plays and pamphlets, but they were not unduly vicious,
doing little worse than to portray doctors as jargon-spouting windbags,
peering into books rather than bodies, dodderers more familiar with
the library than life – and, from time to time, in the old 'Spring and
Winter' topos, being cuckolded by their frustrated young wives.[7] As
characterized by the droll essayist John Earle, the physician was thus a
man whose erudition consisted 'in reckoning up the hard names of
diseases, and the superscriptions of galley pots in his Apothecary's
shoppe' – comical foibles rather than heinous crimes.[8]

The success of Tudor and Stuart physicians in professional image-
building owed much to the fact that few broke ranks: a composite and
collective stereotype was forged of the exemplary physician – high-
minded, dignified and austere – and they stuck to it, as is evident from
the poses adopted by the leaders of the profession in portraits or in
woodcuts on the title pages of their books (illus. 63–6).[9] The effect is
striking, for all convey corresponding qualities: the sobriety of clothes
and countenance bespeak wisdom, gravitas, venerability, while the air
of unworldiness hints that the physician is brother to the clergyman,
both specializing in counsel, one about health, the other about
holiness.[10] How Thomas Linacre, the first notable Tudor physician,
actually looked we cannot be absolutely sure, for there is no securely

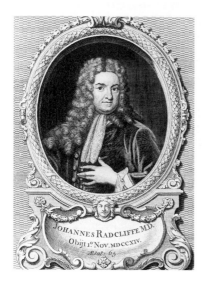

67 Pierre Fourdrinier, line engraving of the Royal Physician John Radcliffe (1652–1714), after a portrait of 1710 by Sir Godfrey Kneller.
Note the full-bottomed wig and sumptuous garb.

authenticated contemporary portrait – any more than there is one of Hippocrates. There are, however, many posthumous paintings and engravings which physicians venerated as the virtual Linacre. In a formulaic manner, all show a lean figure attired in academic robes, suggestive of the seriousness and discretion of a man 'learned and deeply studied in physic'.[11]

A stark contrast is afforded by a later era. In the decades flanking 1700, a bunch of elite metropolitan doctors seem to have enjoyed publicly flaunting themselves as men behaving badly, apparently heedless of what traditionally counted for honour and reputation. On James II's abdication in 1688, for instance, the Royal Physician John Radcliffe (illus. 67) reputedly refused to accompany Princess Anne in her retirement to Nottingham, brazenly insisting that he was detained in London by his patients. A still greater offence followed six years later.[12] The sick Princess sent for the Royal Physician; out quaffing with his bottle-companions, the story goes, he fobbed her off. Summoned anew, he cavalierly declared that 'her Highness's distemper was nothing but the vapours'. This insult got back to her, and when, next day, he finally presented himself at her house, he was refused entry and fired. Gossip also spread about other prominent doctors who, when in their cups, could not be bothered to visit their patients. Reminded that he had failed to keep his appointments, Samuel Garth (illus. 68) supposedly replied: 'It's no great matter whether I see them tonight, or not, for nine of them have such bad constitutions that all the physicians in the world can't save them; and the other

132

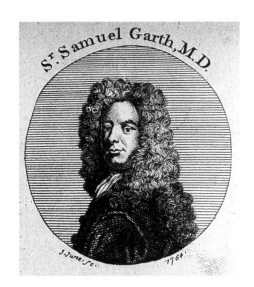

68 John June, line engraving of
Samuel Garth (1661–1719), 1764,
after a portrait by Sir Godfrey
Kneller.

Garth and Radcliffe were both
painted as men of the world by the
most fashionable society portraitist
of the time.

six have such good constitutions that all the physicians in the world
can't kill them.'[13]

All manner of dubious and unscrupulous practices were ascribed to
the supreme manipulator Radcliffe. On his first arrival in London, he
allegedly hired half the porters in town to call for him at coffee-houses,
so as to get his name about – a scam commended in *The Art of Getting
into Practice in Physick, here at Present in London* (1722), an anonymous
satire credited to a rival physician, John Woodward. If 'just arriv'd in
Town ... and an absolute Stranger here', it suggested, 'the first Thing
then I am to advise you just now upon your Arrival, is to make all the
Noise and Bustle you can, to make the whole Town ring of you if possible; So that every one in it may know, that there is in Being, and here in
Town too, such a Physician.'[14] The ruse apparently worked: Radcliffe's
fame and fortune spread, and in due course he could swagger around in
his coach-and-six, an escutcheon on the side, accompanied by running
footmen, corroborating the contemporary jingle:

> The carriage marks the peer's degree
> And almost tells the doctor's fee.

Radcliffe dined off his reputation for arrogance and brutal candour.
At the sight of William III's dropsical ankles, he exclaimed: 'I would
not have your Majesty's legs for your three kingdoms.'[15] He also liked
being known as a good hater. The Covent Garden surgeon John
Bancroft had a son sick with inflammation of the lungs, runs a tale. Dr
William Gibbons was called in, and he prescribed heroic remedies; the
child worsened, whereupon Radcliffe was, at last, sent for. 'I can do

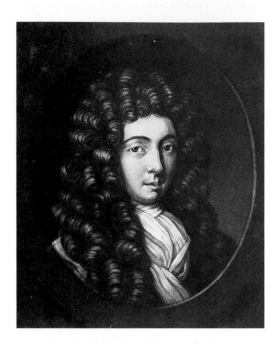

69 William Humphrey,
mezzotint of John Woodward
(1665–1728), from an original
painting in the family of
Dr Woodward's executor.

nothing, sir, he is killed to all intents and purposes,' he remarked, unprofessionally: 'But if you have any thoughts of putting a stone over him, I'll help you to an inscription.' Radcliffe's offer was accepted and, over the grave, a headstone was erected with a figure of a recumbent child, with one hand on his side, saying, '*hic dolor*' [here is the pain], while pointing with the other to a death's head on which was carved, '*ibi medicus*' [there is the doctor].[16]

In an age deafened by pamphlet polemics, pride of place amongst disputatious doctors goes to the aforementioned Woodward, Gresham College professor of physic, natural historian, pioneer geologist, collector, and a fellow of surpassing vanity and pride (illus. 69). In *The State of Physick, and of Diseases*, published in 1718, he dogmatized that good health depended upon maintaining the right balance of 'biliose salts' in the stomach. Too much and there was but one relief: the bilious matter had to be ejected.[17] A satirical retort appeared, in the name of a Dr Byfield – though it was an open secret that it was by John Freind – which in turn drew an instant response from Woodward's old champion, John Harris. Attend to the matter not the man, the latter's *A Letter to the Fatal Triumvirate* (1719) charged Byfield – hypocritically, since he was hardly above the *ad hominem* himself, transforming his rival into 'Don Pedantio Amichi'.

Battle was further joined. In February 1719 there came *A Letter from the Facetious Dr Andrew Tripe at Bath to his Loving Brother the*

Profound Greshamite, revealing that Woodward ('Don Bilioso'), was suffering from *scribendi cacoethes*, that 'Involuntary Propensity in the Hand to write down something without any Manner of Regard to the two Circumstances what or wherefore' – it was, predictably, 'a Distemper arising from a Redundancy of Biliose Salts'. Such salts in the fingers explained his uncontrollable itch for fees.

The Woodward camp hit back, next month, with *The Two Sosias, or the True Dr Byfield*, which outed Byfield as the Jacobite John Freind and Tripe as Richard Mead. There followed the increasingly abusive *A Serious Conference between Scaramouche and Harlequin* by Momophilus Carthusiensis; *An Account of a Strange and Wonderful Dream Dedicated to Dr. Mead;* and *An Appeal to Common Sense* by a 'divine of the Church of England'. Recently guyed on stage as Dr Fossile in John Gay's farce *Three Hours after Marriage*,[18] Woodward now starred as the anti-hero in *Harlequin-Hydaspes: or the Greshamite*, a burlesque opera, performed at Lincoln's Inn Fields.[19]

Such public vituperations became a hallmark of Augustan medicine. 'Anatomists have ever been engaged in contention', William Hunter later reflected on this phenomenon, 'for anything we know, the passive submission of dead bodies, their common objects, may render them less able to bear contradiction.'[20] The scalpel might even lead to the sword. Expelled from the Royal Society's council after a spat with Hans Sloane, on 10 June 1719 the belligerent Woodward actually fought a duel with Richard Mead – fashionable doctors would still in those days sport a sword. Disarming his opponent, Mead (so report went) generously exclaimed: 'Take your life'; to which 'Don Bilioso' responded, 'Anything but your physic'.[21] What is remarkable here is not that, fanned by hotheads like Woodward, controversies blazed, but that leading doctors positively revelled in washing their dirty professional linen in public – easy to do in an age of pamphlets – and basked in becoming the talk of the town or the butt of the wits.

As a strategic ploy in the ongoing sibling rivalry between the College of Physicians and the Society of Apothecaries, in 1696 a number of Fellows of the College set up a dispensary for the sick poor, in a gesture designed to demonstrate its goodwill to Londoners at large.[22] In the skirmishes that ensued – not merely between the two bodies but within the College itself – the big gun was Samuel Garth's *The Dispensary* (1699). The first English poem in the mock-heroic vein, it enjoyed immense popularity, being reissued all through the following century.

The College's dignity has been disturbed, we are told, by discord among the Physicians, resulting in Sloth taking up residence at its headquarters at Warwick Lane in the City. That god's slumbers are rudely disturbed, however, by the din arising from the building of the new Dispensary. Deeply irritated, Sloth sends his servant Phantom to summon help from the goddess Envy. Assuming the guise of the apothecary Colon, Envy then goes to see a fellow apothecary, Horoscope (Barnard),[23] only to find congregating at his shop a gaggle of gullible patients promised by Horoscope 'future health for present fees'. Envy's news of the rise of the Dispensary causes Horoscope to swoon at the threat to his guineas; Colon stirs up resentment against the Dispensary movement; and, after a sleepless night, Horoscope calls the apothecaries to a meeting, and the scene shifts to Apothecaries' Hall at Blackfriars:

> There stands a structure on a rising Hill,
> Where Tyro's take their Freedom out to Kill.[24]

The meeting is addressed, first by the emollient Diasenna, by Colocynthis, who urges a fight to the death, and then by Ascarides – all diseases or remedies personified – who suggests a pact with alienated physicians to sabotage the Dispensary.

Cut next to Covent Garden, where Mirmillo (the anti-dispensarian physician, Dr William Gibbons) has gathered his disaffected cronies, to whom he proclaims:

> Long have I reigned unrivalled in the Town,
> Glutted with Fees and mighty in Renown.
> There's none can die with due Solemnity,
> Unless his Pass-port first be signed by Me.[25]

Having failed to recruit Disease to his cause, Horoscope urges caution, but when the 'Bard' (the physician-poet Sir Richard Blackmore) recites some of his own clodhopping verses, that goddess is finally roused, and determined to promote the contest. Dawn breaks with the apothecaries and their physician confederates assembling to storm Warwick Lane, but, alerted by the goddess Fame, they are prepared. A terrible battle ensues, involving volleys of gallipots, syringes and other medical paraphernalia. The apothecaries' troops begin to gain the day and their leader, Querpo, is on the point of slaying the physicians' chief when Apollo assumes the form of Fee: instinctively Querpo snatches at it instead of striking the fatal blow!

The fray comes to an end when Hygeia, the Goddess of Health, arrives to bid senior physicians accompany her to the Elysian fields to consult with the god-like William Harvey. Referring to the dissent within the faculty:

136

> How Sick'ning Physick hangs her pensive head
> And what was once a Science, now's a Trade,[26]

that divine figure declares that by attending more to science and less to lucre, the College could once again be restored to its former glories, and the poem closes with Hygeia returning to the College with this message – though the reader is left to suppose that there is scant prospect of the great Harvey's advice being heeded.

One of *The Dispensary*'s running jokes is that, although the Collegians, possessed of a 'Right t'Assassinate', enjoy the accolade of being 'The Homicides of Warwick-Lane',[27] each branch of the profession is equally adept at slaughter. Physicians are applauded in Hades, explains Charon, since

> Our awful Monarch and his Consort owe
> To them the Peopl'ing of their Realms below.[28]

'Physician' proverbially became synonymous with 'assassin'.[29] 'This Body of Men, in our own Country', pronounced *The Spectator*,

> may be described like the *British* Army in *Caesar*'s time: Some of them slay in Chariots, and some on Foot. If the Infantry do less execution than the Charioteers, it is because they cannot be carried so soon into all Quarters of the Town, and dispatch so much business in so short a Time.[30]

If Garth's mock epic primarily badmouthed the apothecaries, *The Dispensary* actually mocked all comers in the medical mayhem. Chief butt amongst the physicians was the already-mentioned Dr William Gibbons, who, as the apothecaries' ally, could expect no mercy. The carnage caused by his practice was the subject of a boast issuing from his own mouth:

> Oxford and all her passing bells can tell,
> By this right arm what mighty numbers fell.
> While others meanly ask'd whole months to slay
> I oft dispatch'd the patient in a day: ...
> Some fell by laudanum, and some by steel,
> And Death in ambush lay in every pill ...[31]

The apothecaries, of course, gratefully acknowledged his services:

> ... Each word, Sir, you impart
> Has something killing in it, like your art.[32]

Assailed by the Tory Garth for his dud poetry and politics alike, the

Whig Sir Richard Blackmore parried with *A Satyr Against Wit*, which pilloried his political foe and deplored the cultural malaise springing from Dryden's debased pursuit of 'Wit', which had seduced a whole generation of poets into scorning both religion and virtue.[33]

Drunkenness, disputatiousness, mercenariness, callousness toward patients – all this was capped, not surprisingly, with revelations as to doctors' sexual misdemeanours. Endless innuendoes, for instance, implied that Woodward, with his telltale fondness for enemas and syringes, was a sodomite and a 'great Lover of Boys'. The doctor, gossip had it, had 'attacked [one patient] behind, and made an Evacuation in his Body'.[34]

Tales also circulated of Radcliffe's outrageous misogyny, and the veteran Richard Mead's sex life was splashed in *The Cornutor of 75, being a Genuine Narrative of the Life, Adventures, and Amours of Don Ricardo Honeywater, &c. &c.; Containing, among Other Diverting Particulars, his Intrigue with Donna Maria W——s, of Via Vinculosa, in the City of Madrid*. That impotent old lecher, this pamphlet alleged, had to make do with gazing on the naked charms and combing the red locks of Maria, the daughter of a Fetter Lane (*Via Vinculosa*) black-smith. To please her, Mead had allegedly travelled to Paris to take dancing lessons, using the medical excuse that he required exercise for his health.[35] His susceptibilities were immortalized in *Tristram Shandy* in the guise of Dr Kunastrokius:

> But every man to his own tastes. – Did not Dr Kunastrokius, that great man, at his leisure hours, take the greatest delight imaginable in combing of asses' tails, and plucking the dead hairs out with his teeth, though he had tweezers always in his pocket?[36]

Finally, some of the physicians of that era became embroiled in religious scandal. The Jacobite Radcliffe was deemed by Bishop Burnet an 'impious man',[37] while the Whig Messenger Monsey was a freethinker, hostile to bishops, the Established Church and the Athanasian creed. When, lamenting the unbelieving times, an acquaintance grumbled to him: 'doctor, I talk with people who believe there is no God', Monsey responded: 'And I, Mr. Robinson, talk with people who believe there are three.'[38] He left directions for his body to be dissected, after which 'it may be put into a hole or crammed into a box with holes and thrown into the Thames', and his self-composed epitaph runs:

> Here lie my bones; my vexation now ends;
> I have lived much too long for myself and my friends.
> As to churches and churchyards, which men may call holy,
> 'Tis a rank piece of priestcraft, and founded on folly.

What the next world may be never troubled my pate;
And be what it may, I beseech you, O fate,
When the bodies of millions rise up in a riot;
To let the old carcass of Monsey be quiet.[39]

In short, top Augustan physicians nonchalantly displayed a conspicuous indifference to the hard-won honour of their profession, and were seemingly hell-bent upon defying its prudential etiquette, indeed its elementary moral code, through shock tactics, displays of drunkenness, debauchery, avarice and sexual misconduct. Deriding cherished ideals, elite physicians relished transgressive behaviour and even colluded with Grub Street in trashing their profession and sensationalizing its goings-on. One might perhaps compare the itch of today's film stars, footballers and other celebrities to tell all – their sex lives, drink and drugs problems and psychiatric disasters. Then and now, it appears a self-destructive, or at least high-risk, course of action – so why embark upon it? The answer lies in the mixed bag of anxieties and opportunities typifying the early eighteenth-century metropolitan medical marketplace.

Fears were fuelled, because, corporately speaking, the standing of physicians had grown insecure. The Royal College ended the Stuart era enfeebled, and it was to grow ever more cliquy, clubby and comatose.[40] The legal ruling in the Rose case of 1704 in effect threw the practice of medicine in the capital open to all and sundry,[41] and any subsequent hopes on the part of Collegians of regaining exclusive rights were foredoomed, since Parliament and the public had wearied of medical, as of all other, monopolies. Having little likelihood of being buoyed up by the collective clout of the College, physicians had to sink or swim as individuals. In this *sauve qui peut* climate, they needed to reinvent themselves, displaying talents and traits that would appeal, or at least grab public attention.[42]

Big fish learned to make a splash. Demand for medical services was buoyant in a bubbling commercial and consumer society – indeed in a more secular climate in which the health of the body was perhaps eclipsing concern over the salvation of the soul.[43] Stakes were high, but pickings were rich. In order to thrive in this competitive but lucrative market, a physician had to get his name about: all publicity was good publicity, be it a literary reputation, high political visibility, newsworthiness, entrepreneurship,[44] notoriety, or just a nifty jingle like

Within this place
Lives Dr Case.[45]

139

Charles II's court had launched a cult of cynicism, which then rippled outwards. With its defiant devilry, cavalier wit made it cool to mock revered regal and noble icons. Doctors too got in on the act, mimicking the lifestyles, habits and behaviour of Restoration rakes and play-wrights – maybe in the most literal way. Radcliffe, as mentioned earlier, supposedly paid flunkeys to call for him at coffee-houses to get his name known: doesn't this sound suspiciously like an echo of Petulant in Congreve's *The Way of the World*, who, turning up in disguise in public places, would 'send for himself', for the very same purpose?[46] In the manner of 'life imitating art', physicians may have picked up the ways of the world from fashionable brattish, foppish culture, and learned to glory in the invective, controversialism, physical violence, duelling and theatrical excess cultivated by the smart set.[47]

The louche cynicism of top doctors fed a lasting negative public view of the profession. 'To acquire this Art of Physic', commented Robert Campbell in the 1740s, was in the popular mind supposed to require

> only being acquainted with a few Books, to become Master of a few Aphorisms and Common-place Observations, to purchase a *Latin* Diploma from some Mercenary College, to step into a neat Chariot and put on a grave Face, a Sword, and a long Wig; then *M.D.* is flour-ished to the Name, the pert Coxcomb is dubbed a Doctor, and has a License to kill as many as trust him with their Health.[48]

Later in the century, the hardbitten Bath doctor Dr James Makittrick Adair observed that success reputedly depended on 'sauntering in coffee-houses, or tippling in clubs; the size of their wig ... effusions of unmeaning jargon ... [and] forming dirty connexions with nurses and ladies' women'.[49] Piling on the irony, the pseudonymous Peter MacFlogg'em advised the physician 'never if possible to visit a patient, when he is absolutely so *drunk* that he can neither *walk* nor *stand*'.[50]

Such defamation found endless echoes in literary works that cast doctors as pompous, grasping and lethal. In his play *The Mock Doctor*, and in *Tom Jones*, *Amelia* and *Joseph Andrews*, Henry Fielding paraded meddlesome, vain and greedy practitioners: 'a physician', he wrote, 'can no more prescribe without a full wig, than without a fee.'[51]

The most devastating satire came, however, from one of the tribe itself. In *Ferdinand Count Fathom* (1753), the Scottish surgeon Tobias Smollett laid bare the professional strategies supposedly essential for fame. Having 'read a few books on the subject of medicine', the cash-strapped Fathom sets up in practice at Tunbridge Wells, where he enlists an apothecary to put his name around.[52] Coming up to London, he then finds 'every shabby retainer to physic' must keep a coach 'by way of a travelling sign-post, to draw in customers', and be driven furiously about town to prove how much in demand he was. He also arranged to be puffed by a colleague, ostentatiously dished out free medical advice to the needy, and 'never failed to make his appearance at the medical coffee-house with all ... solemnity of feature and address'.[53] Ever more outlandish devices were becoming necessary because 'the other means to force a trade, such as ordering himself to be called from church ... had been so injudiciously hackneyed by every desperate sculler in physic, that they had lost their effect on the public'.[54] Even bad reviews paid: 'Some of the faculty have been heard to complain, that they never had the good fortune to be publickly accused of homicide.'[55] Crucial, explained the worldly-wise physician Erasmus Darwin, offering advice to a young man about to set up in practice, were visibility and sociability: make your face known:

> At first a parcel of blue and red glasses at the windows might gain part of the retail business on market days, and thus get acquaintance with that class of people. I remember Mr Green, of Lichfield, who is now growing very old, once told me his retail business, by means of his show-shop and many-coloured window, produced him £100 a year.[56]

An exposé of 'Dr Wriggle', subtitled *The Art of Rising in Physic*, dissected the dodges of top doctors:

> His first great maxim is: 'Bring your name before the public; it will, by degrees, become familiar to them and they will at length think you a man of consequence. For this purpose, the doctor contrives to have his name appear every now and then in paragraphs in the newspapers which everybody reads.

The author went on to instance such self-promoting newspaper puffery:

> 'Yesterday as Dr. Wriggle was returning in his chariot from such a place, he was attacked by two highwaymen, who demanded his money, etc', – Or,
> 'On Wednesday last, as Dr. Wriggle and his lady, etc'. But Dr. Wriggle was never robbed.
> No. It was a mere invention: a pretext for bringing his name before the public. There are a variety of other methods by which a man may bring his name before the public in the newspapers, all which Dr. Wriggle has successfully employed.[57]

Unsurprisingly in these circumstances, scepticism ran high. Professionals at large were in bad odour in Augustan England (illus. 52), and medicine notably got it in the neck, for practitioners, so the saying went, fleeced the public first and slew them afterwards: 'When a Nation abounds in Physicians', bantered *The Spectator*, 'it grows thin of people.'[58]

We must not, of course, take this at face value, but anti-doctor diatribes were so common as to suggest disquiet was not just hackneyed. Gravest of all was the charge that, by acts of commission or omission, physicians were fatal. 'While the doctors consult', claimed John Heywood, 'the patient dies.' Should one consult an old or a young physician? Frank Nicholls was asked. 'The difference', replied the doctor, is this: 'The former will kill you, the other will let you die.'[59] Some grew allergic: 'The sight only of her Physician disorders her extremely & throws her into convulsions,' wrote Mary Heber about a companion.[60]

Doctors were also caricatured as sublimely indifferent. Prints portrayed them mouthing their abstruse jargon even as their patients expired – or as too aloof and conceited even to notice. In 'A Going! A Going!!!' (illus. 53) Rowlandson depicted a corpulent doctor, gold-headed cane tucked under his left arm and cocked hat under the other, smiling beatifically over his emaciated dying patient near a table supporting a medicine bottle and a paper lettered 'Prescriptions Bolus and Blisters'. 'My dear Sir,' he booms, 'you look this morning the Picture of Health, I have no doubt at my next visit I shall find you intirely cured of all your earthly infirmitys.'

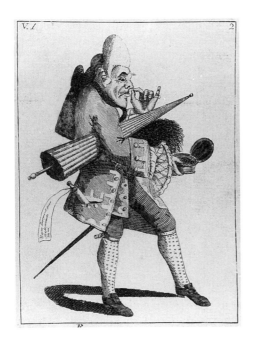

70 Matthew Darly, 'MONᴿ. LE MEDECIN', 1771, engraving.

No English doctor was presented as such a macaroni as the Frenchman. This ridiculous figure is taking snuff while walking; he has a large muff and umbrella, and in his pocket is a syringe labelled 'Une Lavement pour Mademoiselle Mimi'.

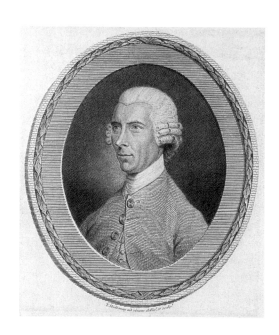

71 Thomas(?) Holloway, line engraving of John Coakley Lettsom (1744–1815), 1792, done from life after himself.

Not just fatuous, the doctor was also mocked for being a pretender to fashion, all got up in his curled and powdered wig, frock coat of satin or brocade, buckled shoes and tricorn hat, and carrying a gold-headed cane and sometimes a muff, to preserve his delicacy of touch (illus. 70).[61] In his *Pompey the Little* (1752), Francis Coventry described the physician as sporting 'a gilt headed cane, a black suit of cloathes, a wise mysterious face, a full-bottomed flowing peruke and all other externals of his profession'. Dressed up to the nines, prattling on, indifferent to their charges – such practitioners seemed offensively full of themselves. Doctor distrust was bound to fester as the profession seemed to be aggrandizing itself and health did not improve in a society in which print increasingly assumed the role of public watchdog.

That was not the whole story, however. Key features of the august presence formerly so assiduously cultivated actually carried over into the post-Restoration era, despite the antics of an elite. If the eighteenth-century surgeon remained archetypically a hefty fellow, handy with the saw and knife, the ideal physician, by contrast, was sublimated, almost disembodied, distinguished by his intellect.[62] In this rather Cartesian professional polarity, it remained, as shown in the previous chapter, the true physician's metier to take the history, frame a diagnosis and formulate a regimen. There being, as yet, no routine physical examination, his job was not hands-on and what counted were acumen, memory and judgment.[63] Signifying the superiority of head over hand, mind over matter, he should appear a model of sagacious self-control.[64] 'I would have the Physician, a Man endowed with Sagacity, Learning and Honesty', declared Robert Campbell in his *London Tradesman* (1747), in a phrase which could just as easily have been written a century or two earlier.[65] Such time-honoured traditional messages come across loud and clear in the self-presentations of many a Georgian physician, who had themselves portrayed as paragons of restraint and sobriety. Take for example the Quaker, John Coakley Lettsom (illus. 71). His portrait shows him as almost incorporeal, entirely untainted by superfluous flesh or flashy display. Indeed, he gave himself out to be almost too busy to take notice of – or even to have – bodily needs. 'Sometimes for the space of a week', he wrote in 1782, 'I cannot command twenty minutes' leisure in my own house,'[66] while on another occasion he declared that his practice 'had not suffered him to sleep in his own bed for thirteen following nights'.[67] The moral was clear: the ascetic Quaker's flesh had been disciplined into utter submission – had almost disappeared.

Similar austerity characterized the public image of William Heberden, a man described as 'tall, thin and spare'.[68] That Cambridge-trained classicist physician was praised by Samuel Johnson as '*ultimus Romanorum*'.[69] The elegiac edge was apt, for new elements in the self-fashioning of the physician were moving to the centre of the Georgian stage, in an updating of the Renaissance scholar-physician into the modern man of the world. In this revamping two interconnected trends stand out. The physician, for one thing, was attempting to doff what was now derided as the fuddy-duddiness of the cloistered and melancholic academic, and don that of the gentleman.[70] This modernization of image – from pedantry to politeness – is captured by many a Georgian portrait: see the fashionable Whig practitioner Messenger Monsey (illus. 54), all assurance, ease and urbanity.[71] In Georgian medicine, the accent newly fell on worldly success. 'In my opinion,' William Hunter taught the students who flocked to his anatomy school, 'a young man cannot cultivate a more important truth than this, that merit is sure of its reward in this world.' Having formed from youth a 'consciousness of the superiority of his talents', William, that Scottish 'lad o' pairts' made good, played the Hogarthian industrious apprentice, and performed word-perfect. Spurred (in his brother John's words) by ambition 'to be at the head of his profession', he drove himself to the top: as early as the 1760s he was raking in more than £10,000 a year – the income of a peer. After toying with the idea of sinking a cool £20,000 into an estate, he chose a more prudent seal to his fame, laying out his fortune on a consummate collection of medals,

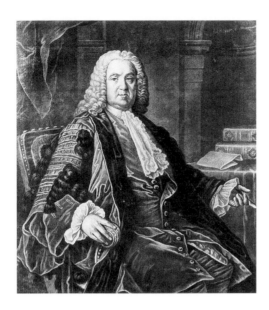

72 Richard Huston, mezzotint of Richard Mead (1673–1754), after an oil of 1740 by Allan Ramsay.

paintings and manuscripts, as well as medical and natural history specimens, and winning an enviable name for connoisseurship. Collecting symbolized his assimilation into superior society, literally through acquiring the trappings of culture and annexing tangible tokens of control – above all, coins. Professional achievement was a means to the end of social prestige, prominence and power.[72]

Belief in *suaviter in modo* marks a significant shift in the physician's image. Hunter had in part modelled himself upon Dr Richard Mead, a man, so Samuel Johnson observed, who 'lived more in the broad sunshine of life than almost any man'. Ensconced in fashionable Bloomsbury Square as the Mycaenas of the Augustan physician collectors, Mead was polished and courtly – such was the message of the portrait of him executed in the grand manner by the Scottish painter Allan Ramsay (illus. 72).[73]

Georgian physicians basked in what Hunter dubbed 'the happiness of riches'.[74] Incomes soared: Radcliffe and Mead apparently made up to £7,000 a year, but two generations later Lettsom's earnings were amounting to as much as £12,000 – far better than the average country gentlemen. Though a Quaker, wealth gave him no qualms, for he laid it out on appropriate improving activities, notably a villa in suburban Camberwell (illus. 55), where he planted five acres of garden, including sixteen types of grapevines, walks, lawns, fountains, ponds, statues and a 'Shakespeare's Walk' – to say nothing of a museum and a library. And he disbursed his surplus income charitably. 'Who will

145

thank us for dying rich!' he exclaimed: 'Not those who get hold of our scrapings. And pray who earns his money with more solicitude than a physician! Who, therefore, has a greater moral right to exchange care for pleasure? especially when those pleasures are the gratification of intellect.'[75]

Worldly success genteelly displayed thus filled the dreams of Georgian physicians. Complementing this ideal, they also displayed new attitudes towards learning that chimed with the broader Enlightenment restyling of the man of letters. Thinking, it was now emphasized, was too important to be left to crabbed or crack-brained dons – it must be rescued from those 'monkish' Oxbridge cells which bred morose pernicketiness; what was needed, according to the enlightened, was discussion not disputatiousness, conversation not crotchets, politeness not pedantry. John Locke's pupil, the third Earl of Shaftesbury, thus denounced 'all that Dinn & Noise of Metaphysicks, all that pretended studdy',[76] claiming that 'to *philosophize*, in a just Signification, is but To carry *Good-Breeding* a step higher'.[77] Proposing, through *The Spectator*, to bring 'Philosophy out of Closets and Libraries, Schools and Colleges, to dwell in Clubs and Assemblies, at Tea-Tables and in Coffee Houses', Joseph Addison, the first great media man, thus sought to turn the philosopher into a man of letters and hence a man of the world.[78]

The Scottish philosopher David Hume applauded this modernization of the intellectual: 'The separation of the learned from the conversable world', he lamented, had been 'the great defect of the last age'; learning had 'been as great a loser by being shut up in colleges', while philosophy had gone to ruin 'by this moping recluse method of study'. Where lay the fault? Thinking had been monopolized by head-in-the-clouds academics 'who never consulted experience in any of their reasonings, or who never searched for that experience, where alone it is to be found, in common life and conversation'. Things, however, were on the mend. 'Men of letters in this age have lost in a great measure that shyness and bashfulness of temper', he noted, 'which kept them at a distance from mankind.'[79]

Just like that philosopher, doctors too wished to come out of the closet and embrace the ways of the world.[80] Old bookishness became discounted in favour of new science: an attachment to facts, experiments and the study of Nature, complemented by that good sense and cultivation of the arts and humanities which would enable the physician to fraternize easily with his patients as friend and fellow.

The greatest clinician of the post-Restoration decades, Thomas Sydenham exalted observation and experience over musty erudition.

Quizzed as to what were the best medical books, he reportedly replied: 'Read "Don Quixote".'[81] Radcliffe too could assume an aggressively anti-intellectual pose, allegedly boasting that he had never even read Hippocrates. Asked where his study was, he answered, pointing to a skeleton, some vials and an herbal: 'Sir, this is Radcliffe's Library.' He published little, and when, in his will, he endowed Oxford with a library, Garth quipped that it was a bit like a eunuch founding a seraglio.[82]

As if taking literally Addison's proposal to bring 'philosophy out of Closets and Libraries ... to dwell in Clubs and ... Coffee Houses', new-style physicians actually conducted their practices from those popular institutions, where they would not merely command maximum visibility as clinicians but also shine as witty men of letters (the two went hand in glove). 'If you can Chat, and be a good Companion', observed the cynical doctor-poet Bernard de Mandeville, 'you may drink yourself into Practice ... [or] you must ... keep a set of Coffee Houses, observe your certain Hours, and take care you are often sent for where you are, and ask'd for where you are not.'[83] Woodward ensconced himself at Nando's; while Radcliffe and his heir Mead attended Tom's in the morning and Batson's in the evening, and Richard Blackmore would hang out at Garraway's. The Falstaffian Scot George Cheyne reported that, once in the capital, he frequented the coffee-house and tavern, 'nothing being necessary for that Purpose, but being able to Eat lustily, and swallow down much Liquor', all of which he did 'to force a Trade, which Method I had observ'd to succeed with some others'.[84] Such coffee-house attendance helps account for the crew of Augustan physicians who also won names as wits and poets, notably Garth, Arbuthnot, Akenside, Blackmore and Mandeville.[85]

These Georgian mutations in the physician's self-image were prudent adaptations to the temper of the times: in a century in which such eminences as Edmund Burke, Sir Joshua Reynolds, Oliver Goldsmith, Sir Joseph Banks, Charles Burney, David Garrick, Edward Gibbon and Adam Smith were proud to be members of Samuel Johnson's club, convening at the Turk's Head in Gerrard Street, it can come as little surprise that physicians too were eager to be seen and shine in elegant, affluent circles – Goldsmith, after all, was trained as a doctor. Clinicians must move with the times, and urbanity became the password to the new polite society of the Enlightenment, promoted by The Spectator.[86]

A Georgian doctor who lacked civility risked censure. 'I doubt not his being a man of great skill', commented Fanny Burney on the celebrated Quaker physician John Fothergill: 'but his manners are stiff, set, and unpleasant ... He is an upright, stern, formal-looking old man.'[87] That may have done very nicely in 1570, but it would no longer serve, at least in the eyes of that lady experienced at Court, two centuries later. Others, by contrast, got the art of the fashionable physician down to a T. 'To a sound judgment and deep observation of men and things', it was said of Richard Warren, physician to the Prince of Wales,

> he added various literary and scientific attainments, which were most advantageously displayed by a talent for conversation that was at once elegant, easy, and natural. Of all men in the world, he had the greatest flexibility of temper, instantaneously accommodating himself to the tone of feeling of the young, the old, the gay, and the sorrowful ... no one ever had recourse to his advice as a Physician, who did not remain desirous of gaining his friendship and enjoying his society as a companion.[88]

Such suavity could, however, be taken too far. 'Never listen to any Doctors' of that kind, Sara Hutchinson warned in 1824, 'London Doctors are, in general, too *polite*, to say disagreeable things.'[89]

Alongside the distinctive 'physical wig', the trademark of the era was the gold-headed cane, that more pacific successor to the sword, sometimes perforated and hollow so that it could contain some sweet-smelling substance to counter the hazards and stinks of the sickroom (illus. 73). With its gold-mounted cross-piece as a handle, Radcliffe's cane was handed down to his successor Dr Richard Mead, and then passed on to other notables until it was presented to the

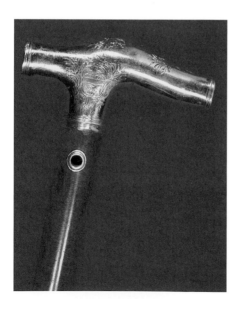

73 An 18th-century gold-headed doctor's cane from the Royal College of Physicians, London.

Royal College, where it is still displayed, traditional medicine's most distinctive prop, symbolizing the public presence of the Georgian physician.[90]

Healing had ceased to be religious, and even royal. It had become, notionally at least, the appurtenance of the polite gentleman. If often exposed as mere show, praise was also forthcoming:

> The medical profession enjoys in Great Britain that degree of estimation and credit, which a science, conferring on mankind the greatest of all comforts except those of religion, justly deserves. Hence Physicians in this kingdom are almost invariably men of liberal education and cultivated minds. Hence too the art of medicine is carried among us to a singular height of excellence.[91]

6 Profiles of Patients

> I find my spirits and my health affect each other reciprocally –
> that is to say, everything that discomposes my mind, produces a
> corresponding disorder in my body.
>
> TOBIAS SMOLLETT, *The Expedition of Humphry Clinker*[1]

The early modern medical drama cast the sick person in the lead role –
at least when he or she was, as commonly, the practitioner's superior in
social origin and status: he who paid the piper called the tune.[2] It was
the sick who authored and (co-)directed their exchanges with the
doctors they summoned, and physicians performed in patient-
controlled space (the sickbed as a set in home theatricals) in storylines
shaped by lay patronage and priorities. The affluent expected to be
heard; they often disregarded their attendants' advice and would feel
no compunction about shopping around for second and third opinions; they made free use of quack and unorthodox remedies, following
a try-anything approach which gave no automatic privilege to regulars;
and they commonly discharged bossy practitioners. In short, the elite
largely carved out their own preferred sick roles, and they it was who
ailed, recovered – or died. 'It is a small thing that the patient knows of
his own state', commented Coleridge, 'yet some things he *does* know
better than his physician.'[3]

In matters of diagnosis, prognosis, regimen and therapy, prudent
practitioners learned the arts of pleasing – even bowing and scraping –
in accordance with the expectations of polite society: what enabled the
occasional Radcliffe to get away with imperiousness was precisely its
novelty value. Notoriously compliant towards his betters was Thomas
Gisborne, a 'member of the *haute noblesse* of medicine'. 'One of the
princesses being taken ill, and Dr. Gisborne in attendance', his
contemporary, the radical Thomas Beddoes (illus. 74) tartly recounted:

> her royal highness enquired of the doctor if she might not indulge in
> the use of a little ice cream, as she thought it would greatly refresh
> her. Dr. G., who never contradicted his royal patients, answered that

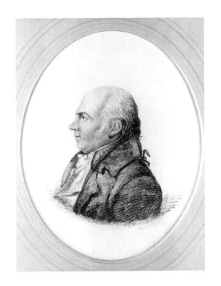

74 Thomas Beddoes (1760–1808),
c. 1790s–1800s, pencil drawing after E. Bird.
   Thick-set, balding and intent, Beddoes
obviously chose not to have himself portrayed
as one of the *haute noblesse* of medicine.

he '*entirely agreed with her royal highness*;' and the ice was accordingly provided. His Majesty [George III], visiting the chamber and observing the glass, with some of the ice still remaining in it, seemed alarmed, on the supposition that it might be improper; but her royal highness assured him that she had the doctor's permission for what she had done. His Majesty ordered the doctor into his presence, and observing to him that he had never heard of ice being recommended in such cases before, expressed his apprehension that it was on some new system. The doctor seemed at first a little confounded, but quickly recovering himself, replied, '*Oh no, please your Majesty, it may well be allowed provided it be taken warm*' – '*Oh well, well, doctor, very well, very warm ice, warm ice.*'[4]

Displays of deference – though not always as extreme as Gisborne's – were appropriate, not least because, as we saw in Chapter 4, in those days before 'scientific medicine' medical know-how was an idiom broadly shared by doctors and patients rather than constituting the kind of esoteric technical monopoly which guarantees professional dominance. Before the cumulative impact of pathological anatomy, diagnostic technology, cell science and the germ theory of disease gave doctors the whip hand, it inevitably fell to the patient to specify his or her 'complaint' – the physician had, as yet, no privileged access to it. And since maladies were held to be essentially constitutional, individual and holistic, the clinical encounter might in large measure be stage-managed by the patient; it would at least involve negotiation and (hopefully) consensus.[5]

All this had important implications. As their reflections show, sufferers paid close attention to sickness and its sources and took energetic steps to avoid it, prompted by an advice culture instructing the public in matters of health and sickness. The body was energetically monitored. The diary of the pioneer experimentalist Robert Hooke logs the kind of unceasing vigilance in physical self-scrutiny that a Puritan might direct towards his soul. Thus Christmas week, 1672:

> (21) At home all day vertiginous, took conserves of Rosemary flowers. took two aloes Rosata pills, ointment in eye from Mr Colwall … (22) Mr Moor here, had been at Portsmouth, told me of a woman in the Tower cured diver of the vertigo by stone horse dung. Mr. Gidley let me blood 7 ounces. Blood windy and melancholly, gave him ½ crown. The vertigo continued but upon snuffing ginger I was much relievd by blowing out of my nose a lump of thick gelly. Went abroad (23) in the morn returned home very guiddy. Refresht by eating Dinner, in the afternoon pretty well. Consulted Dr Goddard, he advisd amber and ale with sage and rosemary, bubbels, caraways and nutmeg steepd and scurvy grasse. (24) Very ill and giddy in the afternoon but pretty well before. I tooke a clyster after which working but once I was very ill and giddy. The worst night I ever yet had, melancholly and giddy, shooting in left side of my head above ear. (25) Christmas day. Slept from 7 to 10, rose pretty well. Upon eating broth, very giddy … Eat plumb broth, went pretty well to bed but slept but little and mightily refresht upon cutting off my hair close to my head and supposed I had been perfectly cured but I was somewhat guiddy (26) next day and tooke Dr Godderds 3 pills which wrought 14 times towards latter end.[6]

Hooke was obviously examining what made him sick (drink, late nights, broth, etc.) and which medicines 'worked' – as Dr Goddard's evidently did with a vengeance.

And, upon falling sick, people ventured diagnostic opinions of their own, rather than leaving such rulings wholly to the doctor. When, early in 1663, Hooke's fellow man of science and diarist, Samuel Pepys, went down with stomach pains and fever, he puzzled over the cause, concluding it was 'some disorder given the blood: but by what I know not, unless it be by my late great Quantitys of Dantzicke-girkins that I have eaten'.[7] Formulating such an account allayed anxiety and assisted in the next important decision: should the doctor be called?

Usually not: being sick often remained a one-man show, and 'primary care' in those days generally meant care by the head of the household, by a cook, nursemaid or neighbours, or, for the poor, recourse to a 'lady bountiful', perhaps the parson's wife. A market was also growing for the self-help books like Buchan's *Domestic Medicine*, earlier discussed.[8] Pursuing self-managed regimens of healthy living, such as those touched upon in Chapter 3, the sick routinely monitored their diet, and dosed themselves with home-brewed diet-drinks, herbal tonics, purges and emetics.[9] Contemporary recipe books and commonplace books are crammed with remedies for disorders from corns to cancer, and the sensible home was stocked with laxatives, vomits, painkillers, cordials, febrifuges (medicines to reduce fever) and other sorts of home-physic. In the emergent 'consumer society', people would also buy in such shop-bought patent and proprietary medicines as Dr James' Powders, the Georgian aspirin,[10] or invest in a ready-to-use medicine chest. Oral health lore was on everyone's lips. 'Prevention is better than cure' dates back at least to the seventeenth century, along with such other gems of proverbial wisdom as

> Agues come on horseback, but go away on foot.
> At forty a man is either a fool or a physician.
> After dinner sit a while, after supper walk a mile.[11]

Health know-how began at home. Commiserating with his friend, John Moody, 'plagu'd with yt cursed Distemper, the Piles', the actor David Garrick told him exactly what to do: 'live abstemiously for a little time, & take Every Night a large tea spoonfull of flower of Brimstone (night & morning) mix'd up with honey or treacle, & you will be ye better for it.'[12] People might be equally eager to pick up tips. 'Read part of *The Universal Magazine* for June', recorded the Sussex grocer Thomas Turner in the summer of 1757,

> wherein I find the following receipt recommended (in an extract from Dr. Lind's Essay on the most effectual means of preserving health of the seamen in the Royal Navy) as a specific against all epidemical and bilious fevers and also against endemic disorders. He first recommends a regular course of life and to abstain as much as possible from animal food, and to confine as much as possible to a vegetable diet. Then he orders about 2 ounces of the following tincture to be taken every day upon an empty stomach (and better if taken at twice):
>   8 ounces of bark
>   4 ounces dried orange peel, which infuse in a gallon of spirits.[13]

The profusion of medical articles, queries, responses and controversies printed in the *Gentleman's Magazine*, that best-selling monthly, and elsewhere, shows that the literate laity, far from being fatalistic, docile or uncomprehending, was medically articulate and expected to have its say, and perhaps its way.

Clinical relations were thus power plays, but trust was often achieved

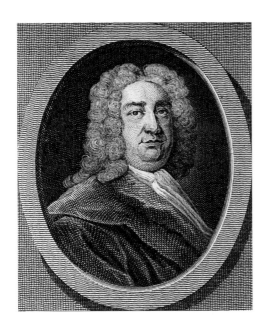

75 J. Tookey, line engraving of
George Cheyne (1671–1743),
1787, after Johann van Diest.

between patients and doctors, as is amply borne out by the extensive correspondence between the Countess of Huntingdon and George Cheyne (illus. 75), and also that between the latter and the novelist Samuel Richardson.[14] A 'staunch Epicure', Richardson unhealthily combined an aversion to exercise with overwork, for which his physician urged him to unwind, work out, and be more sparing with food and alcohol. Appealing to his patient not only as a physician but as a 'sadly experienced' fellow-sufferer – one far more obese than Richardson ever became – the doctor particularly recommended the 'chamber horse', an exercise machine consisting of a long plank supported on each end, with a seat in the middle which bounced up and down.[15] 'I wonder you get not the Chamber-horse which is now so universally known and practiced in all the studious Professions in London', admonished Cheyne, who himself rode upon it daily with 'great Benefit':

> It is certainly admirable and has all the good and beneficial Effects of a hard Trotting Horse except the fresh Air. I ride an Hour every Morning and will do more when the Weather will not permit me to walk in my Garden or ride in my Coach. (Only remember the Board ought to be as long as the Room will permit 18 or 20 Feet 16 at least, and the Chair you sit on with a Cushion on the Board as a Bottom to it with a two armed Hoop and with a Foot-stool that with a sliding Board may be raised higher or lower.) It may be bought for a Couple of Pounds ... You may dictate, direct, or read in it.[16]

Identifying Richardson as 'a true genuine Hyppo' – i.e., hypochondriac – Cheyne attempted, in time-honoured fashion, to devise diversions, recommending him to read 'interesting Stories, Novels or Plays' (if homoeopathic in its basis, it also sounds like coals to Newcastle!). Pious works of devotion had calmed Cheyne in his own crisis, and he supposed that they would also soothe his patient's injured spirits. As well as serving as physician, Cheyne doubled as his patients' friend.[17]

Attentive and courteous doctors like Cheyne in return produced patients eager to show appreciation with all the decorum cultivated by the Augustans. In some lines printed in the *Gentleman's Magazine*, the skill and tenderness of the surgeon William Cheselden were, we are asked to believe, celebrated by a twelve year old, on whom he had operated for the stone:

> The Grateful Patient
> The work was in a moment done,
> If possible, without a groan,
> So swift thy hand, I could not feel
> The progress of the cutting steel ...
> And above all the race of men,
> I'll bless my God for Cheselden.[18]

Unlike their earnest and maudlin Victorian successors, Georgian patients tended to be portrayed in prints and fiction in the comic mode, often caught on the receiving end of some nasty medicine, or involved in ludicrous mix-ups and set-tos with the doctor. Comic patients generally came in one of two guises, the believe-all and the know-all.

'Henry is an excellent patient, lies quietly in bed and is ready to swallow anything': Jane Austen thus teasingly awarded her brother his booby prize as the true English patient.[19] Gullibly duped by physician or quack, the credulous patient enjoyed a popularity that was seemingly universal and never palled. Typical of the edgy humour of misplaced trust is a print (illus. 83) depicting a rustic couple consulting a decrepit, dim-sighted doctor. Accompanied by his anxious wife, the man explains: 'Do you see Doctor my Dame and I be come to ax your advise – we both of us eat well and drink well, and sleep well – yet still we be somehow queerish.' Reinforced – or rebuked – by the bust of Galen on the mantelpiece, the physician replies: 'You eat well – you drink well and you sleep well – very good. — You was perfectly right in coming to me, for depend upon it I will give you something that shall do away all these things.'[20] In reality, few patients can have been so credulous – indeed that is precisely what made the stereotypes such reassuring sources of amusement.

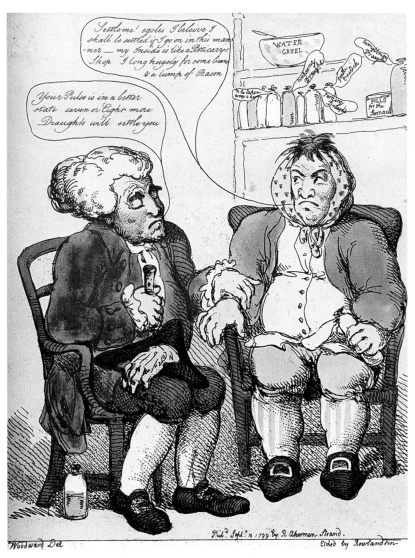

76 Thomas Rowlandson, 'DOCTOR', 1799, coloured etching after George Moutard Woodward. The shelves behind contain gruel and an array of draughts and pills.

The sick and their circles often thought they knew best, and another familiar trope presents plain-man common sense answering the doctor back. Rowlandson depicted a doctor piling on the treatment to his reluctant, and already overdosed, patient (illus. 76). 'Your Pulse is in a better state', explains the doctor, 'seven or eight more Draughts will settle you.' 'Settle me!', explodes the bumpkin, mistaking the meaning, or hearing it only too well: 'Egoles I beleive I shall be settled if I go on in this manner – my Inside is like a Potticarys Shop, I long hugely for

156

Beddoes's dialogue reads like a trial run for a work of fiction he never wrote; George Eliot for her part later conjured up in an actual novel that precise ring of lay (over-)confidence. Middlemarch society was taking tea, when conversation turned to Lady Chettam's 'remarkable health', which she attributed to her 'home made bitters', in the process slighting Mrs Renfrew's preferred 'strengthening medicines'. Everyone then chipped in:

> 'It strengthens the disease', said the Rector's wife, much too well-born not to be an amateur in medicine. 'Everything depends on the constitution; some people make fat, some blood, some bile – that's my view of the matter; and whatever they take is a sort of grist to the mill'.
> 'Then she ought to take medicines that would reduce – reduce the disease, you know, if you are right, my dear. And I think what you say is reasonable'.[23]

Fictional advice and medical narratives were obviously coming closer to each other, and perhaps they shared similar therapeutic ends, for writer and reader, doctor and patient alike.

The classic eighteenth-century joke patient was neither the deceived and defrauded nor the dogmatist, however, but the hypochondriac: the true enlightened egoist grown self-absorbed to the point of sickness, Mr Consumer incarnate as an insatiable medicine consumer or, like Richardson, advice-seeker. Indeed, the age saw the very idea of hypochondria reconfigured.[24]

Originally classed as an organic affliction of the lower abdomen, hypochondriasis was becoming rethought, in that discourse-driven society, as the psychiatric condition of morbid health anxiety (illus. 84). Such growing sensitivity is not hard to explain, since polite mores valued the cultivation of watchfulness, introspection and sensibility; at what point, however, did responsible and sympathetic individualism descend into morbid brooding?

In his *Treatise of the Hypochondriack and Hysterick Diseases* (1730), the enlightened physician Bernard Mandeville pondered the fictional case of 'Misomedon', a liberally educated man of letters possessed of sufficient leisure to dwell upon his pains, and of book-learning enough to launch himself into compulsively fantasizing the workings of disorders and drugs. In better days, he tells his physician Philopirio, he had been a raffish gentleman-scholar. Ruining his constitution by 'good living', he fell to consulting a crew of learned physicians, but none of their treatments worked – indeed their drug cocktails merely made bad worse – and such vexatious consultations reduced him to a

'Hypochondriacus Confirmatus ... a Crazy Valetudinarian'. Seduced by suggestibility into every sickness under the sun, he acquired 'a mind to study Physick' himself – a further fatal step! By consequence he finally convinced himself that he had been infected with venereal disease. 'When I grew better, I found that all this had been occasion'd by reading of the *Lues*, when I began to be ill; which has made me resolve since, never to look in any Book of Physick again, but when my head is in very good order.'[25] Just as talking to the humane Philopirio was meant to cure Misomedon, Mandeville generously offered his book as a corrective for hypochondria. One wonders, however, to revert to a theme by now familiar, how many read the *Treatise* and caught the 'hyp' instead – might that even have been Mandeville's sick joke?

Mandeville's tale mirrored the valetudinarian as depicted almost contemporaneously in *The Spectator*. 'I am one of that sickly Tribe', the magazine's readers were informed by a (presumably fictive) correspondent:

> who are commonly known by the name of Valetudinarians; and do confess to you that I first contracted this ill Habit of Body, or rather of Mind, by the Study of Physick. I no sooner began to peruse Books of this Nature, but I found my Pulse was irregular, and scarce ever read the Account of any Disease that I did not fancy my self afflicted with. Doctor *Sydenham*'s learned Treatise of Fevers threw me into a lingring Hectick, which hung upon me all the while I was reading that excellent Piece. I then applied my self to the Study of several Authors, who have written upon Phthisical Distempers, and by that means fell into a Consumption; till at length, growing very fat, I was in a manner shamed out of that Imagination. Not long after this I found in my self all the Symptoms of the Gout, except Pain; but was cured of it by a Treatise upon the Gravel, written by a very Ingenious Author, who (as it is usual for Physicians to convert one Distemper into another) eased me of the Gout by giving me the Stone. I at length studied my self into a Complication of Distempers.

Boning up on sickness was a health risk in itself: would reading *The Spectator* heighten hypochondria or provide comic relief?[26]

Accused of first making and then milking hypochondriacs, physicians in self-defence were apt to condemn such sufferers as morbid attention-seekers who made rods for their own backs – souls, mocked James Makittrick Adair, 'sick by way of amusement and melancholy to keep up their spirits'.[27] 'No disease is more troublesome either to the Patient or Physician', he noted, 'than hypochondriac Disorders; and it often happens, that, thro' the Fault of both, the Cure is either unnecessarily protracted, or totally frustrated.'[28] Catch 22 indeed, if the cunning of hypochondria lay in the fact that a doctor's intervention would merely reinforce dependency. Hence, stressed John Hill, 'though the physician can do something toward the cure, much more depends upon the patient'.[29] Once again the medical scene becomes an enigma in the case of diseases in which the doctor does more harm than good.

There was thus recognition that the hypochondriac was both the doctors' monstrous brood and their Waterloo, the child of discursive overload from physicians, overdosing by apothecaries, and overcharging by both. The web of words was bewitching. Hypochondria, observed Dr Robert James, was such a tough nut to crack precisely because 'the Patients are so delighted, not only with a Variety of Medicines, but also of Physicians'.[30] The only escape, suggested Dr Peter Shaw, was for the patient to write himself out of the script, or rather into a different role: you must become 'your own physician'.[31] In other words, doctor's orders were ironically: patient, heal thyself.[32]

The first great English stage hypochondriac is the comic hero of Aphra Behn's *Sir Patient Fancy* (1678), a play modelled on Molière's *Le malade imaginaire* (illus. 77). Never out of his nightshirt, Sir Patient swallows twelve purges a month, though his 'Disease', as one acquaintance remarks, 'is nothing but Imagination'.[33] Informed by his wife and friends that he looks under the weather, the ultra-suggestible valetudinarian is immediately seized by 'a kind of shivering', followed by a nervous paroxysm. 'Methought I felt the Contagion steal into my Heart', he exclaims, 'I'm a dead Man, have me to Bed, I die away, undress me instantly, send for my Physicians, I'm poison'd, my Bowels burn, I have within an *Aetna*, my Brains run round, Nature within me reels.'[34]

Spin-offs from Molière and Behn, parades of hypochondriacal buffoons, mouthing pseudo-medical jargon, whine and wheeze their way through Georgian plays and prints. A rather more nuanced version of the bittersweet joys of invalidism and suffering later makes its appearance in sentimental novels like Henry Mackenzie's *The Man of Feeling* (1771), and the genre was thereafter to be deliciously parodied in *Emma* (Mr Woodhouse) and in *Sanditon*.[35] Jane Austen's final fragment – she died before completing it – is set in a newly launched south coast seaside resort, where, alongside a local landowner angling for consumptives so that she can put her milch-asses to profit, we meet the resort's booster, Mr Arthur Parker, and his two hypochondriacal sisters, Diana and Susan.[36] Of that pair, the former suffers from 'spasmodic bile' (it had become chic to be 'bilious'), whereas Susan is a victim of nerves – by then rather *demodé*.[37] Having run through 'the

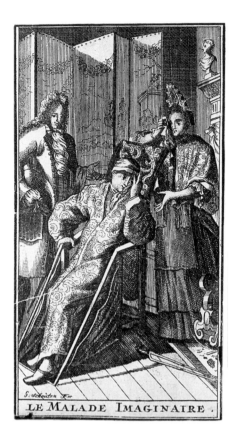

77 Hubert Peter Schoute, undated etching of a scene from Molière, *Le malade imaginaire* (1673).

Argan, the hypochondriac, is attended by Beline, his wife, and Dr Purgon, his physician. Those who did not attend plays could see them virtually through such illustrations.

whole medical tribe' without benefit, the sisters have taken, like Misomedon, to self-medication. 'Six leeches a day for ten days' have not, however, relieved Susan's headaches, leading Diana to conclude that the roots of her sister's troubles lie in her gums, persuading her to have three teeth pulled out.[38]

Their condition pervades their imaginations and dominates their conduct, every waking hour. Indeed the able-bodied but idle Arthur, whose conversation revolves around his rheumatism, nerves and stomach lining, affords an early instance of what would today be called an 'illness career':

> 'I hope you will eat some of this toast', said he, ... 'I hope you like dry toast'.

> 'With a reasonable quantity of butter spread over it, very much – ' said Charlotte [a visitor] – 'but not otherwise – '.

> 'No more do I' – said he exceedingly pleased – 'We think quite alike there. – So far from dry toast being wholesome, I think it a

very bad thing for the stomach. Without a little butter to soften it, it hurts the coats of the stomach. I am sure it does. – I will have the pleasure of spreading some for you directly – and afterwards I will spread some for myself. – Very bad indeed for the coats of the stomach – but there is no convincing some people.'[39]

Had Arthur too been reading Cheyne?

The stomach, as we have seen that British national organ par excellence, starred in another stock moral tale, the Romantic connection between hypochondria and talent: the guts were the cradle of genius. Born into a family modest in means but high in ambition, Thomas Carlyle attended Edinburgh University from 1809, thereafter acting as a schoolmaster for a few years before returning to college in 1818 to study law. And it was in Edinburgh at 23 that he began what he later in his *Reminiscences* called his 'four or five most miserable, dark, sick, and heavy-laden years', being attacked (note the anthropomorphism) by dyspepsia 'like a rat gnawing at the pit of his stomach'.[40]

'Bad health does depress and undermine one more than all other calamities put together,' he observed in 1819. A couple of years later he was complaining of 'coorsed nervous disorders', of 'all my dyspepsias, and nervousness and hypochondrias', which gave him 'my usual share of torture every day'. 'No wish has arisen within me more constantly and fervently for the last half-year', he informed his brother Alick, 'than the wish for a return of sound, vig[or]ous health. I tell you, my boy, all the evils of life are as the small dust of the balance to a diseased stomach.' A torrent of subsequent bellyaching letters relates a similar tale. 'I seem as it were *dying by inches*,' he told that brother in November 1823, 'even porridge has lost its effect on me.' He had 'grown sicker and sicker', he went on: 'I want health, health, health.'[41]

Around this time, Carlyle began to consult doctors 'who made me give up my dear nicotine, and take to mercury'. Whether owing to doctors or self-inflicted, his digestive difficulties surely stemmed from purgatives – from blue pills to castor oil – taken for his constipation. In particular, he discovered a Birmingham practitioner called Badams ('though his business is in chemical manufactures'), writing up that anecdote in black-comedy mode,

> one of the most sensible, clear-headed persons I have ever met with. … After going about for a day or two talking about pictures and stomach disorders, in the cure of which he is famous, and from which he once suffered four years in person, what does the man do but propose that I should go up to Birmingham for a month and live with him that he might find out the make of me, and prescribe for my unfortunate inner man. I have consented.[42]

Eight weeks with the silver-tongued Badams, however, brought no relief. 'I have been bephysicked and bedrugged', he groaned, 'I have swallowed about two stoupfuls of castor oil since I came hither; unless I dose myself with that oil of sorrow I cannot get along at all.' Badams himself, Carlyle later maliciously recorded, took to drink and 'died miserably'.[43]

Following his marriage, Carlyle settled permanently in Cheyne Walk, Chelsea, but no improvement followed. 'Why am I not happy then?', he asked another of his brothers: 'Alas, Jack, I am bilious. I have to swallow salts and oil.' Growing 'sick with sleeplessness, nervous, bilious, splenetic, and all the rest of it', he reflected, 'it is strange how one gets habituated to sickness'.[44]

Mid-life in London brought deepening crisis. 'Weary, dispirited, sick'; 'Bilious, too, in these smothering windless days'; 'Broke down in the park; *könnte nichts mehr*, being sick and weak beyond measure ... I am full of dyspepsia.'[45]

'Why not quit literature? ... I am weary almost of life itself,' he revealed in 1836; 'It is my nerves, my nerves.' 'Dyspepsia working continually ... Dispirited, in miserable health.' 'I shall never be other than ill, wearied, sick-hearted, etc. ... Bilious, heartless and forlorn ... Sick, sleepless, driven half mad.' And so on and on. Correcting proofs could be guaranteed to bring on the bile. On completing his life of Oliver Cromwell he bewailed, 'I have still three weeks of the ugliest labour (correcting proofs), and shall be fit for a hospital then.' Yet at least he had the insight to recognize his troubles were self-inflicted and almost a matter of choice: 'My work needs all to be done with my nerves in a kind of blaze; such a state of soul and body as would soon *kill* me, if not intermitted.' Biliousness was, in other words, one of those ironically therapeutic sicknesses that gave a life a storyline.[46]

The 1830s and 1840s rumble with letters complaining of nausea – 'as for myself I make very bad progress, the work is so chaotic, unimaginably confused, and I am so bilious, irregular in sleep etc. etc.' On attaining the age of 49, he entered in his journal this dismal bulletin: '*Eheu, eheu*! I am very weak in health, too ... Thou art verily growing old, and thou hast never been young.'[47]

Later, when composing his life of Frederick the Great, he was afflicted with terrible nightmares, and soon afterwards, the proofs all too predictably brought on 'villainous headaches'. Heartily disliking doctors, Carlyle had allowed none of them near him except his brother; but in old age he submitted to occasional visits from them, dying in his eighties, a year before his fellow sufferer, Charles Darwin.

Back in the 1830s Carlyle had written indirectly about himself in

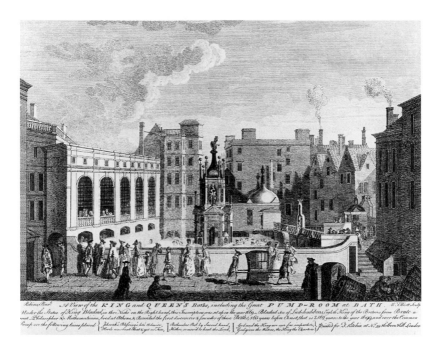

78 William Elliott, 'A View of the KING and QUEEN's Baths, Including the Great PUMP-ROOM at BATH', undated engraving with etching after Thomas Robins.

This print dates from the beginning of the reign of George III (1760–1811). Note how the bath itself is a public spectacle, with promenaders all around.

Sartor Resartus through his romantic hero Teufelsdröckh, thereafter living out the part. Long floundering in spiritual despair, Teufelsdröckh had been cast down into the abyss of religious uncertainty, excluded from hope. Shrouded in darkness, he clung, however, to his belief in Truth and the infinite and absolute nature of Duty, suffering from fears of unbelief, from physical ill health and from failure to find congenial work. That is how Carlyle saw himself and his maladies in his self-dramatization of his body into a living pathognomy.[48] Sickness gave shape to suffering in the soliloquizing of the autobiographies of genius.

Before Sanditon and its ilk, those with means visited inland spas like Bath and Buxton, bathing and taking the waters (illus. 78). Boosted first by royalty and later by the medical profession, English spas enjoyed their halcyon days in the long eighteenth century, as they acquired all the refinements of upper-class recreation: concerts, balls, plays, soirées, gambling and assignations. Their popularity so grew, that by the early years of George III's reign the influx of *nouveaux riches* irked the quality. 'Every upstart of fortune, harnessed to the trappings of the mode, presents himself at Bath,' grumbled Squire Bramble in Tobias Smollett's *Humphry Clinker*, 'because here, without any further qualifications, they can mingle with the princes and nobles of the land.'[49]

By the close of the century, Bath had rocketed to become the seventh largest city in the kingdom, though by then it had passed its apogee, declining gracefully thereafter to become the first great retirement city for the rich. By then, newer spa towns were eclipsing it, especially Cheltenham, which captivated the select with its grand Regency style. And, for the more strenuously sick, there arose such other centres as Malvern, staking claims to superior thermal waters or more rigorously scientific healing regimes. In the shadow of the dark Malvern Hills, the celebrated Dr Gully (illus. 79), the most severe but sincere of the water curers, treated a succession of eminent Victorians – Carlyle himself, but also Charles Darwin, perennially laid up with dyspepsia, migraine and vomiting – with his muscular hydropathic regime before an adultery and murder scandal wrecked his career.[50]

Shooting up during the last third of the eighteenth century, and led by Weymouth, Brighton and Margate (illus. 80), the seaside resort

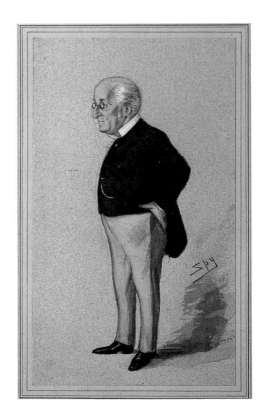

79 Sir Leslie Matthew Ward ('Spy'), watercolour showing James Manby Gully (1808–1883), 1876.
    Unlike their 18th-century precursors, Victorian doctors were eager to get themselves represented in the public press as debonair gentlemen.

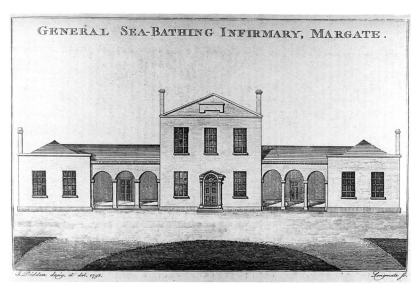

GENERAL SEA-BATHING INFIRMARY, MARGATE.

80 Barak Longmate (the Elder), 'GENERAL SEA-BATHING INFIRMARY, MARGATE', line engraving after J. Pridden.
    This institution was set up, partly through the backing of John Coakley Lettsom, to give sea-bathing opportunities to the tubercular. The seaside resort was launched primarily on the strength of its sanitive qualities.

was destined to become the choice Victorian venue. Claiming great salubrity for coastal environments, Dr Richard Russell at Brighton recommended the *drinking* of sea water; all champions of the seaside encouraged bathing in the ocean and, tuberculosis in mind, doctors contended that the atmosphere of resorts facing the ocean and flanked with bold cliffs were restorative. In *Sanditon*, the hero Mr Parker, owner of various local shops and lodgings, is guyed for his non-stop boosting of the virtues of the sea, holding it to be certain

> that no person could be really well, no person (however upheld for the present by fortuitous aids of exercise and spirits in a semblance of health) could be really in a state of secure and permanent health without spending at least six weeks by the sea every year. – The sea air and sea bathing together were nearly infallible, one or the other of them being a match for every disorder, of the stomach, the lungs or the blood; they were anti-spasmodic, anti-pulmonary, anti-sceptic, anti-bilious and anti-rheumatic. Nobody could catch cold by the sea, nobody wanted appetite by the sea, nobody wanted spirits, nobody wanted strength. They were healing, softening, relaxing – fortifying and bracing – seemingly just as was wanted – sometimes one, sometimes the other. – If the sea breeze failed, the sea-bath was the certain corrective; – and where bathing disagreed, the sea breeze alone was evidently designed by nature for the cure.[51]

Be the resorts inland or coastal, their medical charades attracted caustic comment. 'The Physicians here are very numerous', observed Richard Steele of Bath – adding, with a sting in the tail, that as a consequence 'they had almost killed me with their humanity' ('to these charitable gentlemen I owe, that I was cured, in a week's time, of more distempers than I have ever had in my life').[52]

Spa regimes evolved superstitious rituals redolent of the old popish pilgrim shrines. The Revd John Penrose, a Cornish clergyman who visited Bath in 1766 seeking relief for his gout, thought the waters beneficial but all the palaver of the bathing and drinking instructions ludicrous: 'The Doctor has altered my Regimen: I am now to take Water from the Cross Bath at 7 and 8 o'clock mornings, and from the King's Bath at 12, quarter a Pint each time.'[53] Why such peculiar punctiliousness? 'Every one, who comes in, tells me this exactness as to Time and Quantity is a mere Farce, notwithstanding the Doctors so gravely prescribe.' Yet why not give it all a try? 'It may be so for ought I know; but as it may not be so. I'll try strictly adhere to Rule.'[54]

In one of the letters he wrote almost daily to his daughter back home, Penrose alludes to Christopher Anstey's *The New Bath Guide*. Following the death of a relative, that Anglican clergyman had headed for Bath to recoup his health, and to console himself he wrote a series of 'poetical epistles' penned 'to shoot folly as it flies'. Published in 1766, the *Guide* went through more than twenty editions, and in 1798 Rowlandson produced illustrations for a new edition.[55] This print series, collectively titled COMFORTS OF BATH (illus. 85), satirized the activities, social and medical, taking place at the spa. And his *Dance of Death* series included death at Bath, in a scene entitled *The Pump Room Door*.

Popular partly for its cameos of city celebrities, the *Guide* professed to warn the unwary traveller of the 'whirlpools and rocks' on the voyage of life, but it also served as the comic style sheet as to conduct becoming at the resort. Its climax related the 'bilious' Matthew Blunderhead's reminiscences of the doctor's attendance on himself and his sister whilst taking the waters:

> I'm bilious, I find, and the women are nervous;
> Their systems relax'd, and all turn'd topsy-turvey,
> With hypochondriasis, obstructions and scurvy,
> And these are distempers he must know the whole on,
> For he talk'd of the peritoneum and colon,
> Of phlegmatic humours oppressing the women,
> From feculent matter that swells the abdomen;
> But the noise I have heard in my bowels like thunder,

Is a flatus, I find, in my left hypochonder,
So plenty of med'cines each day does he send
Post singules liquidas sedes sum end
Ad crepitus vesper' & man' promo vend
In English to say, we must swallow a potion,
For driving out wind after every motion ...[56]

The reader is evidently left wondering whether our hero's malaise is not entirely iatrogenic, of the doctors' own making. 'We have read "The New Bath Guide", a series of Poetical Epistles, describing the Manners and Humours of the People', Penrose wrote home: 'Some of it is very well, but upon the whole scarce worth the Price it is sold at, five shillings. But it is the Fashion to read it: and, who would be out of the Fashion?'[57] Indeed. Perhaps the superior sick, above all, had to be conformist.

Medical encounters in Bath – a classic carnivalesque site with rules of its own – became focal points of the theatre of physic that subverted the very idea the medicine was rational rather than frivolous. Smollett's Peregrine Pickle in the novel of that name is so riled by the faculty farce there encountered that he plays a trick. Blaming an incompetent surgeon for his afflictions, a gouty colonel has come to the spa, determined upon a course of self-prescribed treatments. The idea is foolish; his regimen does no good, and he is confined to his bed. Peregrine fixes one morning for a fellow to call on all the physicians in town bidding them to attend the colonel post-haste. Arriving in a rush, only to be told the patient is still asleep, they fill the house and begin to discuss his case with the utmost dogmatism, though none has ever so much as set eyes on his putative patient. He has 'obstinate arthritis', says one: 'a confirmed pox', judges another, and a third hits upon 'an inveterate scurvy', their reflections being 'supported by a variety of quotations from medical authors, ancient as well as modern'. So clamorous the disputatious doctors grew that the patient awakes in great agony, whereupon they burst into his bedchamber. Besieged by all those detested doctors, the colonel 'sprang out of his bed with incredible agility', seized a crutch and laid about them all with great vigour. Is this a shrewd healing stratagem on Peregrine's part – or simply an exposé of universal sham?[58]

Smart spa physic was sent up not only by satirical poets and novelists but also by medical men themselves. Spas, explained Thomas Beddoes, were a scam for the exploitation of the fashionable fool. First the metropolitan practitioner ran through his repertoire of 'amusing prescriptions ... stories, compliments, the small talk ... the whole magazine of expedients by which the patient is diverted from the contemplation of his declining state'.[59] This rigmarole, however, could be spun out only so long. When exhausted, it was high time to pronounce the magic word 'travel', for how could a tender family doctor in the capital 'bear to think, that the son or daughter of a dear friend of his should die at home, just under his nose'?[60] And so patients were 'recommended to go to Dawlish, Exmouth, the Land's End, or God knows how much further off still'.[61] Not least, they were sent to Beddoes's own Bristol as 'Hotwells cases', a genteelism for a corpse – so much so, that one might fix up a sign 'upon Temple gate Bristol, reading "*Lasciate ogni speranza, voi ch'entrate*"'.[62]

This black comedy of the travelling circus was directed by what Hogarth would have called the 'company of undertakers' performing at such spas, their job being to manage the revels. Such impersonators were gratuitously given a helping hand by lay aides-de-camp – there was never a watering place without its 'dowager of quality' who officiated as 'mistresses of the ceremonies of medicine',[63] gaily instructing new pilgrims in the medical marketplace, saying '*Surely, my dear, you won't think of consulting any body but Dr. Such-an-one.*'[64]

So it was all a deadly *danse macabre*, a migratory *ars moriendi*.[65] Your Baths, Scarboroughs and Margates were best viewed as 'institutions of convenience for one part of the faculty and of charity for another', it being handy for the family physician to have 'a sort of charnel-house ready provided into which he may toss a half-animated carcase'.[66] Spas were but vast marketplaces of quackery, regular and irregular alike – with the collusion of hypochondriacs and valetudinarians desperate for attention and anxious to ail fashionably.

What the spa was to the Georgians, the sickroom became in the following century. The former was tailor-made for satire, the latter for sentimentality – and for solitary writing. No small number of eminent Victorians pursued authorship propped up on pillows – the association became a cliché – and many reflected upon the affinity between the state of sickness and the realm of the writer, enchanted through the power of solitude. 'For what else is it but a magnificent dream for a man to lie a-bed, and draw daylight curtains about him; and, shutting out the sun, to induce a total oblivion of all the works which are going on under it?' asked Charles Lamb:

> To become insensible to all the operations of life, except the beating of one feeble pulse?
> If there be a regal solitude, it is a sick bed. How the patient lords it there; what caprices he acts without control! how king-like he sways his pillow – tumbling and tossing, and shifting, and lowering,

and thumping, and flatting, and moulding it, to the ever varying requisitions of his throbbing temples ...

How sickness enlarges the dimensions of a man's self to himself; he is his own exclusive object. Supreme selfishness is inculcated upon him as his only duty.[67]

In Victorian fiction the sickroom (illus. 81) beckons as a haven of sincere feeling and pampered calm: Oliver Twist is 'comfortably deposited' in a bed at Mr Brownlow's, for instance, 'tended with a kindness and solicitude that knew no bounds'.[68] The split personality of illness as both bane and boon became a convention of fictional narratives, and ample testimony is provided as to the therapeutic potential of what Harriet Martineau called 'life in the sickroom'.[69] 'I have not been so happy or so thankful in a long time,' Florence Nightingale wrote from her ailing grandmother's bedside, a remark prescient of her future life in the sickroom as an invalid of 50 years' standing.[70]

Georgian patients were expected to be assertive; hence they left themselves liable to be mocked, through pen or paints, either for obstinacy or feebleness. It was weakness that was to endear the reader of Dickens to the plight of the sick. Bracing laughter gave way to sympathetic tears.

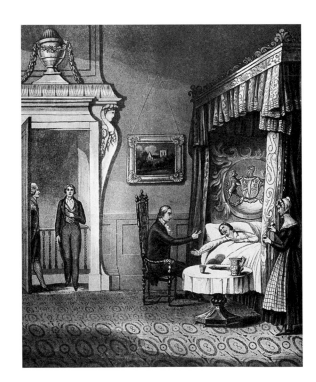

81 'The Sickroom', scene from *The Life of a Nobleman*, 19th century, aquatint.

A man lies ill in bed, a woman pours him a drink, and a doctor sits by the bed.

7 Outsiders and Intruders

In *Worlds Apart: The Market and the Theater in Anglo-American Thought, 1550–1750*, Jean-Christophe Agnew presents two models of the social order prominent in early modern times: the idea of the marketplace on the one hand, and that of the *theatrum mundi* on the other. Were they truly, as suggested by his title, 'worlds apart' – that is, polar opposites – with the latter paradigm in course of time supplanting the former? Or, contrariwise, were they two sides of the same coin – was the theatre itself a matter of salesmanship and the market a performance art? Did medicine market its own stageshow? It is this issue that this chapter explores.

Pre-1800 medicine, I have been arguing, represented itself in rather theatrical terms, with its distinctive branches having their own formally designated parts to play, each distinctively decked out in its own (royally recognized) titles, insignia, paper qualifications, entrance rituals and, indeed, mysteries. But should this public front be accepted at face value, rather than as evidence of strategic attempts to carve out occupational demarcations and affirm order amidst occupational flux during times of turbulence?

Historians formerly played along with this account, picturing a rigid hierarchical profession, with elite physicians – those discussed in Chapter 5 – at the apex, and surgeons and apothecaries on lower levels, each tier being respectively regulated by its own governing body. Physicians commanded the highest prestige and fees because they had been trained at university, 'physic' being thus a learned and liberal profession; the cutter's art carried lesser status because it was a manual art which involved the shedding of blood; and the apothecary's trade was at the foot, being in essence but shopkeeping (illus. 82).

Over the last couple of decades, however, research has revealed that this model of a closed, stable professional pyramid, governed by a corporate hierarchy, sanctioned by the state, was a rhetoric which, however serviceable to some, corresponded only tangentially with reality.

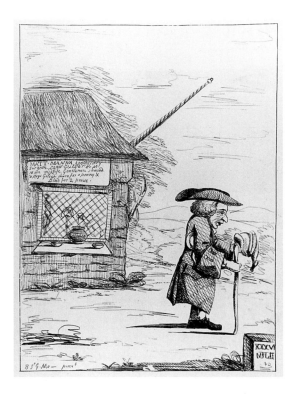

82 Matthew Darly, 'Matthew Manna. A Country Apothecary.', 1773, etching after R. St. G. Mansergh.

The sign above the window of the shop reads: 'MATT. MANNA Apothecary surgeon. CORN Cutter &c. Man midwife. Gentlemen shaved & Hogs gelded. Shave for a penny and Bleed for 2 pence.' Such mockery of the lowly apothecary was standard fare.

English medical practice was in actuality – indeed, increasingly over time – fluid and heterogeneous, with traditional legal demarcations undergoing challenge *de facto* and *de jure*, and being eroded or ignored. This destabilization and marginalization of official structures owed much to the enormous success in the eighteenth century of the Scottish universities, above all Edinburgh and Glasgow, as medical manufactories. Unlike at Oxbridge, Scottish students learned both physic and surgery in combination, in effect being trained to become a new breed of mould-bursting general practitioners. Permeating market towns and the up-and-coming industrial centres, Scottish graduates combined all the medical functions in a single pursuit as the prototype of the 'family doctor' which became dominant in the Victorian era and was still the backbone of British medicine in the twentieth century.[1] The medical practitioners of Georgian England were not, in reality, if they were ceremonially and in some degree statutorily, confined within closed corporations. Be they the London elite discussed in Chapter 5 or common-or-garden provincial workhorses, most acted, willy-nilly, as self-employed entrepreneurs in a medical marketplace in which demand for their services, if unpredictable and fluctuating, was rising, and handsome financial rewards were beckoning for the enterprising, energetic or lucky. Provincial physicians like Erasmus Darwin could accrue over £1,000 a year, enough for comfort, and even humble market-town surgeon-apothecaries might clear £500. In a Georgian England increasingly wedded to laissez-faire, medicine shrugged off legalistic professional and corporate restrictions. In contrast to France or the German principalities, chartered and bureaucratic medical faculties did not dictate who might practise, nor did royal appointees at court have the power to restrict entry to, or license and police the profession. In Britain, doctors operated where opportunity afforded: the laws they obeyed were principally those of supply and demand.[2]

Literary and artistic representations of practitioners should be read in this light. Satirical images of practitioners typically continued, as shown in previous chapters, to depict them vaunting, or caught in, the trappings of an official hierarchy: the pompous physician, with his wig and cane and bust of Galen; the coarse and corpulent surgeon, the aproned apothecary at his counter – all these stereotypes continued to do stout service as shorthands. But these persistent, if increasingly anachronistic, portrayals must not be taken at face value: they are indicative principally of public unease – or at least uncertainty – at who was who, and who was meant to be doing what, within the healing business.

The ensconced image of surgery was as a manual craft, involving hand not head (illus. 86). The surgeon's job was to treat external complaints (skin conditions, boils, wounds and injuries), to set bones, and to perform simple operations. It was also he who was largely responsible for treating venereal infections. Both being arts of the razor, surgery and barbering had long been yoked together, the Barber Surgeons Company of London dating from 1540; not until 1745 did the two trades split and go their separate ways.[3] The uncouth surgeon provided endless cannon-fodder for the caricaturist, comedian and critic: 'Never for God's sake see a d—— d-ct-r again as long as you live,' was the advice given to Lord Herbert in 1786, after he had done with the services of 'butcher Pott': in such cases 'butcher' simply tripped off the tongue, but in reality Percevall Pott, surgeon to St Bartholomew's Hospital, was anything but coarse.[4]

Surgery was suspect in large measure by association: not because of the ineptitude of its practitioners but because much of what the surgeon did was bloody, painful and perforce dangerous, and he had to work on repugnant conditions like venereal sores. Brave folks like Pepys would submit to the knife for the removal of a bladder-stone rather than endure a lifetime's excruciating pain: luckily for him – and for us – the diarist survived unscathed. Internal surgery, however, was virtually impossible before the introduction of anaesthetics and anti-septic procedures in the mid nineteenth century, and before then the only bodies surgeons were accustomed to opening up were dead ones, for post mortem purposes and anatomical instruction.

Enterprising surgeons, however, turned the physical, hands-on quality of their art into a Baconian virtue, by emphasizing the strengths of their no-nonsense approach, in implied contradistinction to the impractical, word-bound physician: 'I am a Practiser, not an Academick,' boasted Richard Wiseman, England's most renowned late Stuart surgeon – a down-to-earth self-image also adopted by the naval surgeon James Handley, who in 1710 pronounced that what the surgeon ought to have was 'a steady Hand, a clear Sight, ... and to be an *honest Man*'.[5]

The low public perception of the craft was partly sustained by the idea that the training and qualifying examinations for would-be surgeons were superficial and perfunctory, as portrayed in Tobias Smollett's first novel, *Roderick Random*. In 1740 poverty drove this young Scot to seek employment as second surgeon's mate on board the *Chichester*, about to be sent to reinforce Admiral Vernon in the West Indies during the War of Jenkin's Ear, and he later projected his personal experiences onto his fictional hero.

To obtain his warrant as surgeon's mate, Random is told to go to Surgeons' Hall, where he is summoned by a beadle before a board of grim-faced examiners (illus. 87) who inquire after his qualifications and quiz him inanely: 'If during an engagement at sea, a man should be brought to you with his head shot off, how would you behave?' The footling examination ends, predictably, with a demand for a fee.[6]

Off to war, a newly qualified surgeon's mate would normally then purchase his chest of drugs at Apothecaries' Hall before proceeding to his ship; but, upon leaving Surgeons' Hall, Roderick was, without further ado, set upon by a press gang:

> As I crossed Tower Wharf, a squat tawny fellow, with a hanger by his side and a cudgel in his hand, came up to me, calling 'Yo, Ho!, brother, you must come along with me'. As I did not like his appear-ance, instead of answering his salutation, I quickened my pace, in hope of ridding myself of his company; upon which he whistled aloud, and immediately another sailor appeared before me, who laid hold of me by the collar and began to drag me along. Not being of a humour to relish such treatment, I disengaged myself of the assailant, and with one blow of my cudgel laid him motionless on the

> ground; and perceiving myself surrounded in a trice by ten or a dozen more, exerted myself with such dexterity and success that some of my opponents were fain to attack me with drawn cutlasses; ... I received a large wound on my head, and another on my left cheek.[7]

The very first military wounds he encountered were thus his own!

Our hero is then dragged aboard the *Thunder*, whose captain espouses a medical philosophy which is simplicity itself: 'Harkee, sir, I'll have no sick people on board, by God!' Shown down to the surgeon's mess, a square no larger than six feet wide, encircled by medicine chests and a canvas screen, a shock awaits him: 'I was much less surprised that people should die on board, than that any sick person should recover.'[8]

A sick-parade follows, conducted according to the Oakum philosophy. So when the servile ship's surgeon Mackshane examines the first fever-stricken patient, he insists that the sailor is perfectly fit 'and the captain delivered him over to the boatswain's mate, with orders that he should receive a round dozen at the gangway immediately for counterfeiting himself sick'.[9]

Truth – or just a good yarn? Whichever, surgery continued to enjoy, in fact and in fiction, a fairly rum reputation. In due course, however, boosts to its image helped endow it with the air of science.[10] Born in 1728, ten years his brother William's junior, John Hunter was the youngest of his parents' ten children. In 1748 he joined William, then establishing himself in London as a teacher of anatomy, and arranged for his younger brother to attend surgical classes at St George's and St Bartholomew's hospitals. At the latter, he was accepted as a pupil of William Cheselden, who had won fame for performing lithotomy with exceptional rapidity, and who, rarely for a surgeon, had formed close connexions in polite society.

For his health's sake, John, not unlike Smollett, then procured an appointment as a military surgeon, and joined the expeditionary force that set sail in 1761 on one of the Seven Years' War campaigns. It was at this time that he gained the experience that he incorporated into his great *Treatise on the Blood, Inflammation and Gun-shot Wounds*, published posthumously in 1794.

In February 1763 John set up in practice in Golden Square, Piccadilly, conducting extensive experimental research, making the acquaintance of many leading scientists and naturalists, and being elected in 1767 a fellow of the Royal Society. The next year he was appointed surgeon to St George's Hospital, Hyde Park. Thereupon he began to give lectures on applied anatomy and surgery, and many leading surgeons and anatomists owed their early training and subsequent success to his teaching, including his star pupil, Edward Jenner, pioneer of smallpox vaccination. Hunter carved out a reputation as more than a mere operative surgeon – as a pioneer of what was later called the new experimental science of physiology, of which he would be nominated a founding father. When, on one occasion, Jenner wrote to his mentor with an inquiry about the behaviour of hedgehogs, Hunter replied: 'why think; why not try the experiment?' The scientific approach counted.[11]

Covering surgical topics such as inflammation, shock, disorders of the vascular system and venereal disease, John Hunter's four main treatises – *Natural History of the Human Teeth* (1771), *On Venereal Disease* (1786), *Observations on Certain Parts of the Animal Oeconomy* (1786) and *Treatise on the Blood, Inflammation and Gun-shot Wounds* (1794) – were reckoned, by champions of the profession, to mark the emergence of surgery from manual craft to scientific discipline.[12] If its actual practice and scope could not radically change before the introduction, in Victorian times, of anaesthesia and Listerian antisepsis, its rhetorical representations were undergoing transformation long before. Homage was habitually paid to John Hunter, after his death, for realizing, in the fullest form, the prized Baconian union of hand and head, of manual and mental labour, thanks to which the surgeon's craft was declared to have been ennobled into a true science. 'Mark what he did for surgeons', proclaimed the Victorian surgeon James Paget, hitting on a founding-father hero:

> Before his time [surgeons] held inferior rank in the profession ...
> they were subject to the physicians, and very justly so, for the physicians were not only better learned in their own proper calling, but men of higher culture, educated gentlemen and the associates of gentlemen. From Hunter's time a marked change may be seen. Physicians worthily maintained their rank, as they do now, and surgeons rose to it ... Yes, more than any man that ever lived, Hunter helped to make us gentlemen ... Surely ... if we are to maintain the rank of gentlemen ... It must be by the highest scientific culture to which we can attain.[13]

The stigma of the butcher was thus to be superseded by the myth of the scientific surgeon.

The apothecary's status was traditionally reckoned lowly because he was a tradesman, his premises both dirty and gaudy, according to Samuel Garth's dismissive verse:

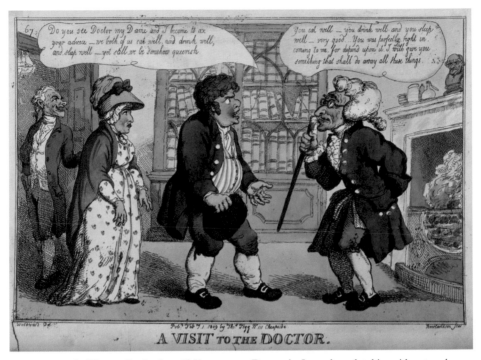

83 Thomas Rowlandson, 'A VISIT TO THE DOCTOR', 1809, coloured etching with watercolour after George Moutard Woodward.

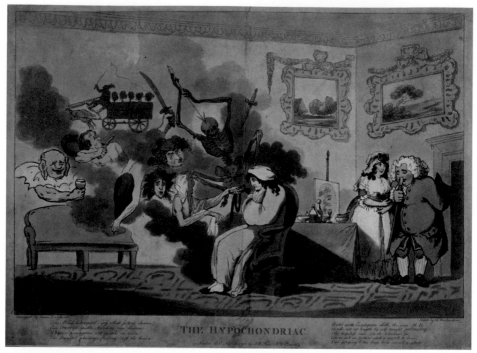

84 Thomas Rowlandson 'THE HYPOCHONDRIAC', 1788, coloured etching after James Dunthorne.

The captioning reads: 'The Mind distemper'd — say, what potent charm, / Can Fancy's spectre — brooding rage disarm? / Physic prescriptive, art assails in vain, / The dreadful phantoms floating 'cross the brain! / Until with Esculapian skill, the sage M. D. / Finds out at length by self-taught palmistry, / The hopeless case — in the reluctant fee: / Then, not in torture such a wretch to keep, / One pitying bolus lays him sound a sleep!' The hypochondriac is haunted by numerous visions: a cauliflower-eared man drinking from a wine glass; a man, haunted by a serpent, preparing to cut his throat; a man driving a hearse whipping his horse; a woman's torso hanging limply upside-down; two lunatic faces; a hand with a sword; a ghoulish old maid holding a cloth and a rope, handing a pistol out of the shadows to the hypochondriac; and a frenzied skeleton preparing to stab with an arrow.

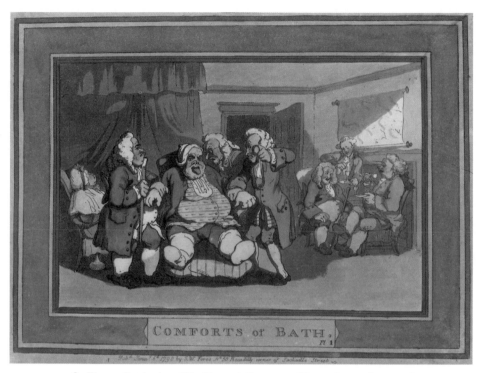

85 Thomas Rowlandson, 'The Doctors', *COMFORTS of BATH*, pl. 1, 1798, watercolour on paper.
Victoria Art Gallery, Bath.

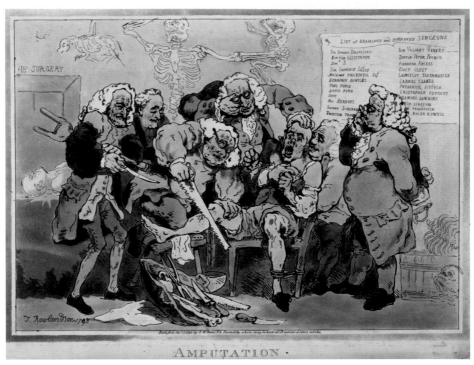

86 Thomas Rowlandson, 'AMPUTATION.', 1793, aquatint and etching with watercolour.

The notice above the door reads: 'The surgery'; skeletons litter the room; on the wall is a 'list of examined and approved surgeons' containing 24 names, including 'Sir Valiant Venery', 'Doctor Peter Putrid', 'Launcelot Slashmuscle' and 'Benjamin Boweles'. Five surgeons participate in the amputation of a man's leg while another oversees them. The surgeon, wearing a carpenter's apron, has set his right knee and left hand on the patient's leg to keep it in position; the other leg is tied to a chair. The absence of a tourniquet is noteworthy.

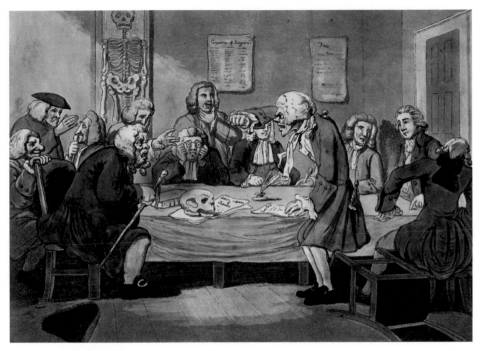

87 Joseph Stadler, 'RODERICK'S EXAMINATION AT SURGEONS HALL', 1800, coloured aquatint after Samuel Collings (based on Tobias Smollett's *Roderick Random*).

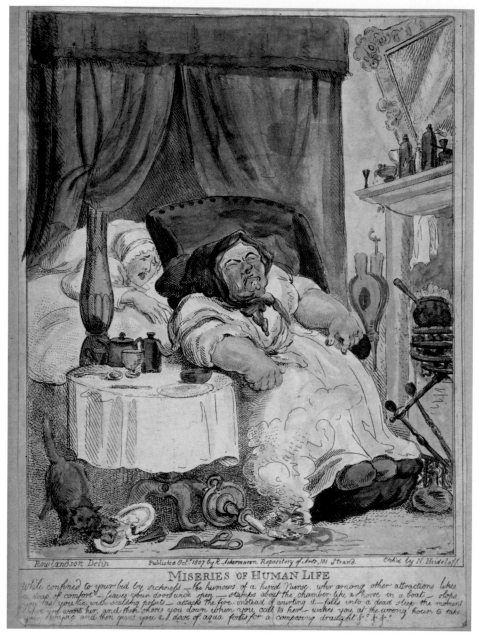

Rowlandson Delin.   Published Oct.r 1807 by R. Ackermann, Repository of Arts, 101 Strand.   Etched by N. Heideloff.

MISERIES OF HUMAN LIFE

While confined to your bed by sickness — the humours of a hired Nurse. who among other attractions likes a drap of comfort — leaves your door wide open — stamps about the chamber like a horse in a boat — slops you as you lie. with scalding possets — attacks the fire. instead of courting it — falls into a dead sleep the moment before you want her. and then snores you down when you call to her — wakes you at the wrong hour to take your clyster, and then gives you a dose of aqua fortis for a composing draught &.c &.c &.c

88 Nicolaus von Heideloff, 'MISERIES OF HUMAN LIFE', 1807, coloured etching after Thomas Rowlandson.

A cat scavenges for food, and a candle sets the carpet on fire.

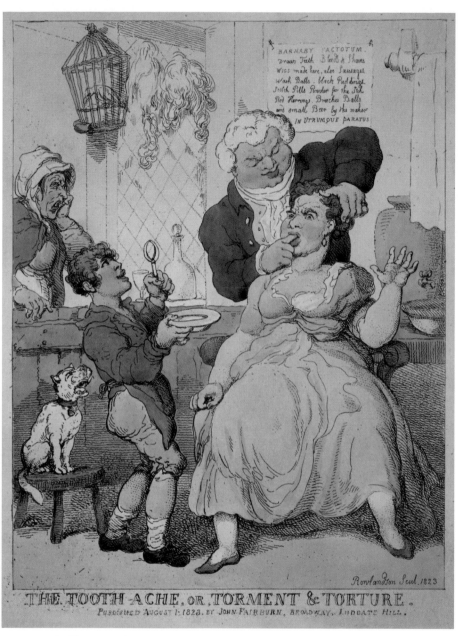

89 Thomas Rowlandson, 'THE TOOTH-ACHE, OR, TORMENT & TORTURE', 1823, coloured etching.

The village jack-of-all-trades is shown drawing a tooth. An old lady, evidently with raging toothache, awaits her turn. On the back wall is a certificate which reads: 'BARNABY FACTOTUM. Draws Teeth, Bleeds & Shaves. WIGS made here, also Sausages, Wash Balls, Black Puddings, Scotch Pills, Powder for the Itch, Red Herrings, Breeches Balls and Small Beer by the Maker. IN UTRUMQUE PARATUS.' A female patient throws out her arm in alarm as a brawny dentist delves into her mouth with a stubby finger. By her side his boy stands ready with a bowl.

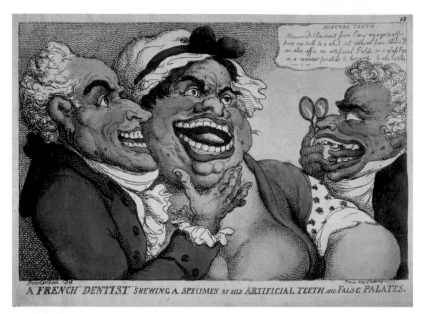

90 Thomas Rowlandson, 'A FRENCH DENTIST SHEWING A SPECIMEN OF HIS ARTIFICIAL TEETH
AND FALSE PALATES', 1811, coloured etching.

M. Dubois de Charmant demonstrates his own, and a grotesque female patient's, false teeth
to a prospective patient. A notice reads: 'MINERAL TEETH. Monsier Dr Charmant from Paris
engages to affix from one tooth to a whole set without pain. Mouns. D can also affix an artificial
Palate or a glass Eye in an manner peculiar to himself. He also distills.'

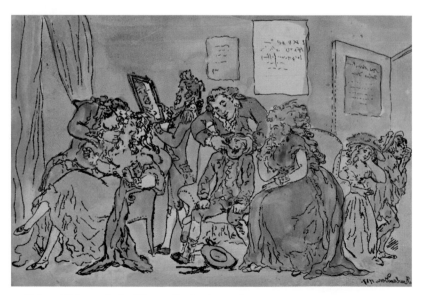

91 Coloured lithograph after Thomas Rowlandson, 1787.

A fashionable dentist's practice: teeth are being extracted from the poor and from children in
order to create dentures for, or to be transplanted into, the wealthy.

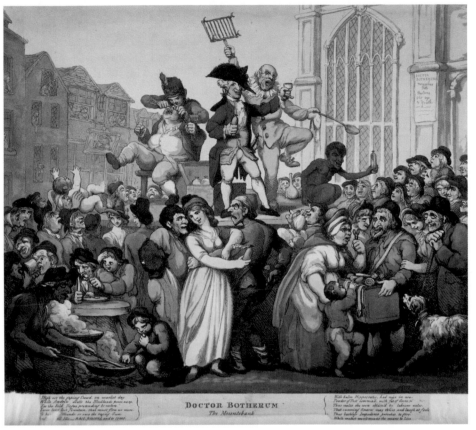

92 Thomas Rowlandson, 'DOCTOR BOTHERUM *The Mountebank*', 1800, etching and aquatint with watercolour.

The captioning continues: 'High oe'r the gaping Crowd, on market day. / While Andrew drolls the Blockheads pence away, / See the bold Rogue pretending to restore, / Loves long lost fountain, that must flow no more. / To heal Wounds, or ease the raging Gum, / And [cure] all Ills — past, present and to come. / With balm Hippocrates had ne'er in use, / Powder of Post commix'd, with fat of Goose. — / Thus melts the coin obtain'd by labours rules. / That cunning Knaves may thrive and laugh at fools / Thus bashless impudence provokes to give, / While modest merit moans the means to live.' Compare the theatrical representations of mountebanks in Chapter 1.

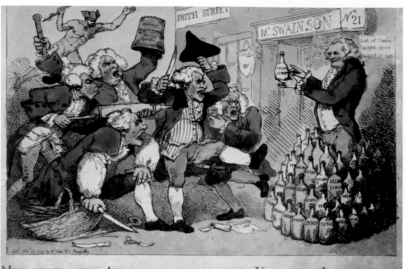

93 Thomas Rowlandson, 'MERCURY and his ADVOCATES DEFEATED, or VEGETABLE
INTRENCHMENT.', 1789, etching with watercolour.

   Isaac Swainson, promoting his 'Velnos Syrup', faces an onslaught of rival practitioners
advocating mercury treatment.

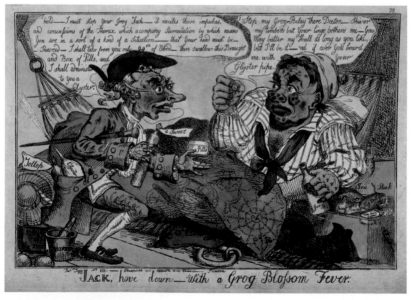

94 William Elmes, 'JACK, hove down — with a Grog Blossom Fever', 1811, coloured etching.

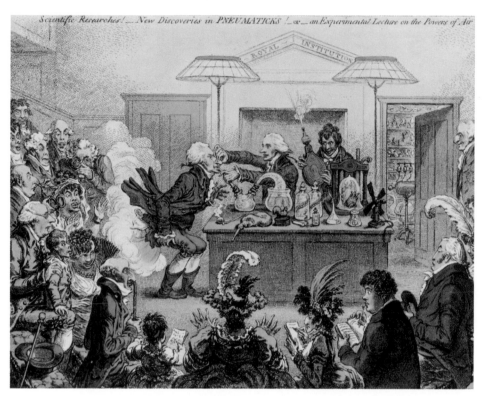

95 James Gillray: 'Scientific Researches! — New Discoveries in PNEUMATICKS! — or — an Experimental Lecture on the Powers of Air—', 1802, coloured etching.

In the premises of the Royal Institution, London, Dr Thomas Garnett demonstrates the effects of nitrous oxide on Sir John Cox Hippisley; Humphry Davy stands by with the bellows. In the audience are Lord Stanhope and Count von Rumford (founder of the Royal Institution).

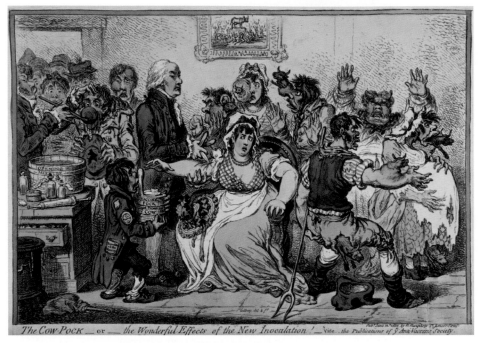

96 James Gillray, 'The COW-POCK — or — The Wonderful Effects of the New Inoculation!:
Vide. the Publications of yᵉ Anti-Vaccine Society', 1802, etching with watercolour.

Scarifier in hand, Edward Jenner is vaccinating an anxious woman in the St Pancras
Smallpox and Inoculation Hospital. Wearing a badge which identifies him as a Charity boy, a lad
bears a tub labelled 'VACCINE POCK hot from ye COW'; poking out of his pocket is a volume
entitled 'Benefits of the Vaccine Process'. Behind him, on top of a chest, is a container of
'OPENING MIXTURE'; an assistant ladles a dose to a client awaiting vaccination. Nearby are
an enema syringe, a box of pills and medicine bottles, one labelled 'VOMIT'. On the wall is a
framed 'Golden Calf'.

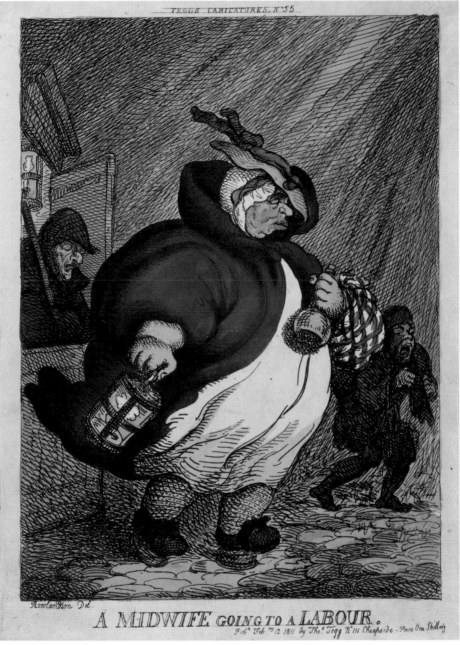

A MIDWIFE GOING TO A LABOUR.

Rowlandson Del.

Feb.ª Feb.ª 12 1811 by Tho.ª Tegg N.º 111 Cheapside. Price One Shilling

97 Thomas Rowlandson, 'A MIDWIFE GOING TO A LABOUR', 1811, etching with watercolour.
An obese midwife battles her way through a storm to go to a labour.

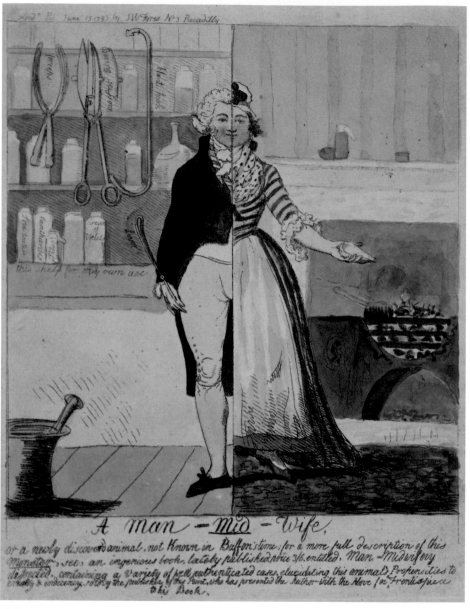

In the image, handwritten text includes:
- Top: *Pub. June 15 1793 by J.W.Fores N⁰3 Pecadilly*
- Caption below image: *A man — mid — Wife,*
- *or a newly discover'd animal, not Known in Buffon's time; for a more full description of this Monster, see, an ingenious book, lately published price 3/6. entitled, Man — Midwifery dissected, containing a Variety of well authenticated cases, elucidating this animals Propensities to cruelty & indecency sold by the publisher of the Print, who has presented the Author with the Above for a Frontispiece to his Book.*

98 Isaac Cruikshank, 'A Man-<u>Mid</u>-Wife', frontispiece to John Blunt [Samuel Fores], *Man-Midwifery Dissected ...* (London, 1793).

The caption reads: 'A man-mid-wife or a newly discover'd animal, not Known in Buffon's time; for a more full description of this <u>Monster</u>, see, an ingenious book, lately published price 3/6 entitled, Man-Midwifery dissected, containing a Variety of well authenticated cases elucidating this animals Propensities to crudity & indecency sold by the publisher of the Print who has presented the Author with the Above for a Frontispiece to his Book.'

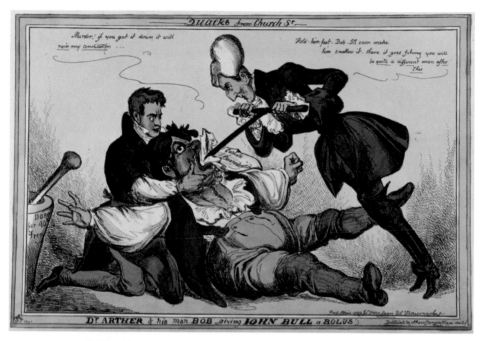

99 William Heath ('Paul Pry'), 'Quacks from Church St. Dʳ ARTHER & his man BOB giving JOHN BULL a BOLUS', 1829, etching with watercolour.

This print satirizes the idea of the Catholic emancipation as a breach of the constitution. It bears the artist's insignia as Paul Pry at the bottom left. John Bull is crying: 'Murder! if you get it down it will <u>ruin</u> my <u>constitution</u> ...'; the paper being forced down his throat is entitled 'Catholic Emancipation'. Prime Minister Arthur Wellesley, Duke of Wellington says to Home Secretary Robert Peel: 'Hold — him fast — Bob — I'll soon make him swallow it — there it goes Johnny you will be <u>quite</u> a <u>different</u> man <u>after this</u>.' The mortar is inscribed: 'DOSE for 40ˢ Free.'

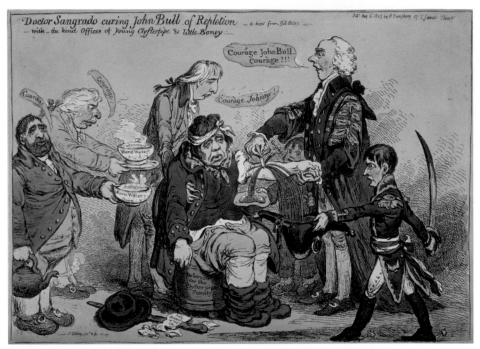

100 James Gillray, 'Doctor Sangrado curing John Bull of Repletion with the kind Offices of Young Clysterpipe & little Boney', 1803, etching with watercolour.

Prime Minister Henry Addington bleeds the exhausted John Bull, seated on a commode. Radical Whigs Richard Brinsley Sheridan and Charles James Fox offer warm water as a palliative; Addington's son ('young Clysterpipe') and Napoleon in the foreground catch the blood, British losses like Malta and the West Indies, in their hats; 'Rule Britannia' lies torn on the ground.

His shop the gazing vulgar's eyes employs
With foreign trinkets and domestick toys.
Here mummies lay most reverently stale,
And there the tortoise hung her coat of mail ...
In this place drugs in musty heaps decayed,
In that dried bladders and drawn teeth were laid.[14]

Hence it was thus perfectly natural to delineate the apothecary as ill bred.

Legally, the apothecary had been the physician's underling: what the latter prescribed, the former dispensed. Such an arrangement was fraught with potential antagonisms; knowing more about drugs than their betters, apothecaries would wish to prescribe on their own say-so and thus please the sick, since the physician's hefty fee was thereby bypassed. In London this led to wrangling between the College of Physicians and the Worshipful Society of Apothecaries – the ensuing 'Dispensary War' has been covered in Chapter 5.[15] The apothecaries' victory in the Rose Case (1704) led to their being empowered to act *de facto* as physicians, and thereafter the apothecary became a figure to be reckoned with in the buoyant medical market (illus. 101). Of that animal Robert Campbell said in 1747 that some 'practise surgery, man-midwifery and many times officiate as Physicians, especially in the country, and often become men of Large Practice and eminent in their way' – that is, apothecaries were the emergent general practitioners to the nation of shopkeepers.[16]

An outmoded historiography implies that women were excluded from medicine until the successful 'storming of the citadel' by Elizabeth

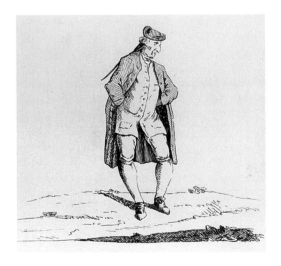

101 Matthew Darly, 'THE MACARONI APOTHECARY', 1772, etching.
Another in Darly's series. Whatever look they adopted – this fashionable image, or the honest-shabby version seen earlier in this chapter – apothecaries remained figures of fun for caricaturists.

Garrett Anderson, Sophia Jex-Blake and other heroines of the mid-Victorian age. In truth, however, they were intimately involved in medical practice throughout the early modern era, being greatly in demand for treating children, servants, family, friends and neighbours alike.[17] 'Agues are much about', observed the Revd George Woodward, 'and my wife being a professed Sangrado for that distemper, has multitude of patients ... and great success she has with her powders.'[18] When Henry Fielding sought 'the best tooth-drawer' for his wife, he ended up with 'a female of great eminence in the art'. Some women achieved fame and fortune, notably Joanna Stephens who sold her 'lithontriptic', a bladder-stone-dissolving nostrum, to Parliament for a cool £5,000, while the 'worm-doctresses' Sarah Hastings and Mrs French of Leicester were immortalized when their treatments were recorded in the *Philosophical Transactions* of the Royal Society. 'That distemper on my tongue ... proceeds from the disease of worms, as you will perceive from the following account,' wrote the Revd Thomas Dent to Sir Edmund King, noting that in M. De la Cross's *Memoirs for the Ingenious* for 1693 he had found an observation concerning the cure of this disease of worms, by one Sarah Hastings:

> I was hence solicitous to enquire out if there were any of the worm-doctresses now in being; and hearing of one famous at Leicester, I was a resolved to write to her, describing all the symptoms, as plain as I could explain them; to which I had a return, that she believed my disease to be worms; and, being resolved to try the experiment, I took coach for Leicester, where being come, my doctress, Mrs. French, no sooner inspected the place, but instantly declared her opinion that the distemper proceeded from worms.
>
> The next day she fell upon her operation ... piercing the part affected with a lancet, she drew some blood, and soon after, with a small spatula, and another instrument, with which she opened the orifices, she picked out five or six worms at a time. She plainly shewed them to the spectators as they came out of the flesh; they were all alive, and moved their heads, and are somewhat less than ordinary maggots.
>
> Thus, in less than eight days, she took out of my tongue more than 100 worms, all nearly of the same size except two very large ones, which she said, were of a cankerous production.[19]

Amongst the best-known Georgian practitioners was the bone-setter, Sarah Mapp, of Epsom, then a fashionable watering-place. At her peak she travelled up to town once a week in a coach-and-four to the Grecian Coffee-House, where she performed her cures, one being upon the niece of Sir Hans Sloane, the President of the Royal College of Physicians. If misogynistically drawing attention *en passant* to her ugliness and obesity, ballads nevertheless sang her praises, one versifier tootling in 1736:

> YOU Surgeons of London, who puzzle your Pates
> To ride in your Coaches, and purchase Estates,
> Give over, for Shame, for your Pride has a Fall,
> And Doctress of Epsom has out-done you all.
>
> Derry Down &.
>
> What signifies Learning, or going to school,
> When a Woman can do, without Reason or Rule,
> What puts you to Nonplus, & baffles your Art;
> For Petticoat Practice has now got the Start.

As with Joanna Southcott, Sally Mapp too packed great power in her corpulent vulgarity.

Nurses too were portrayed, even before Dickens's Sairey Gamp, as elderly slatterns, drunk and negligent, such as the specimen drawn by Rowlandson (illus. 88), to illustrate a passage from the earlier-discussed 'MISERIES OF HUMAN LIFE':

> While confined to your bed by sickness – the humours of a *hired Nurse*, who, among other attractions likes a 'drap of comfort' – leaves your doors wide open – stamps about the chamber like a horse in a boat – slops you as you lie, with scalding posset – *attacks the fire*, instead of courting it, – falls into a dead sleep the moment before you want her, and then snores you down when you call to her – wakes you at the wrong hour to take your physic and then gives you a dose of *aqua fortis* for a *Composing draught* &c. &c.[20]

And the disparaging image of the nurse was mirrored by that of her sister the midwife: as depicted by Rowlandson (Chapter 8), a huge, coarse, battered woman, carrying a telltale bottle. Her repulsive physique suggests, by association, the less than savoury connotations of traditional childbirth.[21]

The challenge to the dignity of regular physicians afforded by the ministrations of women healers and nurses was brought out by Rowlandson in *The English Dance of Death* (illus. 102). In this 'Chamber Scene', an elderly gentleman is being looked after by three physicians plus a nurse. The doctors come daily to prescribe their draughts and pills – such assiduousness was no less lucrative than dutiful; but the moment they withdraw, the old woman tips them away, substituting kitchen physic. When this practice finally comes to their notice, doctors upbraid the nurse's treason. They curse, the nurse

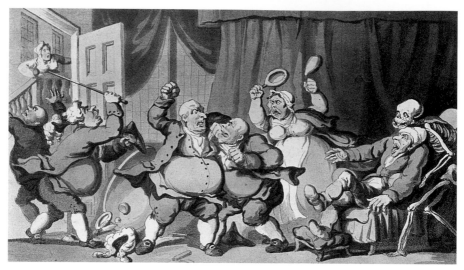

102 Thomas Rowlandson, 'The Dance of Death: The Chamber War', from his *The English Dance of Death*, 1816, coloured aquatint.

The accompanying text (by Rowlandson) reads: 'Sir Samuel, as it appears, / Had reach'd the age of four score years. / Lame, weak and deaf and almost blind, / To his arm chair he was confined: / But while there's Life, there's Hope, they say; / And three physicians every day / Came, gravely, for their daily pay. / A nurse too, who her labours plied / In watching sick men till they died, / Had all that time, and longer, been / The Mistress of the Chamber Scene. / She did the sick man's food prepare, / And nurs'd him with unwearied care. / But still the Doctors came each day, / And bore their golden Fees away.' The text below the image reads: 'When Doctors three the Labour share, / No wonder Death attends them there.'

gives as good as she gets, and a free-for-all results. In the midst of the rout, Death appears to whisper in the shocked patient's ear:

> While these strange people disagree,
> You shall receive my *Recipe*;
> Nor feel a pang, nor give a Fee.[22]

What came to be known as the 'Quack's Charter' was enacted by Parliament in 1542:

> Be it ordered ... that at all times from henceforth it shall be lawful to every person being the King's subject having knowledge and experience of the nature of herbs roots and waters or of the operation of the same by speculation or practice ... to practise use and minister in and to any outward sore, wound, swelling or disease, any herb or herbs ointments bathes poultices and emplasters, according to their cunning experience and knowledge in any of the diseases sores and maladies aforesaid and all other like to the same, or drinks for the stone, strangury or agues.[23]

Evidently it was recognized that traditional practices were ensconced

196

and esteemed – and in any case there were insufficient licensed practitioners to treat the nation. Blessed by this legislative sanction, over the succeeding centuries thousands would devote some of their time to, and top up their income from, medicine: grocers and pedlars retailing drugs, itinerants selling flasks of brightly coloured 'wonder cures', and blacksmiths drawing teeth. Every village, furthermore, had its 'wise women' and wet nurses well-versed in herb lore and in 'secrets' (very few of whom were ever accused of witchcraft), while the gentry and clergy prided themselves upon their knowledge of physic, and treated their servants, households and parishioners out of piety, duty and necessity. In urgent need of medical assistance on a country journey, the politician William Pulteney was told 'that there was no one could do it, but a Man that lived three miles off, who was a good Physician, bled every Man, and Calf, in the neighbourhood, and was a pretty good Surgeon, for he had been originally a Sowgelder'.[24] Makeshift medicine of this kind was not always to be recommended. Parson Woodforde had a frightful experience with a superannuated tooth-drawing farrier:

> sent for one Reeves a man who draws teeth in this parish and about 7 he came and drew my tooth, but shockingly bad indeed, he broke away a great piece of my gum and broke one of the fangs of the tooth … Gave the old man that drew it however 0.2.6. he is too old, I think, to draw teeth, can't see very well.[25]

Yet if some locals were inept, and travelling empirics might be arrant rogues, others possessed genuine skills in treating eye, teeth or ear complaints, performing useful services in the days before business was brisk enough to support permanent resident country-town opticians, truss-fitters, dentists and the like. A few healers, moreover, claimed, and perhaps possessed, extraordinary gifts. The Irish gentleman Valentine Greatrakes discovered he could heal through laying on of hands. His fame spreading, he came to England, holding healing sessions even at the court of Charles II, to the consternation of jealous physicians and sceptical men of science.[26] Georgian England, however, possessed fewer holy healers than France or Italy, largely because of the religious difference between Protestant and Catholic but partly because quacks could make such a killing.[27]

Medical specialization did not systematically evolve and gain legitimacy, not to mention prestige, before the nineteenth century. But certain types of practitioners were carving out niches for themselves. Amongst these, dentists secured a more refined and remunerative trade in the Georgian era. Tooth-pulling, as just discussed, had been a job to which all sorts of people had turned their wrist (illus. 89). Initially in France, however, a new and superior breed developed, who, while keeping up bread-and-butter fang-drawing, pioneered conservation work and specialized in dentures and those aesthetic cosmetic effects – a good face, the right smile – increasingly in demand in polite society. Public perception of the difference between tooth-men old and new was the theme of contrasting prints by Robert Dighton (1785). In *The Country Tooth Drawer* a farrier – perhaps like Woodforde's Reeves – is extracting a tooth in the smithy with a large pair of forceps, assisted by his sturdy workmates. *The Town Tooth Drawer* by contrast shows an elegant lady undergoing extraction in her own home. The smart dentist – reputedly a likeness of the Italian Bartholomew Ruspini, who practised in Paris before setting up in Bath – is conspicuously using a 'modern' instrument, a tooth-key, and is attended by one of those smart black boys so prominent in contemporary prints, carrying his instrument case.[28]

With the new premium on appearances, discussed in Chapter 3, the coming dentist sold the indispensable importance of a good mouth (illus. 90).[29] 'The celebrated Mrs BERNARD and Mr DAVY, DENTISTS from Berlin', fanfared one such team of operators, who sold good looks, 'are just arrived again at Mr Sturdy's Glass-Shop, at the Corner of Goodramgate, YORK, and respectfully acquaint the Public' of their operations. What did they do?

> They transplant Human Teeth, or fix artificial Teeth from one to an entire Sett, in a much easier and by a far superior Method than practised hitherto in this Kingdom. – Their Pearl Lotion is particularly recommended for restoring the Teeth to their native Whiteness and Beauty; (although ever so tarnished) without injuring the Enamel.[30]

There was, however, a class sting in the tail for, as with shady organ transplants nowadays, transplantation meant first removing healthy teeth from the indigent, for a pittance, before they were implanted in the gums of the rich (illus. 91).[31]

To draw notice to themselves while diverting attention from what they actually did, some went in for intense self-publicization. A tapestry-maker's son, born in Flanders in 1736, Martin Van Butchell (alluded to in Chapter 3) (illus. 103) moved to England, he received a good education; and teeth, it seems, attracted his attention after he broke one of his own, whereupon he engaged himself as pupil to none other than John Hunter, author, it will be remembered, of a *Natural History of the Human Teeth* (1771).

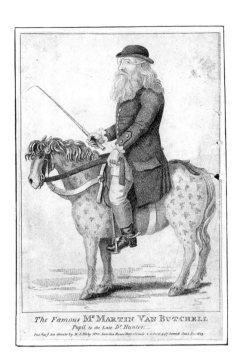

103 'The Famous Mr MARTIN VAN BUTCHELL Pupil to the Late Dr Hunter', 1803, stipple engraving.

The Famous M.ʳ MARTIN VAN BUTCHELL.
Pupil to the Late D.ʳ Hunter.

As his speciality, Van Butchell constructed artificial sets of teeth fitted with springs hinged on gold pivots, professing to fit these complete with gums, sockets and palate without 'drawing stumps or causing pain'. Combining the *dulce* with the *utile*, these were not merely 'useful ornaments' but singularly functional, being 'most helpful to enunciation'.[32]

Like all quacks, Van Butchell was profoundly image-conscious. The *St James Chronicle* for 1 March 1777 trumpeted his fashionable address and practice:

> Van Butchell, Surgeon-Dentist, attends at his House, the upper part of Mount-Street, Grosvenor Square, every day in the Year, from Nine to One o'clock, Sundays excepted.
> Name in Marble on the Door. Advice, £2.2s. Taking out a Tooth or Stump, £1.1s. each. Putting in artificial Teeth, £5.5s. each. A whole under Row, £42. Upper Row £63. An entire set, £105. Natural Teeth, £10.10s. each. The Money paid first.

(He, too, evidently went in for transplantation.)

As well as doubling as a truss-maker, Van Butchell promoted himself as 'the Inventor of Elasticbands (gentlemen wear them, to keep up small-cloathes); also, Cork-bottoms, to Iron-stirrups; Spring-girths for Saddles; and many like things', and he advertised his 'newly-invented Spring band Garters [which] ... will help to make [the ladies] (as they ought to be!) – superlatively happy!' In 1791 Gillray portrayed Mrs Hobart trying on a pair. The painting on the wall behind the rather Swiftian image of this famed but fading actress – mutton dressed up as lamb – reminded viewers of one of her star roles, a scene from *Nina or the Madness of Love*. With the aid of the garters, it was implied, even she might yet be rejuvenated, and recover her languishing glories!

Van Butchell may have appreciated Gillray's attention, but perhaps he hardly needed it, for he was his own publicity machine. He made it his practice to ride through London mounted on a white pony daubed with big black or purple spots, appearing in public with a long white beard and dressed in exotic garb – a one-piece shirt, waistcoat, breeches and stockings, all in white, complete with a large bone in his hand attached to his wrist – a cudgel referred to, in a droll manner, as 'the jaw-bone of an ass'.

'There be many Mountebanks, Quacksalvers, Empiricks, in every street almost, and in every village', whined the Oxford don Robert Burton early in the seventeenth century, 'that take upon them this name, make this noble and profitable Art to be evil spoken of, and contemned, by reason of these base and illiterate Artificers.'[33] The author of *The Anatomy of Melancholy* exaggerated, and his identification of them as 'base and illiterate' is simplistic and biased, but his general point stands: irregular healers were, and remained, plentiful, in town and country alike, right into the nineteenth century (illus. 92). Like whores, it was the sad fate of quacks to be widely used yet ever abused:

> With monstrous promise they delude the mind,
> And thrive on all that tortures human-kind.
> Void of all honour, avaricious, rash,
> The daring tribe compound their boasted trash –
> Tincture or syrup, lotion, drop or pill;
> How strange to add, in this nefarious trade,
> That men of parts are dupes by dunces made:
> That creatures nature meant should clean our streets
> Have purchased lands and mansions, parks and seats ...[34]

Traditionally the mountebank operated as a huckster. Gaudily dressed and assisted by a riddling, drum-banging, pratfall-turning zany and perhaps a monkey, he set up his stage in the marketplace, drew a crowd and then some teeth, doled out a few free bottles of julep and sold a few dozen more, and then rode out of town.[35] Thomas

Holcroft portrayed such a mountebank he saw while a child at Wisbech fair around 1770:

> It was a pleasure so unexpected, so exquisite, so rich and rare, that I followed the 'Merry Andrew' and his drummer through the streets, almost bursting with laughter at his comicality.
>
> When he returned to the stage followed by an eager crowd, and ordered by his master to mount; to see the comical jump he gave, alighting half upright, roaring with pretended pain, pressing his hip declaring he had put out his collar-bone, crying to his master to come and cure it, receiving a kick, springing up and making a somersault; thanking his master kindly for making him well, yet the moment his back was turned, mocking him with wry faces; answering the doctor, whom I should have thought extremely witty, if Andrew had not been there with jokes so apposite and whimsical, as never failed to produce roars of laughter.[36]

Even as late as the end of the Victorian era 'Sequah', an 'American' mountebank, created a stir with the highly theatrical performances he gave up and down the country, vending remedies from the prairie, allegedly based on native Indian wisdom: in actuality, the 'cowboy' hailed from Yorkshire.[37]

In commercial terms, the most innovative and enterprising Georgian irregulars were not Holcroft's face-to-face fairground itinerants – theirs was a traditional act, deriving from medieval Italy – but those who pioneered mass-market, brand-name proprietary and patent medicines, notably by exploiting the new possibilities for high-profile advertising. Cashing in on the opportunities afforded by newspapers and magazines, and on improved communications and distribution networks (turnpike roads, postal services and retail shops), a few such behind-the-scenes entrepreneurs vended their nostrums in astronomical quantities: Anderson's Scots Pills, Hooper's Female Pills, Dr Radcliffe's Famous Purging Elixir, Turlington's Pills, Bateman's Pectoral Drops, Daffy's Elixir, Stoughton's Great Cordial Elixir, and others besides. In just twenty years, some 1,612,800 sachets of James's powders were sold.[38]

Charismatic performers, however, remained very much in evidence, sustained by bravura and theatricality. These were the practitioners endlessly despised and damned by the puritanical temper of English culture for their flagrant, flamboyant showiness: 'Like Mercury, you must always carry a caduceus or conjuring japan in your hand, capt with a civet-box, with which you must walk with Spanish gravity,' snarled some mock-advice to the breed:

> Let your table never be without some old musty Greek or Arabick

author and the fourth Book of Cornelius Agrippa's 'Occult Philosophy,' wide open to amuse spectators, also half a dozen of *gilt shillings*, as so many guineas received that morning for fees.[39]

To be successful a quack had to excel in image-management and keeping his name in the news. When Joshua ('Spot') Ward, pardoned by George II after earlier dabbling in Jacobitism, returned in 1733 from exile in France, he ensured his arrival was widely heralded: 'There was an extraordinary Advertisement this month in the Newspapers', declared a double puff inserted in the *Gentleman's Magazine*, 'concerning the great cures in all Distempers perform'd with one medicine, a Pill or a Drop, by Joshua Ward, Esq; lately arriv'd from Paris, where he had done the like Cures.'[40]

Though lacking medical training, Ward won fame and fortune through his 'Pill or Drop', preparations he succeeded in getting made regulation navy issue. Initially a drysalter, he had got himself elected as a Member of Parliament (another image-sensitive enterprise), but fled at the time of the 1715 Jacobite uprising. Whilst in France, he devised the medicine that made him renowned. Building on the profits of the 'Pill', much remarked and even praised by Henry Fielding – Ward was ever adroit at cultivating the republic of letters – he sanctified himself into the role of respected philanthropist, partly by endowing four London 'hospitals' for the sick poor. On curing Sir Joseph Jekyll, Master of the Rolls, he was given unique personal exemption from the legislation empowering the College of Physicians to inspect medicines; and, having put George II's dislocated thumb back into place (the royal physicians had predictably misdiagnosed gout, whereas Ward was a far better manipulator), he gained entrée at Court and carved out special privileges for himself, including the freedom to drive his ornate coach-and-six through St James's Park. Kings and quacks could see eye-to-eye and do business with each other.[41]

With great assiduity, Ward massaged not only the royal thumb but also his own image. A full-length statue, rather daringly given to the Royal Society of Arts in London, was sculpted by one of his arty friends, Agostini Carlini. Ward supposedly paid the sculptor an annual retainer to keep the statue in his studio and appear to be working at it when patrons were about. An allegorical portrait by Thomas Bardwell, now hanging in the Royal College of Surgeons, captured the potent blend of self-aggrandizement and service characteristic of this enigmatic egoist's public image. 'Britannia' is shown leading a throng of the sick poor to Ward, and presenting him with a purse by way of payment for his benefaction. He, for his part, is pointing to the figure of

'Charity' – a mother nursing her baby, with two children at her side – and instructing that it should go not to himself but to her. Drawing back a curtain, 'Time' reveals that it is Ward who stands between 'Death' and the sick and indigent. An accompanying verse tells all:

> 'Tis Thou, O Gen'rous Ward, thrice bless'd we see
> Crouded with those that seek thy Charity.
> The poor distress'd, the sick, the lame, ye blind,
> Here seek relief, from thee relief they find.[42]

Quacks were boundlessly inventive in devising striking self-publicizing techniques. Having studied under William Cheselden at St Thomas's Hospital, John (Chevalier) Taylor was a skilful oculist, but he eschewed a regular surgical career and preferred to practise as an itinerant, cashing in on a dazzling imagination and cultivating a flamboyant lifestyle. With great flair, he exploited the prestige enjoyed by showman's rhetoric by devising an ingenious English prose style which set grandiloquent terms into the inverted word order of a Latinate syntax ('Of the eye on the wonders lecture will I'), insisting (with some truth) that he held forth in 'the true Ciceronian, prodigiously difficult and never attempted in our language before'. Latinisms still spoke with authority.[43]

Taylor also had himself widely portrayed, sometimes glamorously, sometimes comically. An image by the caricaturist Thomas Patch presents an assistant gripping a patient as the Chevalier surgically removes an eye, which he hoists aloft on a fork. The eyes bejewelling the quack's frock coat broadcast his speciality while hinting that he won his livelihood through his clients' lack of vision. Rather as with the many droll or mocking images of James Graham, this and other graphic send-ups of Taylor may well have been with his own connivance, in line with the axiom that all publicity was good publicity.

Performing the length and breadth of Europe, Taylor achieved an entrée into society, as he chronicled in his three-volume autobiography; and the Scot James Graham also aimed high. Born a saddler's son in Edinburgh in the star-crossed year of the 'forty-five, Graham studied medicine at his home university under Monro Primus, Black, Whytt and Cullen, though never, contrary to his claims, graduating.[44] In 1770 he married and settled in Pontefract, subsequently migrating to America. There, subsidized by Shelley's grandfather, he practised medicine, met Benjamin Franklin, and became a medical-electricity devotee. Travels in Europe were followed in the late 1770s by practice in fashionable Bath, where he won such quality patients as the historian Catharine Macaulay (who was to marry his brother), and

Georgiana, Duchess of Devonshire. Success spurred him to try his fortune in London. Opening his 'Templum Aesculapio Sacrum' in 1780 at the fashionable Adelphi just off the Strand, he combined lectures and multimedia spectacle with a practice touting the newly fashionable electrical therapy.

The Temple's rooms were festooned with electrical machines, Leyden jars, conductors and insulated glass pillars, an 'electrical throne' and chemical apparatus, alongside sculptures, paintings and stained glass windows and other eye-catching paraphernalia. Music and perfumes pervaded the atmosphere. Alluding back to pilgrimage shrines, its entrance hall was decked out with crutches and callipers supposedly discarded as votive offerings by clients who, now healed, no longer needed them. In the 'Great Apollo Apartment' Graham gave lectures, sold his nostrums and mounted displays, assisted by nubile 'goddesses of health', to promote custom.

One of Graham's main claims to fame lay in his 'Celestial Bed', a cure for barrenness, hired out at £50 a night to counter impotence and sterility:

> twelve feet long by nine feet wide, supported by forty pillars of brilliant glass of the most exquisite workmanship in richly variegated colours. The super-celestial dome of the bed, which contains the odoriferous, balmy and ethereal spices, odours and essences, which is the grand reservoir of those reviving invigorating influences which are exhaled by the breath of music and by the exhilarating force of electrical fire, is covered on the other side with brilliant panes of looking glass.[45]

Covered with coloured silk sheets, its mattresses were filled with 'the strongest, most springy hair, produced at vast expense from the tails of English stallions'. Gossip alleged that crowds would form outside the Temple to see which celebrities would be availing themselves of the service – compare the behaviour of fans towards film and pop stars nowadays.

All this glitz was costly and, in due course, cursed by creditors, Graham quit the Adelphi and removed to Pall Mall, where he promoted his 'libidinous' lectures on generation to keep himself in the public eye. And, most colourfully, aided by yet more 'goddesses of health', he championed the omni–curative properties of mudbaths, having himself repeatedly buried, fakir-like, naked, for days on end, fasting and lecturing all the while. The best mud for the purpose was 'fresh, icy, cold earth brought from the top of Hampstead Hill', though for busy folks even a turf strapped to the chest, beneath the shirt, he insisted, was better than nothing.

Rowlandson depicted Graham supervising a corpulent client, relieved of his clothes, crutches and wig so as to relish the pleasures of having his back scrubbed followed by burial in a muddy trench. Other patrons are caught in divers degrees of undress and distress, while a gent descends from a sedan chair and hobbles towards his similar fate. Males and females are separated only by a sheet: the falling drape pantomimes how the curtain is coming down on modesty and virtue.[46]

'I was present at one of his lectures upon the benefits arising from earth bathing (as he called it)', reported the gossip, Henry Angelo, after seeing an Grahamian exhibition of mud-bathing in nearby Panton Street, where had gathered

> a crowded audience of men [and] many ladies ... to listen to his delicate lectures. In the centre of the room was a pile of earth, in the middle of which was a pit where a stool was placed: we waited some time, when much impatience was manifested, and after repeated calls, 'Doctor, Doctor!' he actually made his appearance *en chemise*. After making his bow he seated himself on the stool; when two men with shovels began to place the mound in the cavity: as it approached to the pit of the stomach he kept lifting up his shirt and at last took it entirely off, the earth being up to his chin and the doctor being left *in puris naturalibis*. He then began his lecture, expiating on the excellent qualities of the Earth Bath, how invigorating etc. quite enough to call up the chaste blushes of the modest ladies.[47]

Tattlers like Angelo eagerly colluded in the creation of the quack operators' mystique – until, that is, they chose to drop them for some other media sensation.

Forced by his creditors to sell up, in 1783 Graham put his cures and creeds on the road, just like a troupe of travelling players or indeed an itinerant preacher. Styling himself 'born again', he began to preach an ardent if idiosyncratic evangelical Christianity, adopting the identification: 'the Servant of the Lord O.W.L.' (O Wonderful Love). In course of time, he grew monomaniacal, turning into a veritable vaudeville Messiah; his latter-day Christian guise – stripping off in the street and handing out his clothes to the poor – led some to call him mad. What old age may have had in store for this ardent longevitist – doctor, player, preacher – was pre-empted by his premature death in 1794.

The careers of Graham and his like defy conventional medical-historical analysis because the 'reality' of them is all rhetoric, a foam of fantasy, testimony to their adroitness at image-creation and inflation. Like other media medics, Graham, buoyed up by the froth of tales, cartoons, satires, lampoons and tittle-tattle, throve on outrage and excess, constantly creating and recreating a beguiling believe-it-or-not

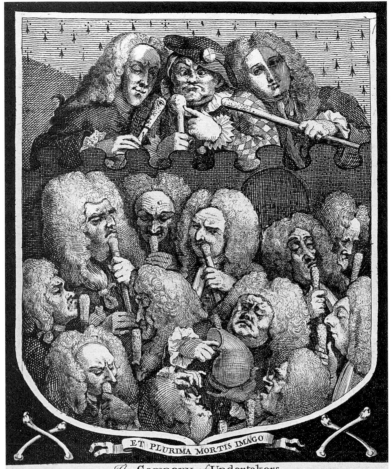

The **Company** *of* Undertakers

Beareth Sable, an Urinal *proper, between* 12 Quack-Heads *of the Second &* 12 Cane Heads *Or,* Consultant . *On a* Chief *Nebulæ,* Ermine, One Compleat D octor *issuant, checkie sustaining in his*
Right Hand a Baton *of the Second . On his* Dexter *&* Sinister *sides two* D emi-Do ctors, *issuant*
of the Second, & two Cane Heads *issuant of the third; The first having* One Eye conchant, *to-*
wards the Dexter Side *of the* Escocheon; *the Second* Faced per pale proper *&* Gules, Guardent . ———
With this Motto ——————— *Et Plurima* Mortis Imago .

Published by W. Hogarth . *March the* 3, 1736.

Price Six pence

104 William Hogarth, '*The* Company *of* Undertakers', 1736, engraving after himself.

In this imaginary coat of arms, Hogarth satirizes physicians and quacks, and their
spurious learning, through the idiocies of heraldry. The three half-figures in the upper
third of the shield design are portraits of notorious quacks. On the left is the absurd
'Chevalier' John Taylor (*c.* 1708–1772), the oculist or 'Ophthalmiator, Pontifical, Imperial,
and Royal', whose cane is marked with an eye and who leers with one eye shut at Mrs
'Crazy Sal' Mapp the bone-setter (dressed as a Harlequin), who points at her bone-shaped
staff. On the right is Dr Joshua 'Spot' Ward (1685–1761), so named from a facial birthmark.
The lower part of the shield is occupied by character studies of twelve pompous doctors,
most of whom sniff the heads of the canes in affectations of profound thought. One holds a
full glass urinal, the contents of which he is about to test by taste, while two colleagues peer
at it through their spectacles. All the medical men wear dark suits and full-bottomed wigs.

air. Scams, scandals and public illusion were the key to their success.

Some irregulars broke into the world of glamour and gossip marked by conspicuous wealth. The uroscopist Theodor Myersbach allegedly enjoyed 'a fortune equal to that of a German prince';[48] starting as a baker, Nathaniel Godbold promoted a successful rejuvenative 'Vegetable Balsam' and eventually bought a country house for £30,000. Originally a woollen draper, Isaac Swainson acquired 'Velno's Vegetable Syrup' and claimed to sell an astonishing 20,000 bottles of the mixture a year (two thirds, he alleged, were ordered directly or indirectly by the faculty), securing him an income of £5,000 per annum.[49]

Such men might hobnob in the looking-glass world of high society. William Read started out as a tailor (another image profession), became a successful oculist, made his fortune, treated Queen Anne, and was knighted in 1705 by the appreciative monarch 'on account of his services to soldiers and seamen for blindness which he gave gratis'. He hired a Grub-Street poet to immortalize himself in *The Oculist* (1705):

> Whilst Britain's Sovereign scales such worth has weighed
> And Anne herself has smiling favours paid,
> That Sacred hand does your fair chaplet twist,
> Great Read her own entitled oculist!

Straddling two worlds, he became host to, while also the butt of, the literati.[50]

It was in the nature of quackery to be thus excoriated and lampooned.[51] But in a free market in which caveat emptor was the watchword, the regulars too, men like Radcliffe and Woodward (as shown in Chapter 5) had no less recourse to commercial and self-promoting antics. Quacks, of course, puffed specifics, but scores of orthodox practitioners did nicely out of patent medicines and nostrum-mongering and had no qualms about advertising, direct and indirect. When Edward Jenner, later immortalized as the humanitarian pioneer of smallpox vaccination, mooted marketing a new proprietary tartar emetic, his mentor, the great John Hunter, told him to go for it: 'I am puffing of your tartar as the tartar of all tartars ... Let it be called Jenner's Tartar Emetic, or anybody's else that you please.'[52] The insinuation that regulars and empirics were two peas in a pod was the moral behind many a skit, or, for instance, a depiction of medical fisticuffs by Rowlandson (illus. 93).[53] The scene is Frith Street, Soho – even then the entertainments capital of London – and it features Isaac Swainson, just discussed. The quack has barricaded himself behind bottles of his 'Velno's Vegetable Syrup' piled up outside his shop. His opponents, an unholy alliance of barber-surgeons and apothecaries, are irate at the loss of trade to the irrepressible empiric. When regulars thus brawled with quacks, they reduced themselves to their level, and so amply justified the charge that they were in reality identical twins, which was also the burden of Hogarth's '*The* Company *of* Under-takers' (illus. 104). Was there truly any difference between the stately, self-important faculty physicians at the foot and the infamous quacks above – Joshua ('Spot') Ward, Sally Mapp, and John ('Chevalier') Taylor, all just discussed? No: because Hogarth's motto was *et plurima mortis imago*: everywhere the face of death.[54]

In a milieu in which quacks were vilified for their self-advertising showmanship, it should come as no surprise that for every anti-quack tirade by 'Misoquackus' and the like, the hocus-pocus of the regulars was the target of *Medicina Flagellata, or the Doctor Scarify'd* (1721), the pseudonymous Gregory Glyster's *A Dose for the Doctor* (1759), and other such quips, with their condemnations of 'medical mystery' and 'large sounds with little meaning'. Quacks were ever denounced as frauds, but cynics took a Shavian view of all the professions; from Ben Jonson, through Butler and Gay, Swift and Pope, to Henry Fielding, it was 'a world of quacks'.[55]

At a time when, amidst the triumph of commercial capitalism and the emergence of a consumer society, the business of medical practitioners was in flux, the official designations and established roles of its diverse branches became objects of public anxiety. Practitioners themselves – and, for very different reasons, satirists too – might wish to highlight distinctive props, emblems and tokens of the trade: the physician's wig, the surgeon's saw, the apothecary's pestle and mortar. In critics' hands, such images served as the means for calling practitioners to order. The imagery of self-promotion provided a clear acknowledge-ment that with change going on all around in a commercial society, professional success, ever of course dependent on fashion, required the revamping of images.

8 Professional Problems

Early modern medicine stirred anxieties and distrust, which were rarely far from the surface, if often displaced into humour. 'Met Mr Forbes the surgeon going to kill a few patients,' diarized William Holland in 1800; yet the parson himself drew routinely upon his fellow professional's 'homicidal' services (and how, one wonders, did the surgeon spoof the clergyman?).[1] No less pointedly, if more politely, one of the Duchess of Gordon's barbs was relayed by the gossipy artist Joseph Farington: 'Our Physician, said she, has lately been confined by indisposition, & sent to know how we did. I returned him an answer that since He was ill, our family had been very well.'[2]

Scepticism was, of course, as old as the profession itself. The New Testament told physicians to heal themselves, while proverbs warned the public that death and the doctors were as thick as thieves. Their legendary reputation for unbelief did not help: *ubi tres medici, ibi duo Athei*: where there are three doctors, there are two atheists.[3] 'A Physician who should be even a *Theist*, still more a *Christian*', mused Coleridge, 'would be a rarity indeed.'[4] Criticism flared as the profession mushroomed and seemed to grow immoderately prosperous.[5]

Medicine's bad public odour was fanned by intra-professional rivalries. The dawn of the eighteenth century brought the Dispensary battle;[6] London's surgeons later divorced from the barbers, while in 1774 there followed the 'Battle of Warwick Lane', the civil war amongst the College of Physicians, set on stage, as we have seen, in Samuel Foote's *The Devil upon Two Sticks*.[7] Rampant quackery and, later, the rise of alternative medicine sects (homoeopathy, for instance) precluded any united front (illus. 105).

Rival doctors seemed ever at cuffs, a situation perpetuated by rich patients' habit of taking second, third, fourth and *n*th opinions: laid low in 1765 with a malignant fever, David Garrick confessed that he 'had no less than Eight Physicians', slyly adding, 'yet I am alive and in Spirits, tho' somewhat ye Worse for Wear and Tear'.[8] 'How strangely the greatest Physicians have disagreed in the most essential Points of

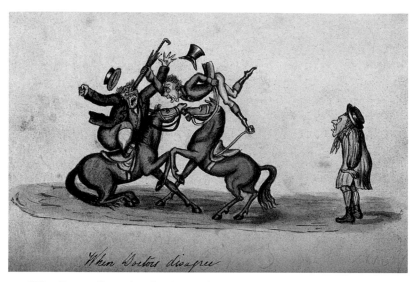

105 'When Doctors disagree', undated watercolour.
Two doctors on horseback in violent confrontation show the hostility provoked when a difference of opinion arises in the medical profession.

their art,' bewailed Mandeville's character Misomedon, rolling his eyes with stagy surprise:[9]

> Who shall decide when doctors disagree,
> And soundest casuists doubt, like you and me?[10]

echoed Pope (answer: Death).

Despite the lip service they paid to *esprit de corps*, doctors notoriously wrangled to each other's faces and whispered behind their backs. Farington recorded the surgeon Sir Anthony Carlisle badmouthing all and sundry at a dinner party:

> He spoke of *Reynolds* as being a weak man, & consequently not a man capable of judging in cases where sagacity & penetration are necessary. Lettsom, He allowed to be above Reynolds in understanding, but yet an inferior man. – Dr. George Fordyce, He sd. killed himself by drinking ... Sir Francis Milman He spoke of as being a man of sense, & very capable; but doubted whether He had sufficient experience. Dr Ash He mentioned as being the best informed man of His profession; with the additional advantage of an extraordinary memory. – Dr. Frazer, who died lately, He sd. had injured His constitution by drinking too much which had hurt some of the Viscera: but He had abstained from it latterly. – Dr. Vaughan He spoke of as being a man amiable in His manners, but one who did not seem to possess any great power of mind.[11]

And on he rabbited: what was a sick person to do?

The various branches of the profession vilified each other with great dedication. 'Every Art has had its Adversarys', disarmingly conceded the early Georgian London surgeon Daniel Turner, before proving his own point by continuing in high dudgeon that it was 'very strange' that surgery, the art which 'gives Sight to the Blind, Hearing to the Deaf: Sets together ... disjoynted and broken Bones, and reduses the Frail Structure of Humane Bodys to their wonted Health and Vigour, should have so much as one [foe]'.[12] Despite that defence of his craft's dignity, Turner nevertheless had no high opinion of those who actually practised it. An 'Abundance of [London's] Inhabitants', candour compelled him to admit, were 'maimed and undone through ... great Numbers of Ignorant, ill designing' surgical pretenders. Among these, street mountebanks were the 'Common Enemy of the People', bone-setters were 'Man-slayers', and barbers the worst of a bad, sad bunch: 'It's almost a Rarity', he revealed, all shock-horror, 'to find one of their Poles without a Frame of Porringers, or some other signal of their Pretension to Chyrurgick Practice' – despite such pretensions, nearly all barbers were actually 'Strangers to Chyrurgery'.[13]

A high-profile case of doctors betrayed – or perhaps basking – in public feuding blew up when George III lost his reason in 1788: 'Great Wars and Rumours of War among the medical Tribe', gasped Betsy Sheridan, shocked at the naked quarrels of the royal physicians, who could not even agree if he was mad or not, let alone whether he would recover. Called in to treat the King, the Tory mad-doctor, the Revd Dr Francis Willis, a mere provincial asylum-keeper and (rather enigmatically) a clergyman to boot, was snubbed by patrician London practitioners including the already discussed ultra-smoothie, Richard Warren, a Whig whose career prospects depended upon the appointment of the pro-Whig Prince of Wales as Prince Regent: their daily health bulletins on the mad monarch diverged completely.[14] Once in a while rivalry even came to a duel, as seen with Mead and Woodward; the nineteenth-century Scottish surgeon Granville Sharpe Pattison was notoriously trigger-happy.[15]

Such brawls threatened the hushed suspension of disbelief essential to the healing arts. So too did utter unintelligibility on the part of practitioners, which ran the risk that a bewildered patient might simply lose the plot. As with stage declamation, professional 'show talk' of course trades on the power to awe with words; yet, taken to extremes, it unleashes the suspicion that medical speech is mere mystifying jargon and pure obfuscation.

Plays themselves afforded the best medium for exposing this trick; set a thief to catch a thief: who better than the dramatist to 'out' the doctor? In Thomas Middleton's early-seventeenth-century *A Faire Quarrell*, the Colonel, wounded in a duel, lies prostrate on a couch. 'What hope is there?', inquires his distraught sister:

> SURGEON Hope, *Chillis* was scapt miraculously lady.
>
> SISTER Whats that sir.
>
> SURGEON *Cava Vena*: I care but little for his wound 'ith *orsophag*, not thus much trust mee, but when they come to *diaphragma* once, the small *intestines*, or the *Spynall medull*, or i' th rootes of the *emunctories* of the noble parts, then straight I feare a *syncope*; the flankes retyring towards the backe, the urine bloody, the exrements *purulent*, and the colour pricking or pungent.
>
> SISTER Alasse, I'm ne'er the better for this answer.[16]

The bristling defensive aggression of the profession there parodied is also captured in Fielding's *Joseph Andrews*, when Parson Adams inquires of the surgeon who has treated the hero: 'What are his wounds?' 'Why, what do you know of wounds?' he retorts testily, before unleashing a battery of sarcasm designed to humiliate the clergyman: had he travelled? practised in a hospital perhaps? studied Galen and Hippocrates? Verbally vanquished, the Parson humbly responds that he would be obliged if the surgeon would let him know 'his opinion of the patient's case'. 'Sir, his case is that of a dead man', he barks back, launching into a pompous account: 'the contusion on his head has perorated the internal membrane of the occiput, and divelicated that radical small minute invisible nerve which coheres to the pericranium.'[17] John Wilson has it said of an injured man, 'as far as I conjecture, the greatest danger ... lies in the chirurgeon's hard words.'[18]

Exchanges between unfathomable practitioners and dumbfounded auditors formed a comic stock-in-trade. In 'JACK, hove down – with a Grog Blossom Fever' (illus. 94), Rowlandson thus dramatized the backfiring of shoptalk, by presenting a stand-off between a sick sailor and his physician, each trapped within his own trade argot. A thin, old-fashioned doctor crouches by a cannon before a drunk seaman lying sick in his hammock. Each pantomimes his occupation, with his (to an outsider's ears) double-Dutch speech and his quirks of attire. The doctor sports a cocked hat, a powdered wig and spectacles. In his left hand he holds a pill box, in his right a bottle labelled 'a Sweat'; the legendary cane is tucked under his arm, and his pocket reveals a clyster and a bottle of 'Jollop', while beside him are a pestle and mortar and two cannonballs (colloquially dubbed 'pills'). 'Hold – I must stop your Grog Jack', exclaims the doctor:

> it excites those impulces, and concussions of the Thorax, which a company Sternutation by which means you are in a sort of a kind of a Situation – that your head must be Shaved – I shall take from you only – 20 ozs of Blood – then swallow this Draught and Box of Pills, and I shall administer to you a Clyster.

Clad in the mariner's regulation striped shirt and neckerchief, the tar rejoins:

> Stop my Grog. – Belay there Doctor – Shiver my timbers but your lingo bothers me – You May batter my Hull as long as you like, but I'll be d—'nd if ever you board me with your Glyster pipe.

The jargoneer thus gets a taste of his own medicine – and each party appears equally absurd.

British doctors, observed the German traveller von Archenholz, were obligingly falling over each other to sell you every conceivable medical service, many of them admittedly sounding rather sinister:

> One person informs you that his Mad-House is at your service; a second keeps a boarding-house for idiots; a good natured man-midwife pays the utmost attention to his ladies in certain situations, and promises to use the most scrupulous secrecy. Physicians offer to cure you of all manner of disorders, for a mere trifle.[19]

The market could be cut-throat; savvy practitioners learned from the secrets of the quacks, proved slick self-publicizers, and exploited such commercial breaks as came their way. An Oxford MD and author of numerous popular medical works, William Rowley was notorious for bugling his name about. 'A few days since', commenced a newspaper story,

> Mr. Hankey, a gentleman of considerable fortune in Harley-street, Cavendish Square, swallowed, by an unfortunate mistake, a tea-cup full of Goulard's extract of lead, one of the most destructive and certain poisons in nature. Mr. Hankey, it seems, sustained himself with an uncommon firmness under this alarming situation, expecting immediate death, from which, however, he has been preserved by the skilful assistance of Dr. Rowley, an eminent physician of the same street; and we have the pleasure to inform the public, Mr. Hankey is now perfectly recovered.[20]

The puff was evidently all Rowley's doing.

Common amongst complaints against doctors, not surprisingly, was

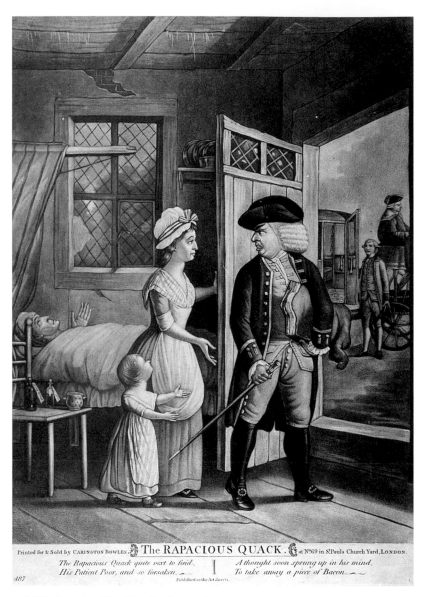

Printed for & Sold by CARINGTON BOWLES, The RAPACIOUS QUACK. at Nº69 in St. Pauls Church Yard, LONDON.

The Rapacious Quack quite vext to find,
His Patient Poor, and so forsaken; —~

A thought soon sprung up in his mind,
To take away a piece of Bacon. —~

487

Published as the Act directs.

106 'The Rapacious Quack', undated mezzotint.

A grasping practitioner demands a leg of bacon from a poor family by way of payment. This image is typical of a genre of sentimental scenes popular in the late 18th century, depicting the poor cottager's family as a hearth of simple virtue exploited by the powerful. The verse reads: 'The Rapacious Quack quite vext to find, / His Patient Poor, and so forsaken; / A thought soon sprung up in his mind, / To take away a piece of Bacon.'

their flagrant mercenariness (illus. 106). 'Paid Myster Forbes Bill', growled the Somerset parson William Holland, 'which he made as much as he could for he is a terrible man for a Bill.'[21]

214

Himself a practitioner, Bernard Mandeville versified the sneer of rapacity:

> Physicians valued Fame and Wealth
> Above the drooping Patient's Health.[22]

while physicians were cast as men on the make:

> You tell your doctor, that y'are ill
> And what does he, but write a bill

– thus Matthew Prior put the matter in a nutshell.[23]

Physicians' incomes excited envious fascination: the fortune of a Radcliffe, Mead or Astley Cooper was the talk of the town, and love of lucre won certain practitioners ignominy. When the medical courtier Richard Warren inspected his tongue in the mirror in the morning, rumour had it, he would, without a second thought, transfer a guinea from one pocket to another; and one could always identify Caleb Parry walking along the streets of Bath, the story ran, from the jingling of his purse. Slightly later, the anecdote circulated of the famous London surgeon, John Abernethy who, when on one occasion given half a guinea as his fee, got down on his knees and searched the floor, as he said, 'for the other half'.[24]

Then as now, in line with the '*primum non nocere*' of the Hippocratic oath, the sick wanted a safe and humane practitioner by the bedside; the thought of one eager to innovate or, worse still, experiment could be unsettling – a fear which was to find its fictional incarnation in characters like Dr Frankenstein, that notorious nocturnal visitor of graveyards. 'I became acquainted with the science of anatomy,' Mary Shelley has her protagonist recall, 'and a churchyard to me was merely the receptacle of bodies deprived of life [which] had become food for the worm.'[25]

Public fears of doctors who set the advancement of science before the relief of humanity were addressed by Thomas Beddoes, a man only too well aware that he was going out on a limb in commending the 'experimentalist' as the model physician, while thereby risking tarring himself with the brush of quackery, via the punning associations of 'empiricism'.[26] Recounting to his old friend Erasmus Darwin his own experiments with gases as healing agents – some are discussed below – he confessed, 'I must expect to be decried by some as a silly projector, and by others as a rapacious empiric.'[27] Reactionary opposition, as he saw it, could masquerade as 'humanitarianism'. 'The protective feeling of indignation against men supposed capable of sporting with life and suffering ... has set the public against experiments, as they are called, in physic.'[28] As the Bristol doctor knew to his cost, scientific originality, particularly anything smacking of 'speculation', had fallen under a cloud of suspicion in the hysterical atmosphere of 'alarm' shrouding Britain in the French Revolutionary era. He became a personal target of lampoons in the reactionary *Anti-Jacobin Review*, which implied that his gas experiments were intoxicatingly orgiastic.[29]

Under Beddoes's supervision, his young assistant Humphry Davy commenced experimenting with nitrous oxide in 1799. By April, he had obtained the pure gas, and decided to try inhaling it. Breathing three quarts on 16 April produced 'a fullness of the heart accompanied by loss of distinct sensation and of voluntary power, a feeling analogous to that produced in the first stage of intoxication.' On the following day he inhaled four quarts, and in half a minute the sensations of the previous day 'were succeeded by ... a highly pleasurable thrilling, particularly in the chest and extremities'.[30] Further experiments later got him high:

> By degrees as the pleasurable sensations increased, I lost all connection with external things; trains of vivid visible images rapidly passed through my mind and were connected with words in such a manner, as to produce perceptions perfectly novel. I existed in a world of newly connected and newly modified ideas. I theorised; I imagined that I made discoveries ... I exclaimed to Dr Kinglake, '*Nothing exists but thoughts! – the universe is composed of impressions, ideas, pleasures and pains!*'[31]

The experiments created quite a stir. On 5 June Robert Southey wrote to an old friend that the 'wonder-working gas ... induces almost a delirium of pleasurable sensations without any subsequent dejection'. And next month the poet – not yet the notorious reactionary – rhapsodized to his brother:

> Oh, Tom! such a gas has Davy discovered, the gaseous oxyd. Oh, Tom! I have had some; it made me laugh and tingle in every toe and finger-tip. Davy has actually invented a new pleasure, for which language has no name ... Tom, I am sure the air in heaven must be this wonder-working gas of delight![32]

All this gaseous enthusiasm was naturally easily parodied as hot air,[33] especially once Davy moved up from Bristol to fashionable London to take up a post at the newly founded Royal Institution in Albemarle Street. In 'Scientific Researches!' (1802) (illus. 95) Gillray satirized such experiments. The scene is the Institution, its lecture-bench littered with air pumps and pneumatic devices. The chemistry lecturer Dr Garnett is illustrating his talk by experimenting upon Sir James Hippisley, whose breeches are burst asunder by a fiery explosion. Next to the lecturer stands Davy, holding the bellows, and before him are an air pump containing a frog, two vessels marked 'Hydrogen' and 'Oxygen', a windmill, a pig's bladder, and an electrostatic machine. Farts of all kinds, as we shall see in the next chapter, had become a stock-in-trade of the political cartoon.[34]

Variolation was another innovation which attracted public suspicion, and Jennerian anti-smallpox vaccination could particularly be represented as perilous, because it threatened the boundary between animals and humans (illus. 96). Those who have just undergone the procedure are displaying signs of grotesque bovine tumours instantaneously issuing from diverse parts of their bodies, presumably aided by the rapid-acting 'Opening Mixture'. A pregnant woman – echoes of Mary Toft! – is already delivering a midget cow from beneath her skirt. Hands raised in horror, her husband is sprouting horns: his cuckolding has evidently resulted (in the time-honoured 'imaginist' way, discussed in Chapter 2) in this monstrous delivery. A painting on the wall represents worshippers abasing themselves before an altar upon which a cow is perched, referring to the biblical story of Aaron making a Golden Calf for the Israelites to idolize – another topos much exploited in political cartoons.[35] As so often, the print encodes an anti-idolatrous, iconoclastic message. If nowadays Jenner is set on a pedestal as one of medicine's great heroes, such was not always his reputation. Byron, for instance, thought nothing of lumping him together with the shameless Elisha Perkins:

> What varied wonders tempt us as they pass!
> The Cow-pox, Tractors, Galvanism, Gas
> In turns appear to make the vulgar stare,
> In the swoll'n bubble bursts – and all is air.[36]

Another late-eighteenth-century development, medico-electrical experimentation, further inflamed fears that doctors were violating taboos and arrogating to themselves a power over life which was God's alone. Especially in cases of insanity, violent shock treatments were being tested. 'On a supposition that the obstruction of the bile might be owing to paralysis or torpid action of the common bile-duct', Beddoes's friend Erasmus Darwin wrote of his approach to one of his patients, 'and the stimulants taken into the stomach seeming to have no effect, I directed half a score smart electric shocks from a coated bottle, which held about a quart, to be passed through the liver.'[37] Such forays signal a new Promethean aspiration that artificial means could revitalize the failing body – paralleling the new faith in artificial respiration promoted by the Royal Humane Society.[38]

In this connexion Galvani's celebrated experiments proved particularly 'galvanizing'. In *De Viribus Electricitatis in Motu Musculari* [On Electrical Powers in the Movement of Muscles], published in 1792, that Italian naturalist described experiments in which the legs of dead frogs were suspended by copper wire from an iron balcony; as the feet touched the iron uprights, the legs twitched. These sensational experiments – life seemingly being restored to the dead – were followed up by his younger contemporary, the Pavian professor Alessandro Volta, whose *Letters on Animal Electricity* appeared in the same year. Volta showed that a muscle could be thrown into continuous contraction by successive electric stimulations. The connexions between electricity and the stuff of life implied by such researches proved highly charged, to say nothing of the apparent blasphemy involved in the possibility of 'resurrection'.

And they came to experimental fruition on humans in London on 17 January 1803, when Giovanni Aldini applied galvanic electricity to the corpse of the murderer Thomas Forster, whose newly hanged body had been rescued from Newgate and rushed to Wilson's anatomical theatre. When wires attached to a galvanic pile composed of 240 plates of zinc and copper were hooked up to the criminal's mouth and ear, 'the jaw began to quiver', it was reported, 'the adjoining muscles were horribly contorted, and the left eye actually opened'. Applied to the ear and rectum, the wires 'excited in the muscles contractions much stronger ... as almost to give an appearance of re-animation'.[39] Such experiments encouraged literary and artistic fantasies in both the comic and the Gothic terror mode, most luridly in *Frankenstein* (1818).

It 'proved a wet, ungenial summer, and incessant rain often confined us for days to the house', Mary Shelley recalled of the months she spent in the Genevan countryside in 1816 with her lover, Percy Bysshe Shelley; her step-sister, Claire Clairmont; Claire's lover, Lord Byron; and Byron's physician, John Polidori. Trapped indoors by downpours, the group got high on German ghost stories. 'These tales excited in us a playful desire of imitation. Two other friends (a tale from the pen of one of whom would be far more acceptable to the public than any thing I can ever hope to produce) and myself agreed to write each a story, founded on some super-natural occurrence.' Shelley and Byron readily came up with their yarns; the eighteen-year-old Mary Godwin, as she then was, found composing harder. But talk of the electrical experiments of Darwin and others led to scary speculations that 'the component parts of a creature might be manufactured, brought together and endued with vital warmth'. With such thoughts racing through her mind she went to bed, but 'when I placed my head on my pillow, I did not sleep, nor could I be said to think. My imagination, unbidden, possessed and guided me, gifting the successive images that arose in my mind with a vividness far beyond the usual bounds of reverie.' There she lay, casting around for a tale 'which would speak to the mysterious fears of our nature, and awaken thrilling horror ... one to ... curdle the blood, and quicken the beatings of the heart':

> I saw – with shut eyes, but acute mental vision – I saw the pale student of unhallowed arts kneeling beside the thing he had put together. I saw the hideous phantasm of a man stretched out, and then, on the working of some powerful engine, show signs of life, and stir with an uneasy, half-vital motion ... he would rush away from his odious handy-work, horror-stricken. He would hope that, left to itself, the slight spark of life which he had communicated would fade; that this thing, which had received such imperfect animation, would subside into dead matter; and he might sleep in the belief that the silence of the grave would quench for ever the transient exis-tence of the hideous corpse which he had looked upon as the cradle of life. He sleeps; but he is awakened ... behold the horrid thing stands at his bedside, opening his curtains, and looking on him with yellow, watery, but speculative eyes.[40]

Thus, via the spark of life, the birth of what Mary called her 'hideous progeny': *Frankenstein*. Thereafter the very name became a shorthand for medico-scientific inordinacy of every kind – if also, ironically, yet one more proof of the riot of the female imagination.

Public disquiet also mounted against the practice of dissection, partly in view of the sordid and illegal involvement of anatomists with 'resur-rection men'. The frequently staged 'Tyburn riot' against the surgeons shows the deep and fierce resistance of common people to having their deceased comrades carted off to Surgeons' Hall and subjected to the profanations of the dissectors – a revulsion caught by Hogarth in the final engraving of his *Four Stages of Cruelty* series (Chapter 2): was not medical dissection but brutality writ large and given an official blessing?[41]

Quality cadavers were much less likely to meet such a fate – they seldom dug up the rich, resurrectionists explained to a Parliamentary committee, 'because they were buried so deep'. Yet that didn't stop scare stories about the illegal procurement of bodies and grave robbing. 'A man going to take up a load of dung in St George's fields', reported the *Gentleman's Magazine*, 'found at the dunghill the bodies of a woman and eight children, cut and mangled in a shocking manner, the handywork, probably, of some young anatomist, who deserves a rigorous punishment for this carelessness and indiscretion.'[42]

By way of solution, a correspondent proposed that, if doctors truly needed to carry out dissections, why should not physicians' and surgeons' corpses be the ones laid open to the knife:

> Since ... these gentlemen think cutting, slashing and scraping, a matter of such indifference, I would humbly propose a method whereby they may be very amply supplied with opportunities of improving anatomical knowledge.
>
> First, That Surgeons' Hall should be the public academy or school for the whole faculty of this great metropolis.
>
> Secondly, That all physicians, men and women midwives (for I would not exclude any old woman of the faculty,) surgeons, apothecaries, quacks, tooth-drawers, their pupils, journeymen, apprentices and labourers, shall, as soon as they are dead, be carried to the said hall, and there dissected.
>
> [signed] L.R.

Southey's 'The Surgeon's Warning' (1796) was to afford an oblique comment on that suggestion:

> All kinds of carcases I have cut up,
> And now my turn will be;
> But, brothers, I took care of you,
> So pray take care of me ...
>
> And my Prentices now will surely come
> And carve me bone from bone,
> And I who have rifled the dead man's grave
> Shall never have rest in my own.
>
> Bury me in lead when I am dead,
> My brethren, I entreat,
> And see the coffin weigh'd, I beg,
> Lest the plumber should be a cheat.[43]

Grave robbing perfectly lent itself to shock-horror exposés in the Gothic mode. One typical print shows a nightwatchman disturbing a bodysnatcher who has dropped the stolen corpse he had been carrying in a hamper, while the anatomist William Hunter runs away (illus. 107).[44] Violation, menace and revenge join in a single ambiguous image.

The 'death and the doctors' trope was repeated by pen and paint as the unseemly intimacy between the 'sack-'em-up' men and anatomy

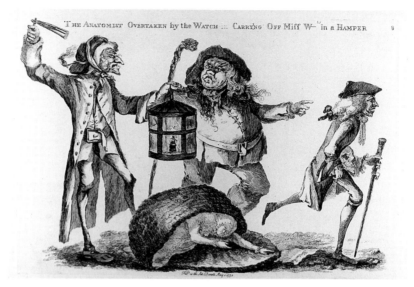

107 William Austin, 'THE ANATOMIST OVERTAKEN by the WATCH IN CARRYING OFF Miss W—
ts in a HAMPER', 1773, etching with engraving.

    A sheet of paper which has fallen to the ground bears the words 'Hunters Lectu[res]'. The
rise of private anatomy schools in 18th-century London saw an increase in the demand for
cadavers for dissection. This in turn led to the employ of Resurrectionists, bodysnatchers who
would steal corpses for use in the new schools. Carrying a large lantern, the nightwatchman has
grabbed the bodysnatcher by the shoulder and is sounding his alarm rattle. A female corpse in
its burial shroud tumbles out of the hamper. The bodysnatcher tries to pass on the blame by
pointing to the fleeing anatomist William Hunter, who is carrying a skull.

school proprietors became hot news: the surgeon Bransby Cooper
admitted that 'resurrection men' could be seen 'flitting about' dissecting rooms, 'complacently bowing to the lecturers'. Such revelations
provoked Thomas Hood's 'Mary's Ghost, a Pathetic Ballad'. Her
grave rifled and her remains dealt out amongst the anatomists, poor
Mary's ghost addresses her fiancé:

> I vowed that you should have my hand,
>   But Fate gives us denial;
> You'll find it there at Mr Bell's
>   In spirits in a phial.
>
> I can't tell where my head has gone,
>   But Dr Carpue can;
> As for my trunk it's all packed up
>   To go by Pickford's van.
>
> The cock it crows, I must be gone,
>   My William we must part;
> And I'll be yours in death although
>   Sir Astley has my heart.[45]

The Anatomy Act of 1832 put an end for sure to the threat of grave robbing and murder Burke-and-Hare style. But it made working people at large feel all the more vulnerable to their possible fate, were they to die in the workhouse or a charity hospital.[46]

Whilst medicine had been, time out of mind, inescapably associated in the public imagination with carnal knowledge, from the Restoration the sexual equivocation of medical practice became highlighted and problematized. Erotic prints and poems exploited 'medicine' as a double entendre, cover or euphemism for sexual opportunism. The parallels between medicine and lechery became staples of bawdy, as, for instance, in John Ellis's *The Surprize*. A maid awaits an apothecary who is coming to administer an enema. Instead, an admirer steals into her chamber and takes upon himself 'the apothecary's duty':

> Up stairs Timante gently came
> (One well acquainted with the Dame)
> And finding all the passage free
> While none perceiv'd him, in bolts he ...

> He spy'd an Engine on a Chair,
> Which he, good Man, with harmless Mind
> Took up, and guess'd the Use design'd,
> Resolv'd The Task himself would dare he
> And so he did, and play'd the Part.[47]

Certain medical trends heightened perceptions of sexual risk, notably the mesmerism craze at the close of the eighteenth century, which threatened the collapse of normal body distance. Critics grew apoplectic about hypnotic 'suggestion', hinting at the slippery slope from 'touching' to 'touching up', and the ambivalence of the mesmeric art of 'making passes'. The anonymous *A Letter to a Physician in the Country on Animal Magnetism* (1786) thus reported the author's experiences of healing at the hands of a mesmerist's assistant, a 'singularly gifted damsel', who was said to have

> supported herself by leaning on me with one hand, while she employed the other in feeling, and wandering lightly, with no unpleasant friction, over the region of the thorax: occasionally straying down the sternum, towards the ensiform-cartilage, and short ribs; and then at times insensibly creeping along the abdomen, in a direction to the os-pubis; which, as my sensations of every kind are naturally rather acute, produced nearly the complicated, and semi-painful effect of tickling. Not willing, however, to interrupt her interesting researches, I bore her tantalizing touches with determined resignation.

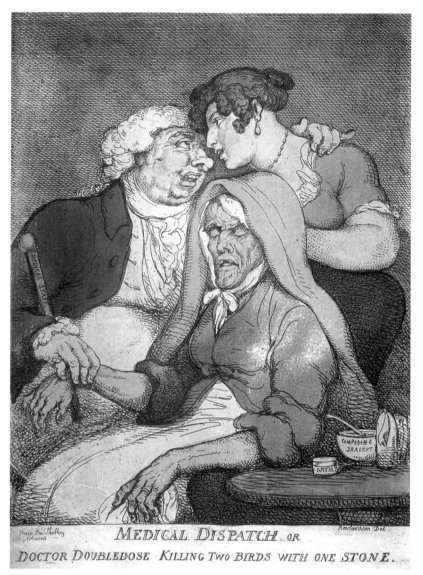

MEDICAL DISPATCH.OR
DOCTOR DOUBLEDOSE KILLING TWO BIRDS WITH ONE STONE.

108 Thomas Rowlandson, 'MEDICAL DESPATCH OR DOCTOR DOUBLEDOSE KILLING TWO BIRDS WITH ONE STONE.', 1810, etching with watercolour.

Who could resist the 'meltings', intuitive 'vibrations', 'fatal fascinations' and 'ecstatic deliriums' of the 'crisis'?[48]

Doctors and their assistants thus represented threats to one's body, not just through therapeutic violence (as explored in Chapter 4) but sexually too. Scores of sketches and playlets feature the physician as lecher and clinical consultations as erotic skirmishes. Rowlandson's doctors gawp, grope and clyster their patients in a most un-Hippocratic

223

manner. In his 'MEDICAL DISPATCH OR DOCTOR DOUBLEDOSE KILL-
ING TWO BIRDS WITH ONE STONE' (illus. 108), with one hand the
physician takes the pulse of his ghastly old patient seated in the chair,
while, behind her back, his arm is thrown around the neck of the
blooming maiden (is she maid or daughter?) into whose eyes he gazes,
his podgy features expressing adoration. The crone's impending end is
made still more certain by the opium and composing draughts placed
ready to hand. The buxom girl hovers between rapture and grief, tears
for the departing and admiration for the attention of the practitioner.
Sex and medicine thus dissolve in a masquerade; physical examination
becomes a motif for fornication, and the practitioner's tackle – his
cane, enemas, lancets, squirts and clyster-pipes – assumes an erotic
air, sometimes bawdily comic. As in *Tristram Shandy*, lewd double
entendres proliferate – though occasionally as doctors gaze upon and
inject the contents of syringes into patients' private parts, the porno-
graphy is overt and nothing is left to the imagination.

Grub-Street revelations exposed doctors abetting sexually shady
practices, notably illicit abortions and undercover childbirths.[49] When
the Duchess of Grafton became pregnant by her lover Lord Ossory,
she made clandestine advances to William Hunter, who had earlier
acted as her obstetrician, to secure his services: no names were
mentioned, but Hunter deduced her identity. He was sworn to the
strictest secrecy. As her term came on, the duchess retired to Combe in
Surrey. Going into labour, she summoned him. He arrived shortly
after the baby was born and confirmed its and the mother's good
health. His duty was then to take the baby back with him, without
arousing suspicions, to his London house, where he had fixed up a suitable wet nurse. Hunter had agreed to take responsibility for the infant's
health and for ensuring that the wet nurse received regular payment.
All this came out at her sensational London divorce trial and in the
lurid pamphlets that followed.

Hunter performed similar undercover services for Lady Boling-
broke, when she became pregnant by Topham Beauclerk (the surgeon
had earlier delivered her legitimate children). Once again, cloak-and-
dagger operations were involved. 'Every means were made use of', he
put it at her subsequent divorce trial, 'to keep her being brought to bed
a secret.' All his visits were under cover of darkness, and he

> always went on foot though it rained, that his own servants might not
> know he was going there; and the said Lady Bolingbroke, still to preserve
> the secret, told the deponent, that when he wrote, or she should
> write to him upon her illness, that they should make use of a feigned
> name in such letters, lest any of them should by accident be lost.

Hunter visited her several times during her pregnancy, was present to deliver her child, and sent her medicines. Medicine thus turned into high melodrama, as was revealed in the divorce-trial publications, which proved riveting reading.[50]

Amongst the recognized branches of the healing profession was the authorized midwife, whose practice required a bishop's licence, attesting her good character. Unblemished morals and religious orthodoxy rather than medical skill were the criteria of fitness to attend births, because midwives so easily fell under suspicion of colluding in illegitimacy, abortion and infanticide (illus. 97).[51]

The male accoucheurs or obstetricians who challenged and supplanted them in eighteenth-century polite society blackened the traditional 'granny midwife' as ignorant and inept. Midwives fought back. In *A Treatise on the Art of Midwifery* (1760), a diatribe against male practice, Elizabeth Nihell held her art was a gift exclusive to women: certain employments were properly exclusive to the sex.[52]

The rise of the man–midwife thus created tensions.[53] In *The Parish Register* (1807), George Crabbe, that practitioner turned parson and poet, related the battle between the old village midwife and the new Doctor Glibb, accentuating the polarity between female and male, nature and science, rural and urban. The egregious Glibb demeaned the midwife by associating her with foolish old Dame Nature:

> And what is Nature? One who acts in aid
> Of gossips half asleep and half afraid;
> With such allies I scorn my fame to blend,
> Skill is my luck and courage is my friend:
> No slave to Nature, 'tis my chief delight
> To win my way and act in her despite ... [54]

The accoucheur in his turn became a satirical target. Books and pamphlets, not just by midwives but above all by male critics, thundered against man-midwifery, casting it as little better than a front for adulterous wives and lubricious operators, and, in particular, an outrageous usurpation of the rights of husbands. Frank Nicholls' anonymous *The Petition of the Unborn Babes to the Censors of the Royal College of Physicians* depicted a kind of Hogarthian Man-midwives' Progress. Accoucheurs, he complained, are allowed 'to treat our wives in such a manner, as frequently ends in their destruction, and to have such intercourse with our women, as easily shifts itself into indecency, from indecency into obscenity, and from obscenity into debauchery'.[55]

The gravest offence, according to Philip Thicknesse's *Man-Midwifery Analysed* (1764), was the digital manipulation of women's private parts, which such influential operators as William Smellie had urged as integral to their 'superior' techniques of diagnosis and delivery.[56] For Thicknesse, merely to quote such authors was enough to condemn them. How could indecencies such as this be justified?

> Dr Smellie in his 'Treatise on Midwifery', page 91, speaking of the parts of generation in women, observes that 'The Clitoris, with its Praeputium, is found between the Labia on the middle and fore part of the Pubis; and from the lower part of the Clitoris, the Nymphae rising, spreads outwards and downwards to the sides of the Os Externum, forming a kind of Sulcus or furrow, called the Fossa magna, or Navicularis, for the direction of the Penis in coition, or of the Finger in touching, into the Vagina'.[57]

Was Smellie suggesting, snarled Thicknesse, that female anatomy had been divinely designed precisely to suit the convenience of the man-midwife's finger? Women, he insisted, had been performing deliveries successfully ever since antiquity, and 'little did the poor Egyptian ladies think, that it would be three thousand years, before Doctor Smellie would be born, and the art of touching be brought to perfection'.[58] What needed doing could perfectly well be done by women. So why resort to light-fingered male operators? Obviously something sinister was afoot, indeed the whole business was a smokescreen, hiding the designs both of these 'touching gentry' and of lascivious ladies. How could it fail to inflame the passions? – 'if men-midwives under these circumstances stand unmoved, they are part of the human species I am stranger to!'[59]

Similar views unfold in other works fulminating against obstetricians. *The Man Midwife Unmasqu'd* (1738) versifies what was purportedly a true case, in which a pregnant woman applied to a man-midwife for an examination:

> She wanted some money
> 'Tis true, and some ...,
> She fail'd of the first,
> But the latter had Luck in.[60]

She offered him temptation. He fell for it, telling her:

> ... I'll do what I can,
> And may venture to say, you will find me a Man;
> A Man both of Judgement and Skill I do mean,
> By Judgement and Skill my Credit maintain;
> But then in each Point you must follow Direction,
> And as your Case lies, must admit of Inspection.
> To give Demonstration that he did respect Her,
> He kneel'd down before her, and then did Inspect Her.[61]

Post coitum, however, she played the wronged innocent, demanded money and, when he refused, brought the doctor to court on a rape charge.

The culmination of the confusion and controversy surrounding the obstetrician's challenge lay in his being stigmatized as a herm-aphroditic freak, half-man, half-woman. That was an image used as a frontispiece for Samuel Fores's *Man-Midwifery Dissected; or, The Obstetric Family Instructor. For the Use of Both Sexes. Containing a Display of the Management of every Class of labour by Men and Boy Mid-Wives; also of their Cunning, Indecent and Cruel Practices. Instructions to Husbands how to Counteract them. A Plan for the Complete Instruction of Women who Possess Promising Talents, in Order to Supersede Male-practice. Various Arguments and Quotations, Proving, that Man-midwifery is a Personal, Domestic and a National Evil.* Fores distrusted accoucheurs as fiercely as he distrusted women (illus. 98). Divided vertically into two halves, the print contrasts the practice of the homely midwife – significantly on the right side – with the man-midwife on the left (sinister). The former works with her hand, which grasps a pap vessel or feeding cup. In stark contrast, the left half portrays the male with all his suspicious accoutrements – horrific instruments such as described by Smellie – and medicaments, plus love potions and philtres on a shelf marked for the practitioner's 'own use', thereby casting aspersions upon his intentions.[62]

Fores and Cruickshank shrewdly played upon the 'mid' in midwife, insinuating that a man-midwife was a hermaphrodite, a contradiction in terms, an unseemly, abnormal mixture of incompatible elements, in short, yet another monster, this time conceived by the evil imagination of the medical profession.[63] Sexual innuendos and accusations thus turned medicine into a scandalous travesty at the crossroads between fear and farce, and a subset of the newly emergent genre of the porno-graphic.[64]

All the topics aired in this chapter caused alarm, especially when presented or sensationalized by the press and in prints. It should hence come as no surprise that the latter part of the eighteenth century brought, by way of a defensive professional rejoinder, the emergence of formal bodies of medical ethics, notably John Gregory's *Lectures on the Duties and Qualifications of a Physician* (1772) and Thomas Percival's *Medical Ethics* (1803) – the profession answering back, developing its own public relations, or getting its act together.[65] For the public the key question was that of medical trustworthiness – indeed, specifically of medical honesty. 'I deny the lawfulness of telling a lie to a sick man for

fear of alarming him,' insisted Samuel Johnson, ever the Christian
rigorist:

> You have no business with consequences: you are to tell the truth.
> Besides, you are not sure what effect your telling him that he is in
> danger may have. It may bring his distemper to a crisis, and that may
> cure him. Of all lying I have the greatest abhorrence of this, because
> I believe it has been frequently practised on myself.[66]

Johnson's stringency was largely upheld in Thomas Gisborne's *An
Enquiry into the Duties of Men in the Higher and Middle Classes of Society
in Great Britain* (1794), which contained a substantial section on the
duties of doctors. Significantly, however, this was the work of an
Evangelical clergyman not a physician.[67] How did the practitioners
respond?

The Manchester physician Thomas Percival's *Medical Ethics* was
rather more equivocal on that issue. Stiff-necked and rigid candour,
deemed Percival, was not required of the physician who, for optimum
therapeutic results, must adapt himself to the world. The doctor must
not lie but could, for therapeutic benefit, in the case of the seriously
sick, be slightly economical of the truth: 'a physician', he advised,
aware of the power of the tongue and its placebo effect, 'should not be
forward to make gloomy prognostications', but rather 'should be the
minister of hope and comfort to the sick' for 'by such cordials to the
drooping spirit, he may ... revive expiring life.' What was crucial was
that the physician should assume that air of honesty and candour
which would inspire in the patient 'gratitude, respect and confidence'.
At bottom the good doctor remained he who put on the finest show and
best acted the part.[68]

9 The Medical Politician and the Body Politic

Previous chapters have been exploring the role of visual images, as well as sayings and stories, plays and proverbs, in the production of meanings about disease, death and the doctors. Such lore provided guides to life in centuries when health was ever at hazard and control over one's destiny tenuous.

Precisely like sickness and the practice of medicine, politics too generated polysemic verbal and visual idioms steeped in ambivalence and irony. Especially in societies overshadowed by censorship, discussion and, above all, criticism of princes and power involves acts of transgression: breaking customs and the law, asserting or insinuating the unspeakable. Under such circumstances pictures may say more than is permitted in words. When the medical and the political concatenate, the subversive potential of the message is reinforced. The verbal and visual language of the body politicized and of politics medicalized forms the subject of what follows.

Through metaphor, language itself, we have seen in Chapter 2, fleshes out our compelling need to figure the world through the body and the body through the world. In the political arena, centuries of habitual allusion to Members of Parliament and parliamentary motions, factional purges (like 'Pride's Purge', leaving behind the 'Rump'), and, above all, talk of the 'Constitution', have left us deaf and blind to the omnipresent figurative political topography incorporated in such phrases.[1]

Conscripting the human frame to emblematize, legitimize or criticize the *status quo* has ever been a favourite device. 'The state [*res publica*] is a body [*corpus quoddam*]', pronounced John of Salisbury back in the twelfth century, setting out the monarch's place:

> Within that state, the prince occupies the place of the head ... The senate occupies the place of the heart, which gives good and bad deeds their impulses. The function of the eyes, the ears and the tongue is assured by the judges and the provincial governors. The

'officers' and 'soldiers' can be compared to the hands. The prince's regular assistants are the flanks ... The feet that always touch the soil are the peasants.[2]

In that medieval account of the body politic, the monarch was figured and legitimated in politico-anatomical terms as the 'head' of state. That was a bodily correlation which was capital but not unchallengeable: after all, for Aristotle and his followers the *heart* not the head was not only the prime mover of all vital processes but the seat of intelligence besides. Drawing upon Aristotelian concepts, it was that organ, insisted Thomas Vicary, which was 'the principal of all other members and the beginning of life'; reversing the metaphorical arrow, that Elizabethan surgeon drew upon the political order to explicate the physiological:

> he [the heart] is set in the middest of the brest seuerally by him selfe, as Lord and King of al members. And as a Lorde or King ought to be serued of his subiectes that haue their liuing of him, So are al other members of the body subiectes to the Hart, for they receyue their liuing of him, and they doo seruice many wayes vnto him agayne.[3]

Such a view of the supremacy of the heart was further endorsed under James I by the anatomist of melancholy Robert Burton:

> Of the noble [organs] there be three principal parts, to which all three belong, and whom they serve, *brain, heart, liver*; according to whose site, three regions, on a threefold division, is made of the whole body. As first of the *head*, in which the animal organs are contained, and brain itself, which by his nerves give sense and motion to the rest, and is (as it were) a Privy Counsellor, and Chancellor, to the *Heart*.[4]

Vicary's and Burton's model of the heart as sovereign was unsurprisingly reiterated by William Harvey, who was not merely the elucidator of the circulation of the blood but a staunch royalist to boot. 'The heart of animals is the foundation of their life', maintained his *De Motu Cordis* (1628), tellingly dedicated to that upholder of divine right monarchy, Charles I:

> the sun of their microcosm, that on which all growth depends, from which all strength and vigour flow. In like manner, the King is the foundation of his kingdom, the sun of his microcosm, the heart of his commonwealth, from whom all power and all mercy proceeds.[5]

Reading the body in such staunchly royalist and absolutist terms lost favour and credibility post-1688 in the more critical and constitutionalist climate of the Enlightenment.[6] When Adam Smith in due

course re-invoked the body metaphor, it was significantly not to conse-
crate the king but to ratify the free-market economics advanced in his
An Inquiry into the Nature and Causes of the Wealth of Nations (1776)
against the more the centralist, *dirigiste* mercantilist models favoured
in France by the Physiocrats. 'Some speculative physicians seem to
have imagined that the health of the human body could be preserved
only by a certain precise regimen of diet and exercise', observed the
Glasgow professor,

> of which every, the smallest, violation necessarily occasioned some
> degree of disease or disorder proportioned to the degree of viola-
> tion. Experience, however, would seem to show that the human body
> frequently preserves, to all appearance at least, the most perfect state
> of health under a vast variety of different regiments; even under
> some which are generally believed to be very far from being perfectly
> wholesome. But the healthful state of the human body, it would
> seem, contains in itself some unknown principle of preservation,
> capable either of preventing or of correcting, in many respects, the
> bad effects even of a very faulty regimen.[7]

In other words, so ran Smith's counter-contention, just as, according
to best bio-medical thinking, the physiological economy of the human
body would, on balance, maintain its own natural state of health if
spared the bombardment of stimulants and purgatives all too often
prescribed by physicians, the market too was, in the long run, self-
adjusting and worked best if left to its own homoeostatic processes –
the economic analogue of the 'healing power of nature'. Smith took
pleasure in pointing out to his French counterpart the follies of
medical meddlesomeness:

> Mr. Quesnai, who was himself a physician, and a very speculative
> physician, seems to have entertained a notion ... concerning the
> political body ... that it would thrive and prosper only under a certain
> precise regimen, the exact regimen of perfect liberty and perfect
> justice. He seems not to have considered that in the political body,
> the natural effort which every man is continually making to better
> his own condition, is a principle of preservation capable of prevent-
> ing and correcting, in many respect, the bad effects of a political
> oeconomy, in some degree, both partial and oppressive.[8]

The body has thus been endlessly drafted over the centuries to
teach politics. Not surprisingly, it has also provided a versatile
armoury of weapons for political satire.[9] This has been facilitated by
the conventions of art itself – before the twentieth-century plunge into
Abstraction, art drew instinctively the charged idioms of the human
form[10] – but it is one also consequent upon habits of mind and figures

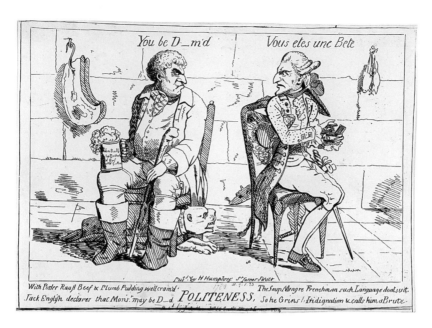

Within the image: "You be D—m'd" / "Vous etes une Bete" / "POLITENESS" / "With Porter Roast Beef & Plumb Pudding well cram'd / Jack English declares that Monsr. may be D—d / The Soup Meagre Frenchman such Language dont suit, / So he Grins Indignation & calls him a Brute."

109 James Gillray(?), 'Politeness', engraving, 1779(?). British Museum, London.

The verses read: 'With Porter Roast Beef & Plumb Pudding well cramm'd / Jack English declares that Monsr. may be D—d / The Soup Meagre Frenchman such Language dont suit / So he Grins Indignation & calls him a Brute.'

of speech.[11] Through synecdoche and metonymy, the human body readily speaks for the subject or citizen, the nation, and humanity itself: if a cartoonist wants to exemplify war between Britain and France (illus. 109), how easy to boil the idea down into contrasting physiques – the fat John Bull figure squaring up against the starveling Frenchie![12] Through rather more inventive cartographical cartoon wizardry, Britain easily turns into a person, the map of the realm doubling as a portrait of George III, literally identified with the nation (illus. 110) – and Portsmouth the anus of England.[13]

As our earlier invocation of Bakhtin would suggest, the legible body can be seen as a double agent in the conventions of the political cartoon. It may be the innocent target of medico-political brutality; contrariwise, it may serve as an explosive organ expressive of retaliatory hatred and contempt – hence the power of the fart in grotesque prints and low humour generally, and many other 'kiss my arse' tropes.[14]

Political prints drew upon artistic repertoires which were practically immemorial. As touched upon in Chapter 2, caricature juxtaposes and conflates the human and the monstrous, man and beast – even man and fruit, as demonstrated by that celebrated descent of

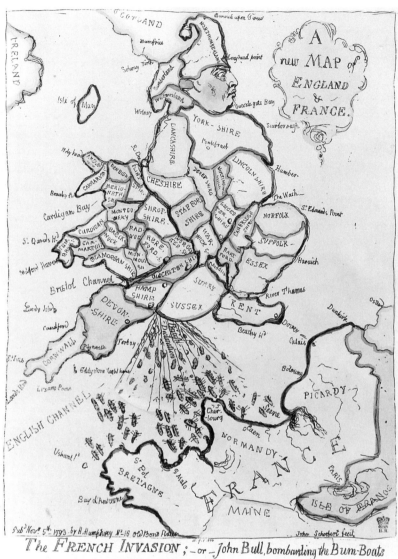

110 James Gillray after John Schoebert, 'A New Map of England & France', 1793, coloured engraving. British Museum, London.

The caption to the map of Britain (which is also a scatological portrait of George III) reads 'The French Invasion; —or— John Bull, bombarding the Bum-Boats'.

Louis Philippe into a pear revealed by Philipon, founder of Paris' *Le Charivari*. In such conventions incongruities of size, scale, and hence power, are meat and drink to the caricaturist as well as the satirical writer: small wonder that Hogarth illustrated *Gulliver's Travels*.

Hogarth, however, played a somewhat equivocal role in the development of the political cartoon, for he cast himself not as a caricaturist but as the engraver of 'moral subjects'. Supreme as a moral commentator, he seldom dabbled overtly in party politics or in Westminster personalities and, when he did, it was mainly to settle personal scores, as in his vendetta against the maverick radical libertarian, John Wilkes.[15]

The establishing of political caricature in England owed less to Hogarth than to George Townshend, later first Marquess Townshend, whom Horace Walpole credited with being the first to apply portrait caricature to politics using a free and relaxed style. Thomas Rowlandson and James Gillray learnt from both, Rowlandson commenting on human foibles with zesty good humour, while the savage, and probably finally demented, Gillray concentrated on high-political satire, blending symbolism with portrait caricature and supplementing both with elaborate bubble captions and legends.

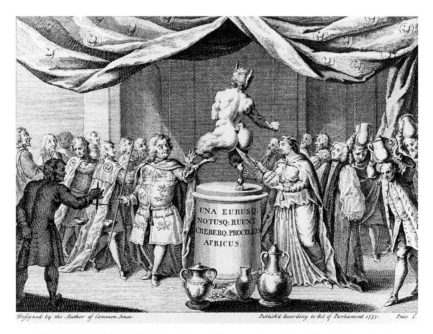

Defigned by the Author of Common Sense.   *Publish'd according to Act of Parliament 1737.*   *Price 1.*

111 'The Festival of the Golden Rump', 1737, line engraving with etching 'designed by the author of Common Sense'.
   A satyr on a pedestal kicks out at a magician while a priestess attempts to insert a clyster-pipe. The print depicts a play called 'The Golden Rump', satirizing King George II, Queen Caroline and Prime Minister Sir Robert Walpole. The priestess (Queen Caroline) injects 'Aurum potabile' (drinkable gold) into her royal husband with a clyster. Behind her is the lame Benjamin Hoadly, Bishop of Winchester and prominent supporter of the Crown (another contemporary Benjamin Hoadly was a comic playwright); balancing scales on the left is Walpole, 'the Balance-Master of Europe'. Attendants bearing urns deposit them at the feet of the idol; the room is filled by peers bearing the 'Golden Rump' emblem, which also embellishes the canopy.

Fervently patriotic in the French Revolutionary and Napoleonic era, and devastating in his grotesques of subhuman *sans culottes* and 'Little Boney' – yet further anatomical double entendres – Gillray was contemptuous of party infighting at home, lashing Pittites and Foxites alike, while conjuring up shocking images of the moronic mob.[16]

A punchy cartoon-idiom thus emerged. Though initially hiero-glyphic, arcane and abstract, perhaps so as to outflank prosecution, political prints grew barbed and biting, rendered into a body language that revelled in coarseness and indecency. In offensively scatological mode, for instance, cartoonists expressed the slanderous Swiftian 'deflating' humour of 'Magna Farta'. Ever-popular, the fart proved adaptable, for instance to the ballooning era as in images of 'Inflatable Hot Air', with politicians rising up into the sky. Use of the epithet 'Broad Bottoms' as a label for broad-based political coalitions proved an irresistible invitation to visual punning, especially with a view to conveying the notion that the one thing 'Broad Bottom' politicians could always be relied upon to do was to shit upon the nation.[17]

Somewhat more arcane and far more scandalous was the iconogra-phy of the royal Rump (illus. 111), a savage travesty of the court cere-monials of His Highness – or rather His Backside – George II. The rebus of the rump served as a favourite opposition icon under the second Hanoverian, the Rump-Steak Club being formed by peers who had the royal backside turned upon them at Court. Waving a wand of office, Walpole may be seen presiding over the ritual, while Queen Caroline, here a priestess, shoves an enema up her bilious husband.

In an era in which politics endlessly turned into public theatre,[18] the backside formed one of the great symbols of politics, and brown-nosing became a hot issue as Walpole consolidated his regime, as in 'Idol-Worship or The Way to Preferment' (1740) (illus. 112) which contained a double assault. Its picture showed one could get on only by kissing the prime ministerial arse, while its caption blamed it all on George II. But if Walpole's butt symbolized filthy lucre and dirty power, the Prime Minister was himself also maliciously portrayed as on the receiving end of an 'up yours' in another print in which Cardinal Fleury of France was shown administering a humiliating clyster from the rear, while Walpole's illegitimate daughter Lady Churchill incestu-ously fondled her father's privy purse.

Bums remained formidable and outrageous totems of power – standing either for the obscene might of ministers or as instruments of impudent protest.[19] An American cartoon of 1775, *The Congress of the Necessary Politicians*, features two men easing themselves in a public privy. One is tearing up the resolutions of Congress for bumf, while the

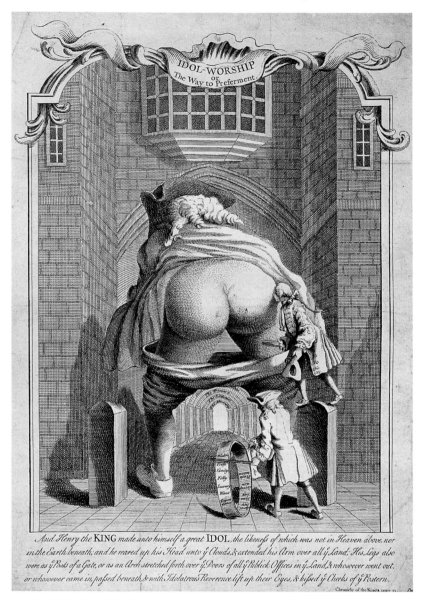

And Henry the KING made unto himself a great IDOL, the likeness of which was not in Heaven above, nor in the Earth beneath; and he reared up his Head unto ỹ Clouds, & extended his Arm over all ỹ Land; His Legs also were as ỹ Posts of a Gate, or as an Arch stretched forth over ỹ Doors of all ỹ Publick Offices in ỹ Land, & whosoever went out, or whosoever came in, passed beneath, & with Idolatrous Reverence lift up their Eyes, & kissed ỹ Cheeks of ỹ Postern.

Chronicle of the Kings, page 51.

112 'Idol-Worship or The Way to Preferment.', 1740, engraving. British Museum, London.

The quotation parallels George II and Henry VIII to make the king bear responsibility for his minister's actions: 'And Henry the KING made unto himself a great IDOL, the likeness of which was not in Heaven above, nor in the Earth beneath; and he reared up his Head unto ye Clouds, and extended his Arm over all ye Land; His Legs also were as yet Posts of a Gate, or as an Arch stretched forth over y^e Doors of all ye Publick Offices in y^e Land, and whosoever went out, or whosoever came in, passed beneath, and with Idolatrous Reverence lift up their Eyes, & kissed y^e Cheeks of y^e Postern' (*Chronicle of the Kings*).

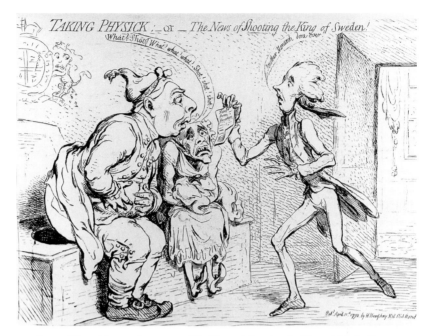

113 James Gillray, 'TAKING PHYSICK: or The News of Shooting the King of Sweden!', 1792, etching.

    The grossly agitated King and Queen seated in a latrine receive a message from the emaciated Prime Minister, William Pitt, who rushes in bearing 'news from Sweden' and exclaiming 'Another Monarch done over!' The horrified King clutching his bloated stomach stammers 'What? Shot? What? what? Shot! shot! shot!' The band of the King's nightcap reads 'Honi soit qui m...', the motto of the Order of the Garter.

other is reading a pamphlet confuting Samuel Johnson's *Taxation No Tyranny*. Lord Chatham, tarred and feathered, figures in the graffiti adorning the wall.

    Festering anti-Scot prejudice was likewise sustained by images in prints like *Sawney in the Boghouse*, in which Sawney, the stage Scot, shows what a barbarian he is by sticking his legs into the holes in a communal lavatory seat. The scatological overtones served to sharpen the humour when the throne's occupant was none other than the King. Gillray (illus. 113) depicted the royal couple relieving themselves as a frantic Prime Minister Pitt dashes in bearing the 'News from Sweden', shrieking 'Another Monarch done over!' Wearing a crown which twins as a fool's cap, George III, displaying his distinctive speech tic, can only utter: 'What? Shot? What? what? what? Shot! shot! shot!' while uncontrollably evacuating his bowels, as is treasonably mimed by the lion on the royal arms on the privy wall. In that surrealist comedy of inversion and subversion perfected by Gillray, boghouse and royal throne merge, reminding us of Swift's jingle

> We read of kings, who in a fright,
> Though on a throne, would fall to shite.[20]

and calling to mind an aphorism of Benjamin Franklin's: 'The greatest monarch on the proudest throne, is oblig'd to sit upon his own arse.'[21]

In the cartoon-world, in short, the body – that is, by association, the body politic – is perpetually pummelled and punished; torsos which serve as national emblems are racked; and carcasses maimed and butchered. A print titled *The Colonies Reduced* thus depicts Britannia mutilated by the loss of her limbs, the American Colonies.

Yet the body political may be, in true Bakhtinian fashion, a monster in itself, deformed, atrocious and terrifying. The grotesque body often signifies the mob or, in Revolutionary France, the *sans culottes*. Ghoulish English audiences took *schadenfreude* from spine-chilling images of the Terror; and its hideous props lived on in the counter-revolutionary imagination, encouraging George Cruikshank to produce 'A Radical Reformer, i.e., a Neck or Nothing Man' (illus. 114), a deeply ambivalent image in which reform is utterly sanguinary but the bloodshed just. The leaders of the political nation – the Prince Regent and Lords Liverpool, Castlereagh and Eldon – are shown in that print abandoning their money bags as they flee from a repulsive monster whose torso is a guillotine armed with daggers shooting flames after the fugitives.

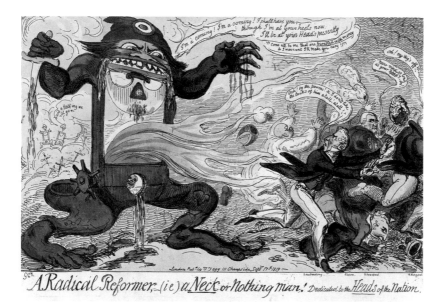

114 George Cruikshank, 'A Radical Reformer, i.e., a <u>Neck</u> or Nothing Man! Dedicated to the <u>Heads</u> of the Nation', 1819, engraving (coloured impression). British Museum, London.

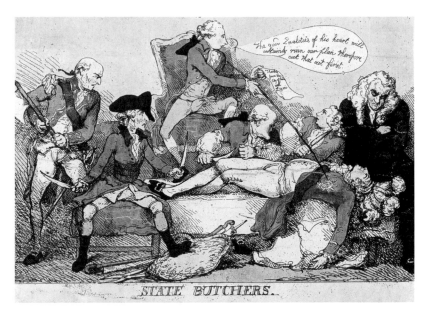

115 Thomas Rowlandson, 'STATE BUTCHERS', 1789, etching with watercolour.
    The Prince of Wales on an operating table surrounded by the knife-wielding Ministry directed by William Pitt; satirizing the crisis over the question of a Regency for the insane George III. Pitt says to his supporter Henry Dundas: 'The good Qualities of his heart will certainly ruin our plan therefore cut that out first', holding out a paper which reads: 'Thanks from the City of London with £50,000.'

Monsters and dismemberment could conjure up a still worse nightmare: dissection. Public execution was a calculated degradation,[22] and, as we have seen in the finale of Hogarth's *Four Stages of Cruelty*, dissection was suffused with all the solemn yet profane connotations of the gallows. Rowlandson rang the changes on these macabre and gory elements. In the 'STATE BUTCHERS' (illus. 115), produced at the height of the Regency crisis of 1789, a ruthless Pitt the Younger is enthroned in the seat of the President of the Company of Surgeons, somewhat echoing Hogarth's setting of his surgeon in *The Reward of Cruelty*. His wand is directed towards the Prince's heart, indicating that this should be excised: 'the good qualities of his heart will utterly ruin our plan therefore cut that our first.'[23] Other ministers have their knives ready sharpened; amongst them, at the Prince's feet, the Duke of Grafton, blade in each hand, and one foot set on a surgeon's bag from which a saw and pair of shears are spilling.[24]

'Political anatomy' was a perennial favourite. Amongst the most striking examples is a print headed *The Conduct of the two B*****rs*. The title, of course, draws attention to a pun, which may signify 'Brothers', or 'Butchers', or what you will. The Whig Prime Minister Henry

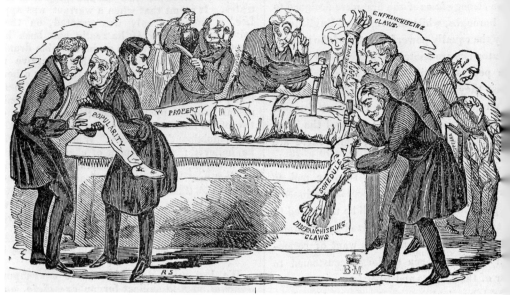

116 Robert Seymour, 'INTERIOR OF THE TORY CHARNEL HOUSE. DISSECTION OF THE BILL', 1832, wood engraving. British Museum, London.

John Bull, laid out on a slab, is divided between supporters and opponents of the extension of electoral franchise marked by the 1832 Great Reform Bill. The Duke of Buckingham holds – and cuts off – the left arm, labelled 'Schedule A', 'Disenfranchiseing Claws'; the left leg, 'Popularity', has been amputated by Lord Harrowby (who shows it to the Henry Pelham, later Duke of Newcastle). Lord Wharncliffe, who helped the Bill to pass, holds and severs the right arm (inscribed 'Schedule B', 'Enfranchiseing Claws'), while the right leg, 'Property', remains as yet untouched. The Duke of Wellington (formerly Prime Minister, an opponent of the Bill) adjusts his pince-nez and plunges a knife into John Bull's breast; Cumberland has already removed the heart. Another, older doctor (the Chancellor, Lord Eldon, a wealthy opponent of reform) rifles the patient's trouser pockets.

Pelham is performing an 'anatomy' – disembowelling Britannia – while his elder brother the Duke of Newcastle sports a ribbon identifying him as 'Undertaker General' (another pun, as 'undertaker' meant political manager as well as funeral director). In the background, the white horse of Hanover drinks Britannia's blood, while limbs imprinted 'Gibraltar' and 'Cape Breton' litter the ground – the latter had just been ceded to France under the Treaty of Aix-la-Chapelle (1748). The anti-Hanoverian thrust of the print is clinched by the German mercenary on the left, pointing to the bust of a Roman emperor, and so incriminating George II.

The trope of politician as state butcher, knifing the people, received its most cutting treatment in 1832, the year not just of the Great Reform Bill but also of the Anatomy Act, which, as noted in the previous chapter, put an end to the Burke-and-Hare business of grave robbing by 'resurrectionists' by giving surgeons legal sanction to dissect unclaimed hospital corpses.[25] Medically speaking a progressive measure, it could, however, be condemned for offering carte blanche to the profession to carve up the populace – and, *mutatis mutandis*, in cartoon terms, to the politicians to unloose carnage. In a print by Robert Seymour (illus. 116), a cabal of Tory peers clusters round a corpse representing the Reform Bill and dissects it, precisely as they were mutilating it in the House of Lords. Buckingham cuts off the left arm, Wharncliffe the right; Lord Harrowby hacks off the left leg and shows it to Newcastle; Cumberland excises the heart, and Wellington plunges his knife into the breast. While two bishops turn a blind eye, Lord Eldon picks the victim's pockets.[26]

The one thing more sacrilegious than dissection was cannibalism, and its cartoon *locus classicus* was 'Un petit Souper, a la Parisiènne' (illus. 117). Prompted by the September massacres of 1792, Gillray depicts a hideously subhuman *sans culotte* household. Anthropophagic

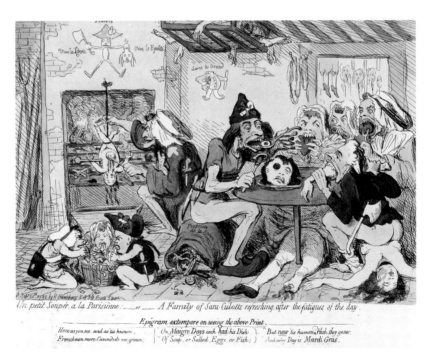

117 James Gillray, 'Un petit Souper, a la Parisiènne; – or – a Family of Sans-Culotts refreshing after the fatigues of the day', 1792, engraving (coloured impression). British Museum, London.
  'Epigram extempore on seeing the above Print. Here as you see, and as 'tis known, / Frenchmen mere Cannibals are grown; / On Maigre Days each had his Dish / Of Soup, or Sallad, Eggs, or fish; / But now 'tis human flesh they gnaw, And ev'ry Day is Mardi Gras.' A graffito on the wall acclaims the regicide Pétion.

Parisians stuff themselves with human vitals, while bloodthirstily basting a baby over an open fire: in an echo, one surmises, of Swift's *A Modest Proposal*, the Revolution is literally devouring its own children. It was Gillray's genius – and, argues Paulson, also his morbid streak – to reduce the politics of revolution to the bestial and the elemental: gorging and being eaten, shitting and being shat upon. Food and faeces haunted his tortured imagination and governed his artistic repertoire.[27]

Cartoonists thus anatomized politics, revealing it to be a theatre of cruelty in which the body was incessantly battered. A more specific idiom was also being articulated, however: politics was encoded through certain medical analogues, via metaphors and models expressive of that distrust of the doctors dealt with at length in this book. Politicians in these tropes became practitioners, and the populace patients, plagued by the diseases of war and impressment, poverty and taxation. Languishing and sick, the body politic is seen being 'heroically' physicked – usually disastrously – by its doctor leaders; surgery is being performed, blood let, the patient purged or vomited, and, if all else fails, as all too often, a post mortem is finally on the cards.

The chief sufferer in all this was John Bull. 'The portrayal of the common people in eighteenth-century cartoon and caricature', explains John Brewer,

> seems inextricably associated with two powerful images: John Bull and the sans culottes or Jacobin. Bull was portrayed as a stout countryman (usually a yokel) who laboured manfully beneath the burdens of British political life, while the sans culottes, emaciated, fiendish, and with a grin that conveyed both concupiscence and folly, personified the threat of the radical plebeian, looking utterly satanic or perhaps foolish and comic.[28]

Unlike the bumptious, corpulent, complacent mid-Victorian stereotype, his precursor was rarely heroized or sentimentalized. Typically a yokel with a peasant's low cunning, the Georgian Bull was coarse, foolish and often drunk. Endlessly put upon and humiliated, if he had any sterling qualities at all they were those of a dumb brute. Not surprisingly, therefore, he frequently appeared sick and suffering. Above all, he was made to submit to the ministrations of the physicians of state (illus. 99), treating him with such odd panaceas as 'Musket Balls', 'Wellington Drops', 'Catholic Pills' and 'Total Defeat for Bonaparte' pills.[29]

Taxation suggested numerous medical metaphors. Sometimes, as in a 1793 anatomy by William Dent (illus. 118), John Bull's very skeleton is depicted transformed into a diagnostic chart for the

242

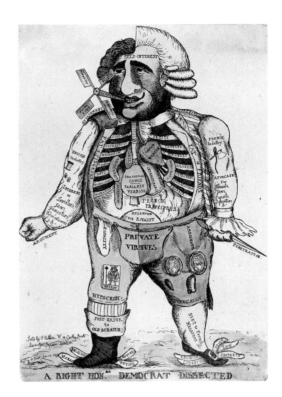

118 William(?) Dent, 'A
RIGHT HON^BLE. DEMOCRAT
DISSECTED', 1793, engraving
(coloured impression).

The various portions of
his anatomy display every
form of hypocrisy and
immorality, personal and
political. British Museum,
London.

A RIGHT HON. DEMOCRAT DISSECTED.

epidemic of taxes, duties and imposts levied by Pitt: the patient is
understandably bellowing with rage. Pitt was also the culprit in a
parody of Henry Fuseli's *Nightmare*, which showed the King's
Minister appearing as an incubus sucking the very lifeblood out of the
traumatized victim.

There are other ways besides bloodsucking to wring the vitality out
of a nation. *Johnny in a Flatting Mill* shows Bull being fed through a
mangle, to squeeze out extra taxes in a year (1796) when war, inflation
and vast military subsidies to Britain's war allies were emptying the
Treasury. Normally so plump, Bull is squashed flat by Pitt and the
Treasurer of the Navy Viscount Melville between rollers labelled
profligacy and taxation.[30]

A joke which never palled – because it obviously rang true – was
John Bull undergoing bloodletting (illus. 100). Sangrado (literally
Dr Blood, the venesecting physician in Le Sage's novel *Gil Blas*), here
metaphorizes the Ministry, which, wielding lancets, is relieving the
nation of its lifeblood, that is, its guineas. Therapeutic phlebotomy
(bloodletting) was justified by philosophies that warned that a plethora
of blood caused apoplexy and fever; physician-politicians evidently
thought the nation likewise could be too well off for its own health. A

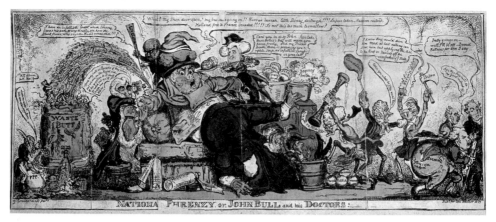

119 George Cruikshank, 'NATIONAL PHRENZY or JOHN BULL and his DOCTORS', 1813, etching with watercolour.

The Chancellor, Lord Eldon, feels John Bull's pulse; Lord Liverpool, the Prime Minister, bleeds him in the arm with a lancet; the ensuing torrent of pensions, subsidies and other expenditure lands in a 'waste butt'. A bottle at Bull's feet is labelled 'Wellington drops' (the Duke of Wellington was busy defeating the French in the Spanish Peninsula). Castlereagh, the Foreign Secretary, shovels in boluses labelled 'cheap bread' and 'total defeat for Bonaparte', to be washed down with 'Regency Froth'. Death, a doctor wielding an 'Allied pestle', is about to crush Napoleon in a mortar into 'reptile soup, an infallible specific'. The radical philanthropist Francis Burdett holds a surgeon's saw and an axe, both labelled 'Reform', declaring that nothing can save John Bull but 'applying the axe to the Root or sawing off the excrescences of State'; he is opposed by a bewigged judge (Burdett had gone to law over his first attempt to enter the House of Commons, and had recently been jailed in the Tower of London by the Speaker of the House). Pitt's supporter Willian Grenville, his large rear labelled 'fat sinecures', is leaving, carrying a doctor's gold-topped cane and declaring these to be 'pretty goings on'.

parallel appears in George Cruikshank's engraving of state physicians bleeding John Bull (illus. 119), who gapes while being bled of all his gold, which goes to subsidize grasping allies. 'You have open'd so many veins', he groans, 'and drained me so incessantly that I fear my constitution is impaired forever. My friends say that I am declining fast and will certainly die of a galloping consumption.' Bull's blood was a cartoonist's standby: in the 1810s, George Cruikshank returned to the 'John Bull and his doctors' theme on at least six occasions.[31]

If it was generally at ministerial hands that John Bull suffered medical violation, that was not always so. Popular politicians also lent themselves to lampooning as adepts of radical surgery. In *Radical Quacks Giving a New Constitution to John Bull*, George Cruikshank drew the nation's hero with both legs already chopped off, one wooden peg being labelled 'Universal Suffrage', the other 'Religious Freedom'. He is undergoing bleeding by the aristocratic radical Sir Francis Burdett, while his supporter, the MP John Cam Hobhouse, presents him with a restorative cordial. John Bull's pillow is inscribed 'False

Promises' and 'Reformers Opinions', while his armchair speaks of 'Mistaken Confidence'. 'Mr Bull, you have lived too well', the radicals explain: 'but when we have renovated your Constitution according to our plan the reform will be so complete — ! that you will never again be troubled with any fullness whatsoever!' Replies the long-suffering Bull:

> May be, gentlemen, but you have taken all the honest good blood out of my veins; deprived me of my real supporters & stuck two bad props in their place, & if you go back on this, I shall die before ever my Constitution can be improved.

The radical surgeons are ready with their answer:

> Never mind Mr Bull, if we have thought it necessary to take off both your legs you will find the others very good substitutes, this Revolutionary Bolus and decoction of disloyalty, are very harmless but they will restore the *general equality* of the intestines & remove any obstruction which may prevent us from effecting a Radical Reform in the System.[32]

On the table drastic political purgatives await – Cobbett's Helebore Ratsbane, Wooler's Black Drops, Cartwright's Universal Grease, Hunt's Powders, and Dr Watson's White and Comfort (Watson was an apothecary and agitator; his son headed the Cato Street Conspiracy). A magnum of Burdett's Mixture is made up of 'Whitbread's Intire', and nearby are two further nostrums, a 'sudorific' (sweat) and an 'opiate for Mr. Bull' – lethal polypharmacy indeed, named after the leading radicals of the day!

Radicals were also vulnerable to a further graphic device: portrayal as arrant quacks. This gag ran and ran. In context, for example, of the Catholic emancipation crisis of 1812, Cruikshank put out *The Mountebanks, or Opposition Show Box*, in which John Bull appears as a farmer and the mountebank doctors are Samuel Whitbread, offering an 'infallible panacea – reform', Sheridan (as a zany), and Lords Grenville and Grey, about to muzzle Bull with a 'Catholic Emancipation' bandage. Whitbread's pockets bulge with medicine bottles, including, once again, 'Whitbread's Intire', alluding of course to his original career as a brewer.[33]

Mountebanks tended to hail (or pretend to hail) from abroad – uroscopists from Germany, for instance, and vendors of poison-antidotes from Italy. For that reason, non-English politicians were routinely portrayed as quacks. The victim-in-chief of that identification was the Scot, Lord Bute, who, as the young George III's favourite, had been appointed in 1762 First Lord of the Treasury. Already alluded to in Chapter 1, *The State Quack* was one of hundreds of attacks on this 'impostor', and on his supposed mistress, George III's mother, the Princess Dowager, depicted falling as the rope-walker. To the right of the print, a sailor assaults a kilted Scot.[34] Elsewhere Bute figured as a mountebank selling nostrums. 'Awa wi ye to the Dee'l ye Soothern Loons', he announces:

> I ken fu' weel yr distemper; I donne mean that, so peculiar to our Country, occasion'd by ye immoderate use of Oatmeal; But it is the Gowden Itch, we' which ye are troobled ... See here my bra Lads, in these bags are contain'd ye Gowden Lozenges, a never failing remedy, that gives Preesent ease.[35]

In that print, the Princess Dowager has wisely given up rope-walking and figures wearing a Welsh hat and peeping through the curtains (the political arras).

Around 1800, satirists were granted a gift from the gods in the guise of Henry Addington, later Lord Sidmouth, who served, in a weirdly back-to-front career, briefly as Prime Minister and later lengthily as Home Secretary. Son of a physician who ran a madhouse, Addington inevitably acquired the soubriquet of 'political doctor', featuring in over 130 prints in the guises of pharmacist, physician, apothecary, nurse and mountebank. He it is who, in Gillray's *Doctor Sangrado Curing John Bull of Repletion*, is the doctor bleeding John Bull, who sits depleted upon a commode labelled 'Reservoir for the Clysterpipe family!' The cartoon makes twin points: it protests against the exorbitant taxes levied to support the French war, while it also ridicules, via the 'Clysterpipe family' associations, a lucrative sinecure swung by Addington for his teenage son.[36]

Cruikshank went to town at Addington's expense, drawing upon the insuperable ludicrousness of a top politician being a doctor's son:[37]

> *My name's THE DOCTOR; on the Berkshire hills*
> *My father purged his patients* – a wise man,
> Whose constant care was to increase his store,
> And keep his eldest son – myself – at home.
> But I *had heard of Politics, and long'd*
> *To sit within the Commons' House, and get*
> *A place*, and luck gave what my sire denied.
> Some thirteen years ago, or ere my fingers
> Had learn'd to mix a potion, or to bleed,
> *I flatter'd Pitt; I cring'd, and sneak'd and fawned,*
> And thus became the Speaker. I alone,
> With pompous gait, and peruke full of wisdom,
> Th' unruly members could control, or call

The House to order ...
My ends attain'd my only aim has been
To keep my place – and gild my humble name![38]

Many medical devices were used to disparage Dr Clysterpipe, popularly slurred as a nobody ('Pitt is to Addington/As London is to Paddington'). Sometimes, as for instance in the Cruikshank brothers' *Blockheads*, Addington was ridiculed through being made to wear on his head an apothecary's mortar tagged 'Drugs for John Bull' and 'Circular Pills', an allusion to an infamous circular sent round in July 1819 by him as Home Secretary, calling on Lords-Lieutenants to adopt all measures necessary to preserve order and to keep the yeomanry at the ready – a command later seen as precipitating the Peterloo Massacre of the following month. That name stuck and it appears in subsequent prints, as for instance in *A Kick Up in a Great House*, where he is seen flying through the air: 'The d____d Bull has given my poor Brain such a Circular Twist – I fear all the Pills, Clysters, Emetics, Draughts, and Bolus's in my shop – will never put right again.' Finally, in William Hone's relentlessly ferocious pamphlet, *The Political House that Jack Built* (1819), George Cruikshank showed Sidmouth, Castlereagh, and Canning huddled together in a small woodcut, *The Doctor*, which opens,

This is The Doctor of Circular Fame
A Driv'ller, A Bigot, A Knave without shame.[39]

If Addington was often portrayed as state physician or quack, doomed to deplete his patients to destruction, other politicians were depicted on the receiving end, as the sick men of Westminster. Classic was Charles James Fox, the caricaturist's dream come true, for his very name afforded endless Aesopian possibilities for animal physiognomy.[40] The Whig's gambling, philandering, drinking and demagogic propensities licensed artists to portray him as a kind of double personage, both patrician and plebeian, the patrician Member turned into the 'lost member' of some roué. And as a lost member, it was appropriate that in another print by William Dent, Fox's corpse, laid bare for dissection, was found to be riddled with every conceivable personal and political weakness. Not least, his unkempt aspect and dishevelled locks, his impetuous switches of political orientation and, after 1789, his vocal support for the French Revolution, induced cartoonists to represent him as not merely a lost member but a lost mind, quite out of his wits. One engraving (illus. 120) pictures him wrapped in a blanket in a Bedlam cell.[41] Wearing a crown of straw and clutching a straw

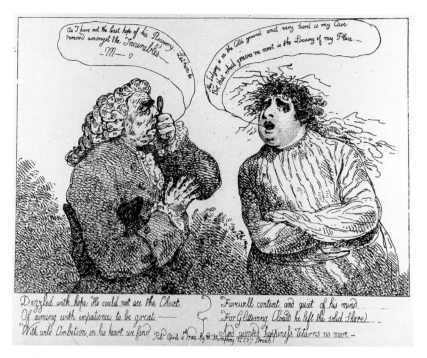

120 Thomas Rowlandson, 1784, untitled etching.

Dr Monro (physician to Bedlam) examines the straight-jacketed and dishevelled Charles James Fox in this satire of the fall of the short-lived Fox-North Coalition, 1784. Fox sings: 'My Lodging is on the Cold ground and very hard is my Case / But that which grieves me most is the Loosing of my Place.' Dr Monro declares: 'As I have not the least hope of his Recovery, let him be remov'd amongst the Incurable's –' The lettering continues: '– Dazzled with hope He could not see the Cheat / Of aiming with impatience to be Great / With wild Ambition in his heart we find / Farewell content and quiet of his mind / For Glittering Clouds he left the solid Shore / And wonted happiness returns no more.'

sceptre, he is a victim of delusions of grandeur: 'Do you not behold friend Sam I have obtained the height of all my wishes?', he button-holes a visitor gaping at him through the cell door. With the Fox-North Coalition utterly discredited, the Whig's future hopes of power and success were evidently mere delusions, thus earning him his 'place' in Bedlam alone.[42] Just five years later, Pitt was set in similar circumstances by Rowlandson, in an etching entitled *The Hospital for Lunatics*. Crouching on a chamber pot in a hospital cell, the Prime Minister, crowned by a twig coronet, is holding a toy sceptre. Above him is inscribed 'went mad supposing himself next heir to a Crown'. With implied sexual innuendos, a female in the next cell has been driven out of her wits by 'Political itching', and each 'victim' is pronounced 'INCURABLE'.

248

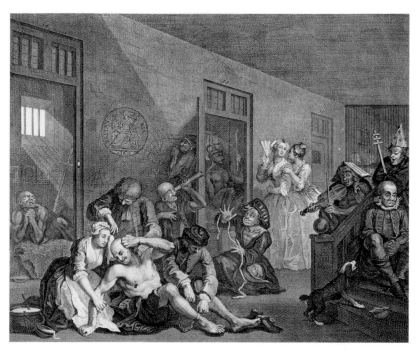

121 William Hogarth, *The Rake's Progress*, scene VIII, engraving of 1763 after one of 1735. The mad artist at the rear draws a halfpenny with the figure of Britannia on it on the back wall.

Madness aptly rounds off this tale of political maladies. It was, after all, the era in which George III tumbled over into insanity, Edmund Burke was regarded as well-nigh certifiable – 'the most eloquent madman I know', quipped Gibbon – and Lord Castlereagh, Samuel Romilly and Samuel Whitbread all slit their throats, while the French Revolution and Napoleonic politics were diagnosed as raging epidemics. Small surprise, as hinted earlier in Chapter 4, that the state was renamed Bedlam by Hogarth who, in the 1763 version of the final print of *The Rake's Progress* (illus. 121), presented what looked like the interior of Bethlem but, through a subtle trick of signwriting, made it 'Britannia'.[43] Politics was thus a disease, and politicians were Dr Death in a territory where statecraft dissolved into sickness and heroic if all too often lethal surgery.

10 Victorian Developments

Nineteenth-century Englishmen prided themselves upon spearheading an age of reform. A typical expression of this was the founding in 1823 of the radical journal *Lancet* by the surgeon and democrat Thomas Wakley (illus. 122), who proceeded less like a blade than a blunderbuss, blasting the entire medical establishment, accusing it of neglecting its duties even as it abused it powers and pocketed its fees. Medical corporations and London's hospitals, charged the belligerent Wakley, were nests of ineptitude and nepotism, and the sick suffered neglect, mistreatment and hamfisted surgery. Readers might be pardoned if they got the impression from its pages that English medicine was a terminal case.[1]

And if it was no wonder, under such circumstances, that people patronized sharks and swindlers, Wakley took aim not only at orthodoxy but also at what he called 'quacks, *regular* and *irregular*' alike.[2] Of

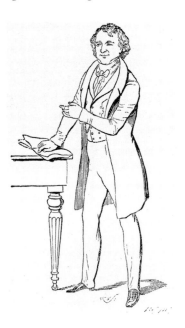

122 W. W., 'Thomas Wakley, Esq., m.p.', wood engraving.
    This print shows Wakley (1793–1862), founder of *Lancet*.

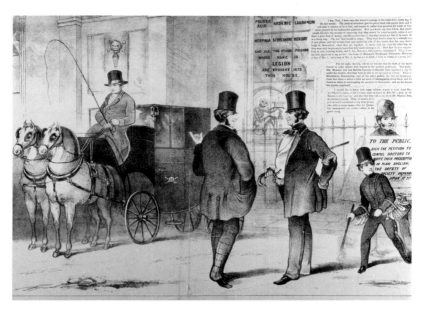

123 'Hygeian llustration No. 5', *c.* 1848, lithograph.

This is a representation of the desperate state of the medical establishment according to James Morison, pill-vendor and self-styled 'Hygeian'. In the background is a dispensary window, with a skeleton next to an urn labelled 'PHARMACOPIÆ'. The captioning states: 'The doctors will no more reform themselves than those who profit by abuses of any kind', before going on to spell out the key principles of Morisonian medicine. The speech bubbles emanating from the two gentlemen run: 'I say, Tom, I have seen this doctor's carriage at the same door, every day, for the last month. The medical attendant gets his purse lined with guinea fees, and the rich man is content to lie in bed, and remain ill, rather than question the mode of treatment pursued by his fashionable physician. Now you know, my dear fellow, that wealthy people fall into the mistake of supposing that they cannot be cured properly unless it costs them a great deal of money, and the positive fact is, that they would not like to be made well in a cheap way. Oh, no! that would be vulgar. They must have it done by a scientific man, if you please, and like to have their ears tickled by a lot of fine words that the very doctors laugh at, themselves, when they get together. A doctor told me, only the other day, that they were only beginning to learn that they knew nothing at all. Now how do you suppose I keep in such stunning health, and I, too, that am a little rackety, sometimes? Why, I carry my true physician in my pocket; my two boxes of MORISON'S VEGETABLE UNIVERSAL MEDICINE, a box of No. 1 and a box of No. 2, by the use of which, I keep as strong as a young bull.' The other man responds: 'You are right, my boy, but let me tell you that the faith of the wealthy classes is sadly shaken with respect to the medical profession. The works of MR. MORISON and THE BRITISH COLLEGE OF HEALTH have knocked a leg from under the doctors, that they wont be able to set up again in a hurry. What with Mesmerism, Homeopathy, and all the other *pathies*, the rich are beginning to think that there is rather little too much *humbugapathy* about them, and have therefore taken to investigating the question for themselves, and are throwing the doctors overboard.' Replies the first: 'I should like to know how many millions a-year it costs JOHN BULL for physic? – some of the Doctors make as much as 20,000 pounds a-year by this Guinea-trade humbug; and after that they talk to us about Mr. Morison being an interested party. Why, of course, he is just as much interested as any other person who sells a GOOD THING, – but his System has emancipated our minds, – which is the grand thing.' On the sandwich board is written: 'TO THE PUBLIC. SIGN THE PETITION TO COMPEL DOCTORS TO WRITE THEIR PRESCRIPTIONS IN PLAIN ENGLISH; THE SAFETY OF SOCIETY DEPENDS UPON IT!!!'

all those he targeted none was so excoriated as James Morison, the most successful of his tribe – his 'poison is swallowed by *bushels*'.[3] 'Murder by Morison's pills' (illus. 123) was his lurid line in 1836, after a coroner's inquest had found the deceased had been swallowing that particular nostrum. The *Lancet* bristled with condemnation of the arch-quack's 'life-destroying career', expressing horror at the public's endorsement of his claims, which was no less than a 'hallucination of the human mind'.[4]

Just like those medical grandees of the day whom, as we shall see, he vilified mercilessly, Morison swanked it up, the *Lancet* pointed out, by having himself driven round in a carriage with a coronet on top and livery servants flanking. 'Nearly every country paper contains columns of advertisements, all puffing the wondrous efficacy of the "Universal Pills"' – and, worse still, Morison's publicity bulged with testimonials from '*certificated* members of the medical profession'.[5]

What was so distinctive about Morison's medicine circus? A businessman, James Morison had suffered ill health, tried any number of regular doctors and their remedies without benefit, and had despaired of physic. That was a familiar enough storyline – how many others had undergone precisely the same experience? Morison's response, however, made him unique. For he came to despise the profession with a positively evangelical hatred, touting a total revolution in medicine – one of his publications has on the title page the characteristic slogan, 'The old medical science is completely wrong.' Doctors were simply useless – his own medical history proved that: they knew nothing about the true principles of health and disease; they concealed their ignorance behind a fancy jargon larded with obscurities and neologisms, designed to dazzle the laity. It was high time the faculty's parasitical restrictive practices were utterly exploded, for once and all. Doctors were not merely ignorant and mercenary: they were dangerous. Their polypharmacy and inordinate dosing habits (therein, after all, lay their profits), and, above all, their reckless indulgence in *poisonous* medicines – heavy metals and artificial chemicals – were little short of criminal.[6]

So far, there was nothing especially original in Morison's iconoclasm, indeed, it sounded remarkably similar to Wakley's own assault on the profession – hence perhaps the editor's resentment at having his radical clothes snatched off his back. It was his positive prescriptions that made Morison novel. Drawing upon his comprehension of his own recovery, Morison proposed a new decalogue for medicine. Ten commandments told all there was to know:

1   The vital principle is contained in the blood.
2   Blood makes blood.
3   Everything in the body is derived from the blood.
4   All constitutions are radically the same.
5   All diseases arise from the impurity of the blood, or in other words, from acrimonious humours lodged in the body.
6   This humour which degenerates the blood has three sources, the maternine, the contagious and the personal.
7   Pain and disease have the same origin; and may therefore be considered synonymous terms.
8   Purgation by vegetables is the only effectual mode of eradicating disease.
9   The stomach and bowels cannot be purged too much.
10 From the intimate connexion subsisting between the mind and the body, the health of the one must conduce to the serenity of the other.

In a nutshell, in Morison's protestant reformation of health, there was a single cause for each and every disease – bad blood (how symbolic!) – and a single therapeutics: heavy and frequent purgation, using vegetable laxatives.

In response to his diagnosis, Morison produced the perfect purge, his 'Vegetable Universal Pills'. Available in two strengths (nos 1 and 2), these contained only natural products – aloes, jalap, colocynth, gamboge, cream of tartar, rhubarb and myrrh. They would cure all diseases (not least, Morison insisted, cholera, which had struck in 1831), and they were so safe that, if need be, they could (ironic to relate) be taken in heroic quantities – up to 30 pills a day.

Insofar as he made his living by marketing a high-dosage nostrum, Morison was a quack of the old school. But he was also creating a new mould, in various ways proleptic of future medical developments. More insistently, consistently and persistently than previous heretics, he taught the public to avoid regular medicine like the plague, and to do so, not merely on pragmatic grounds, but on principle, as a point of faith. Professions were self-aggrandizing ramps, and the medical profession a conspiracy for the expropriation of health. Though mystified by official medicine, health care was in truth simple and, repudiating orthodox physiology and disease theory, he enunciated a radical alternative, dinning into the public mind the inextricable association between his true philosophy of health and his own specific. Previous nostrum-mongers had done little more than to persuade the sick to swallow their panaceas; Morison wanted the public to swallow his philosophy too. He wooed his age with a simple, attractive vision of healthy living which all could understand.

Not least, Morison became a proselytizing medical missionary, turning medical spectacle into evangelism in that early Victorian era of populist tub-thumpers. Establishing the 'British College of Health', he was the first quack to exploit the nineteenth-century reformist passion for organizations and institutions. Terming himself 'the Hygeist' – an epithet that allowed him to dissociate himself from the quack practice of assuming the doctor's mantle – he made the further innovation of publishing a magazine, the *Hygeian Journal*, bombarding the public with heaps of books and pamphlets besides. Unlike any Georgian quack, Morison attempted – with enormous success – to turn selling health into a crusade. His was medicine for the Barnum and Bailey age. Both Wakley and Morison exposed the medicine show of the times: Wakley rested content with performing as the time-honoured iconoclast, sticking the lancet in; Morison created a new theatre of this own.

Wakley's whipping of medicine was evidently self-interested and so must be taken with a pinch of salt, but one element of his diagnosis was spot on. He deplored the fact that medicine was a house divided against itself. The profession would never enjoy its proper authority – indeed would never seize and retain the moral high ground against quackery – while it remained fragmented into the obsolescent and antagonistic branches of physic, surgery and pharmacy, each headed by a self-perpetuating cabal. Until the profession, like Parliament, was officially and constitutionally reorganized, the sick could not be protected, fraudulent practitioners silenced, or the public served. Numerous parliamentary bills intended to alter the statutory regulation of medicine were, indeed, introduced in the early decades of the century, but few were passed, and most which did get through were the work of MPs sympathetic to the wishes of the College of Physicians, which recognized, in a Burkean manner, that a degree of reform was essential to the preservation of the status quo.

Characteristic was the Apothecaries Act of 1815. This specified that the normal qualification for practice as an apothecary should be possession of a licence issued by the Society of Apothecaries (the LSA), which involved apprenticeship, taking stipulated courses, some hospital experience, and passing examinations. It represented a minor victory for general practitioners, since it established a distinct legal boundary demarcating the qualified apothecary from retail druggists and other such lowly medical tradesmen treading on their tails. The aftermath of the Act, however, was recrimination rather than reconciliation, and the divisions within the profession remained, with the Corporations happy to chug along as before.

In the 1830s, in an atmosphere dominated by Parliamentary reform and by the cholera pandemic of 1831–2, the British Medical

Association emerged as a ginger group for GPs, with the aim of opening up the medical corporations on a democratic basis to all their members. But still the medical old guard carried sufficient parliamentary clout to sustain the status quo.[7]

The reconstitution of the medical profession was not achieved until after mid-century, when the Medical Act of 1858 proved an ingenious compromise, placating the reformers, protecting the profession, and ensuring that no branch came out as a loser. To satisfy the Royal Colleges, the tripartite division of English medicine was not abolished, and they themselves survived unscathed. To placate general practitioners, however, these distinctions became for practical purposes meaningless. In future there would be one single public list, the Medical Register, set up under the auspices of a General Medical Council (GMC). It demarcated the 'regular' profession from its competitors, and gave it significant privileges. It contained all legally recognized practitioners; all names would appear equally on it, from the upholstered Harley Street consultant down to the threadbare village LSA. The Register's significance lay, of course, in its exclusions. For all ranks of regular practitioners now appeared together, cheek-by-jowl, as 'insiders', lined up against all the 'outsiders' – the homoeopaths, medical botanists, quacks, bone-setters, itinerants and the like, who were automatically constituted, by the very fact of their exclusion, as the 'fringe'. Parliament had achieved what the doctors never could; it had, formally and symbolically at least, united the divided profession, by defining them over and against a common other, not to say enemy.

That reorganization proved durable, partly because it registered changes the profession was already undergoing. New professional groupings were taking shape. London's elite physicians and surgeons had ceased to require the creaking armour which Collegiate privileges appeared to provide, for they were establishing themselves in plush positions of professional authority and eminence. The distinction of a Harley Street practice, combined with a consultancy at a leading London hospital (illus. 124), with patients referred by one's former pupils for whom one had found preferable practices: these features ensured that medicine continued hierarchical even after the old corporations finally had their teeth drawn.[8]

For the general practitioner in Rotherhithe or Rotherham, however, the professional recognition – the semi-closed shop – offered by the mid-Victorian legislation might amount to little of tangible value. His prospects (till the 1870s professional medicine remained men-only) depended almost wholly upon the market forces of supply and

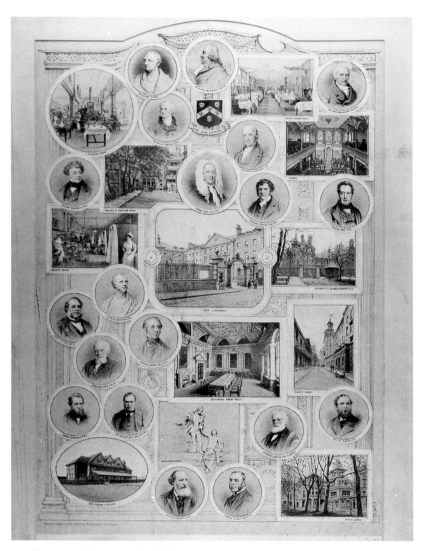

124 Beynon and Company, colour lithograph after Michael Hanhart (*fl.* 1870–82) showing the past surgeons and physicians of Guy's Hospital, Southwark, London, with views of the building.

The view contains pictures (from the top left) of a clinical ward, Astley Cooper ward, a balcony of Martha ward, the chapel, Bright ward, the front quadrangle, the residential college and student's club, the governors court room, William Hunt's house, the club ground and pavilion, and the dental school. Those featured are William Hunt (*b.* 1645); William Saunders (1743–1817); William Babington (1765–1833); Sir Astley Paston Cooper (1768–1841); Benjamin Harrison the elder (1777–1856); James Blundell (1790–1878); Thomas Guy (1645–1724); Richard Bright (1789–1858); Thomas Bell (1792–1880); Thomas Addison (1793–1860); John Hilton (1804–1878); Charles Aston Key (1793–1849); Edward Cock (1805–1892); James Hinton (1822–1875); Sir William Gull (1816–1890); Sir Samuel Wilks (1824–1911); Walter Moxon (1836–1886); Arthur Durham (1833–1895); and Charles Hilton Fagge (1838–1883). Images such as this, increasingly common in the late Victorian era, convey a sense of pride in the lineage and traditions of ancient institutions with a new, reformed professional consciousness.

WHY I DON'T WRITE PLAYS.

(From the Common-place Book of a Novelist.)

BECAUSE it is so much pleasanter to read one's work than to hear it on the Stage.

Because Publishers are far more amiable to deal with than Actor-Managers.

Because "behind the scenes" is such a disappointing place—except in Novels.

Because why waste three weeks on writing a Play, when it takes only three years to compose a Novel?

Because Critics who send articles to Magazines inviting one to contribute to the Stage, have no right to dictate to us.

Because a fairly successful Novel means five hundred pounds, and a fairly successful Play yields as many thousands — why be influenced by mercenary motives?

Because all Novelists hire their pens in advance for years, and have no time left for outside labour.

And last, and (perhaps) not least, Why don't I send in a Play? Because I *have* tried to write *one*, and find I can't quite manage it!

ACCORDING to recent accounts, the attitude of the Salvation Army in Canada may be fairly described as "Revolting."

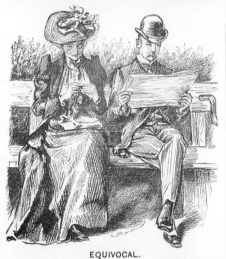

EQUIVOCAL.

Rising Young Physician (who cured so many Patients in last year's Epidemic). "NOT MUCH CHANCE OF MORE INFLUENZA IN ENGLAND *THIS* WINTER, I FANCY!"
His Wife. "LET US HOPE FOR THE BEST, DEAREST!"

A DIARY OF THE DEAD SEASON.

(Suggested by the Contents Bills.)

Monday.—First appearance of "the Epidemic." Good bold line with reference to Russia. Not of sufficient importance to head the Bill, but still distinctly taking.

Tuesday.—Quite a feature. Centre of the Bill with sub-lines of "Horrible Disclosures," and "Painful Scenes." Becoming a boom. To be further developed to-morrow.

Wednesday.— Bill all "Epidemic." Even Cricket sacrificed to make room for it. "News from Abroad." "Horrors at Hamburg." No idea it would turn out so well. A perfect treasure-trove at this quiet season of the year !

Thursday.—Nothing but "Epidemic"—"Arrival in England" — "Precautions Everywhere." Let the boom go! It feeds itself! Nearly as good as a foreign war !

Friday.—Still "the Epidemic," but requires strengthening. "Spreading in the Provinces," but still, not like it was. Falling flat.

Saturday.—A good sensational Murder ! The very thing for the Contents Bills. Exit "the Epidemic," until again wanted.

125   George Du Maurier 'EQUIVOCAL', wood engraving, from *Punch*, 10 September 1892.

The captioning reads: '*Rising Young Physician (who cured so many Patients in last year's Epidemic).* "NOT MUCH CHANCE OF MORE INFLUENZA IN ENGLAND *THIS* WINTER, I FANCY!" *His Wife.* "LET US HOPE FOR THE BEST, DEAREST!".'

demand. For some things worked out nicely; a senior practitioner in a cathedral city, serving as honorary physician to the local voluntary hospital, might be fortunate both in income and in status. But such were in a minority. For many GPs the winds blew chill in Victorian times, since the profession was growing overstocked (illus. 125). As a young GP in Southsea, Arthur Conan Doyle took to writing detective stories because he had so few patients. Not many doctors secured a competent living and all that entailed, including the ability to marry respectably and raise a family, before they were middle-aged. Most remained overworked, on call at all hours, 52 weeks a year. They had to be unfailingly civil – or, as they all too often experienced it, servile – to socially superior patients, willing to bear with snobs and slow payers, and inured to bad debts. The nineteenth century thus produced a paradox. The fortunes of the rank-and-file remained precarious at precisely the time when the state finally recognized the crucial importance to the nation's well-being of medicine and public health.

The Victorian era was an age of idealism and hero-worship, if also, inevitably, one strewn with fallen idols.[9] 'Of the three learned professions, the medical has attained the highest character for disinterestedness', ventured *The Times*, in a somewhat backhanded compliment, on 25 January 1856:

> Hard things are being said of the cupidity of the clergy, the wealth of certain benefices affording a strange contrast to the poverty of the primitive church; still harder things are being said of the lawyers ... but there is probably no class of the community so free from mercenary motives as the members of the medical and surgical profession.[10]

In Victorian fiction the Smollettian brute was replaced by the medical man of the highest ideals, if also tragic flaws. A product of the 1815 Apothecaries Act, the general practitioner – a man like Anthony Trollope's Dr Thorne in the novel of that name – was elevated heroically onto a pedestal in fictions and essays.[11]

Published in 1838, Harriet Martineau's *Deerbrook* centres on Edward Hope, a bachelor practitioner described by a local as being 'one of the two greatest boosts of the town'.[12] His services are valued by all strata of the community from the squire – intriguingly called Sir William Hunter! – down to the scold. His approach is always cheerful and positive; all confide in him and he never betrays a confidence. When cholera strikes, the squire, petrified of infection, barricades himself in on his estate, and no one offers moral leadership but Hope and the parson. Although there is little he can do medically to stay the epidemic, the practitioner sets an inspiring example and vigorously applies such relief as he can, through hygiene, quarantine, wholesome food and clean clothing.

At the novel's climax, Hope hauls himself off his own sickbed to visit Matilda, the dying daughter of the spiteful gossip who has laboured to ruin his practice. A personification of Christian charity – the doctor as the new pastor – he declares he will do everything in his power to save her. She perishes nevertheless, but her stricken mother, reading her daughter's death as a judgment on herself, repents. After the cholera's purgatorial visitation, the town is healed and united, and the good doctor, more popular than ever, is reinstalled in his practice.

Edward Hope embodies the personal qualities of the Victorian doctor-hero, a figure, as we have seen, quite unknown to earlier fiction. He transcends his own suffering to heal his community through selfless dedication, demonstrates moral leadership in a vacuum, while being attacked by the unworthy – as well as being unlucky in love.

Tertius Lydgate, the doctor-hero of *Middlemarch*, written in the 1870s but set in those crucial years of cholera and reform, 1829–31, believes that 'the medical profession as it might be was the finest in the world, presenting the most direct alliance between intellectual

258

conquest and social good'.[13] Soaring above prejudice and gossip, George Eliot's protagonist is an idealist, as hard on himself as he is on others. A humanitarian reformer, Lydgate uncompromisingly tries to work independently of a corrupt town and its old-fashioned medical establishment. He too is unlucky in love.

As is demonstrated by his commitment to medical research, Lydgate is a man of intellectual promise, who strives to do 'great work for the world' by pursuing experimentation into tissue pathology in the new French research medicine style, and 'good small work for Middlemarch' by directing a new fever hospital. His dream is to make a great discovery whilst working in the provinces, like his hero Edward Jenner, so as to keep 'away from the ranges of London intrigues, jealousies, and social truckling'. In advance of his times in using a stethoscope (another foreign innovation) as well as being an experimentalist (see the discussion in Chapters 4 and 8), he also has novel ideas about the treatment of cholera.[14] But his judgment is flawed by naivety, pride and overconfidence.

Casting himself in the roles of medical reformer, scientist and pillar of public spiritedness, Lydgate has complete faith in his own perspicacity. Bluntly deriding and overriding their diagnoses, he makes no attempt to conciliate his fellow professionals; and he also scorns routine drug-dispensing, that standby of the other practitioners, to say nothing of the lay medical folklore of Lady Chetham's circle (see Chapter 6) – in that sense, he may be seen as Thomas Beddoes reincarnate, zealous for modern medical science. 'A young doctor', Lydgate is told, 'has to please his patients in Middlemarch': he will have none of that.[15] In place of traditional therapies, those entrenched strengthening and lowering treatments, he prefers expectant therapy and the healing power of nature.[16]

His idealistic schemes are shattered, however, by debt and a miserable marriage and, even as he tries to distance himself from the ways of the world, he succumbs to the tyrannical power of vested interests. His association with the banker Bulstrode blights him professionally after the latter has been exposed as a humbug, swindler and possible homicide. And because his wife Rosamund is determined to go places, Lydgate cannot remain in Middlemarch to outface his critics. Though wishing to stay on, so as to re-establish his reputation, he admits defeat: 'I am no longer sure enough of myself ... I must do as other men do.' His subsequent living death as a modish London specialist is portrayed as a tragic waste, because he began so nobly and was not 'like other men'. Instead of a 'great work', his gift to the world turns out to be a treatise on gout, that footling aristocratic complaint, and he 'always regarded himself as a failure: he had not done what he once meant to do'.[17] If doctors in Georgian novels, Smollett's for instance, were riddled with personal vices, in Victorian novels they were much more likely to be used to exemplify the towering obstacles to noble attempts to reform the world.

In that hero-worshipping century, the profession was increasingly biographized, a tradition launched by John Aikin's *Biographical Memoirs of Medicine in Great Britain* (1780), Benjamin Hutchinson's *Biographia Medica* (1799) and other works of reference.[18] The new idealization of, and quest for, professional respectability were also reflected in portraiture, in due course through the medium of photography. Eminent Victorian doctors got their faces into popular general photograph albums, for example Fry's *National Gallery of Photographic Portraits* (1858).

There were also two exclusively medical series that achieved prominence, *Photographs of Eminent Medical Men of All Countries with Brief Analytical Notices of their Works* (1867-8) and *The Medical Profession of All Countries Containing Photographic Portraits from Life* (1873-5).[19] In all such works, as well as in the portraits that lined the corridors and stairwells of the London Colleges, medics (now, for the first time since the Stuarts, sporting dignifying facial hair) were invariably depicted as soberly respectable, clad in greys and blacks with the exception of their academic scarlet.[20] There was a return, as in so many respects, to the moral aesthetics of Tudor and Stuart times, newly aided by mass-reproduction.

Yet while such engravings and photograph albums were praised for making likenesses of contemporary notables widely available, they were also liable to be attacked in squalls that blew up over the ethical guidelines for professional behaviour. Showiness, as ever, was suspect to puritan stricture, and the publication of portraits of practising medical men was condemned in some quarters as a reprehensible form of ostentation, self-advertisement and professional cheapening.

Qualms over self-promotion had a history. Back in March 1838, the *Lancet* had launched a short-lived 'Gallery of Medical Portraits', which featured biographical essays illustrated with lithographs. During the next couple of years Thomas Joseph Pettigrew brought out his *Medical Portrait Gallery: Biographies of the Most Celebrated Physicians, Surgeons etc. Who Have Contributed to the Advancement of Medical Science*, which offered 60 biographies and portraits of historical and contemporary figures. In the wake of Pettigrew's success, the *Lancet* ran a second series from 1850 to 1851. A rival, the

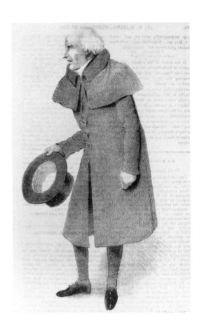

126 J. K. Meadows, portrait of Sir William Blizard, from *Lancet*, 15 June 1833.

Born in 1743, and living through to 1835, Blizard, who was surgeon to the London Hospital, was a practitioner of the old school noted for his formalities of dress.

Medical Circular, began a series of its own in 1852, using daguerreotypes.

The first of these graphic series devoted to medical men was polemical and pernickety: unsurprisingly, Wakley used the pen-portraits accompanying the 1838 *Lancet* pictures to trounce corruption and incompetence in medical institutions – the potted biographies were widely thought libellous. Sir William Blizard (illus. 126), for instance, senior surgeon to the London Hospital, was paraded as a 'sorry spectacle', well known for his 'collegiate scowl' and 'hospital vulgarity'.

By contrast to Wakley's censures, Pettigrew adopted a far more neutral, indeed lofty, tone for the biographies in the *Medical Portrait Gallery*, his stated aim being to write 'professional' rather than 'personal' biography, avoiding both sycophancy and spite.

What worried those who made a parade of ethical concerns was that journal editors and publishers, to say nothing of the individuals featured, stood to profit from such celebrity series: advantage would be taken of interest in the profession's leaders, it was alleged, in order to boost circulation, while, by design or not, the individuals featured would also benefit financially from such publicity. These were matters of consequence to a profession under scrutiny, newly anxious, particularly after the founding of the General Medical Council in 1858, about occupational ethics, etiquette and its own public image.[21] Despite such criticisms and condemnations, portrait series continued to make their appearance, however, the elite of the profession in effect endorsing the publications by cooperating in their compilation.

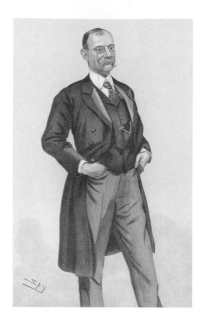

127 Sir Leslie Matthew Ward ('Spy'), portrait of Sir Frederick Treves (1853–1923), 1900, colour lithograph.

Treves was one of the most fashionable surgeons of the late Victorian and Edwardian eras, a man of letters as well as a celebrated doctor. He famously performed an appendectomy on Edward VII just before his coronation and was the 'protector' of Joseph Merrick, the 'Elephant Man'.

Overall, the practitioner emerged in the Victorian novel and in Victorian art as a sympathetic and honourable figure, to be looked up to, or at least to be accepted socially. Harley Street was becoming a name to conjure with; and Victorian media-mongers set the profession on a pedestal, as is further evident in the handsome and flattering caricature portraits of society doctors which appeared in *Vanity Fair* and elsewhere, the work of such distinguished caricaturists as 'Ape' and 'Spy' (illus. 127).[22] Though the late Georgian era, the Regency in particular, was the golden age of satirical caricature, it did not create a regular magazine specializing in the genre. The advent of such a publication was prompted by the appearance in 1830 across the Channel of Charles Philipon's *La Caricature*, and the subsequent daily *Charivari*.[23] First hitting the news-stands on 17 July 1841, *Punch*, in homage to its French precursor, carried as its subtitle *The London Charivari*.[24] It was a significant departure from its English satirical predecessors. One major factor in its success was its innovative layout. Whereas Henry Mayhew's earlier *Figaro in London* had dished up a rather dreary and samey diet of single fonts, from the outset *Punch* displayed greater variety, with comic drawings liberally scattered throughout.[25] Furthermore, as Regency ribaldry gave way to the Victorian ideal of domestic propriety – 'the comic works of past years', observed William Thackeray, 'are sealed to our wives and daughters' – opportunities opened up for a good-humoured and respectable family publication. *Punch* filled that gap. Unlike earlier publications, it avoided coarseness and vulgarity if, at least in its early days, satisfying the craving for a critical political platform in tune with an age of reform.[26] The tastes, preoccupations and anxieties of the growing middle class were Mr Punch's too, who specified as his three self-appointed tasks 'teaching', 'reforming' and 'jollifying'.

At first the illustrations, mainly little black cuts, served as adjuncts to the articles: recourse to freestanding caricature, independent of text, came later. Artwork was initially regarded as secondary to the printed word – indeed the draughtsmen were not treated as socially on a par with the writers.[27]

In addition to such 'blackies', *Punch* featured 'the Big-Cut', an entire page devoted to a humorous drawing, its model being the Paris *Charivari*. Initially titled 'Mr. Punch's Pencillings' – the term 'cartoon' was not adopted until July 1843 – this regular satirical sketch proved immensely popular. The subjects for the small cuts and 'pencillings' alike were various: politicians, the Crown, professional men, street life and social mores, and a favourite motif was the domestic scene: the parlour, the nursery, the family and the everyday pursuits and passions of the bourgeoisie. The first 'big-cut' of a medico-political nature appeared in the opening volume. In *Animal-Magnetism: Sir Rhubarb*

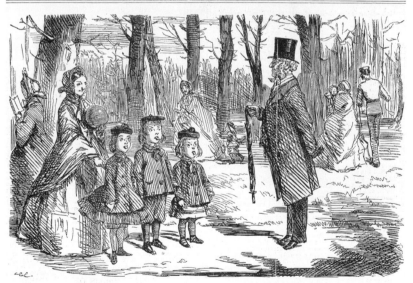

146   PUNCH, OR THE LONDON CHARIVARI.   [APRIL 6, 1861.

FORCE OF HABIT.—(A TABLEAU FOR FAMILY PEOPLE ONLY.)

ADOLPHUS, GEORGE, AND LOUISA, ARE PLAYING IN KENSINGTON GARDENS—TO THEM THE FAMILY DOCTOR UNEXPECTEDLY. A. AND G. AND L. GO THROUGH THE EXPRESSIVE PANTOMIME OF PUTTING OUT THEIR TONGUES AS A MATTER OF COURSE.

128 'FORCE OF HABIT. — (A TABLEAU FOR FAMILY PEOPLE ONLY)', wood engraving (after John Leech), from *Punch*, 6 April 1861.

Pill Mesmerising the British Lion, Robert Peel was transformed by the serendipitous verbal echoes of his moniker into 'Rhubarb Pill'.[28] Behind this image of a frock-coated quack there stands a container labelled 'Grand Electric Politico Battery', imprinted with the names of the various topical issues, such as the 'pension list' and 'new taxes', which 'Rhubarb Pill' would have to settle on succeeding Lord Melbourne as Prime Minister.

Also in the first volume Peel was elevated, in highly traditional manner, to the status of 'state physician' in William Newman's *Mr. Sancho Bull and his State Physician*, where, elaborately cloaked and bewigged, he stops the corpulent John Bull from enjoying victuals being presented to him. The caption, 'A Quote from Don Quixote', reads: 'Though surrounded with luxuries, the Doctor would not allow Sancho to partake of them, and dismissed each dish as it was brought in by the servants' – the roguish servant in this case being a villainous-looking Lord John Russell. The founder of the modern Conservative Party thereafter materialized in *Punch* in many guises; as a child and a nurse, not to speak of a doctor of state.

While espousing broadly middle-class values and opinions, *Punch* expressed no single medical party line. Its take on doctors and medical issues was, in large measure, left to the taste of its stream of talented draughtsmen. It is worth briefly differentiating them and their distinctive styles.

The arrival of John Leech in 1844 marked a new era for the periodical's artists, and he eclipsed all who came before him, his prodigious output over the course of two decades approaching 3,000 drawings, including some 600 cartoons.[29] Leech did not relish churning out political sketches, and by the 1850s he was moving away from them and beginning to embrace his true loves, which he made the great *Punch* staples: family life and the servants, hunting and holidays.[30] Characteristic of these tastes was a cartoon carried in the April 1861 issue, 'FORCE OF HABIT – (A TABLEAU FOR FAMILY PEOPLE ONLY)' (illus. 128). The composition features a bunch of youngsters. At play in Kensington Gardens, Adolphus, George and Louisa are caught poking out their tongues not rudely but courteously, as a matter of habit when the family doctor happens to pass by. What lends this drawing some poignancy is the fact that the physician could just as easily have been Leech himself. He had studied medicine at St Bartholomew's where he won some repute for his superb anatomical drawings. Constrained by his father's straitened circumstances, however, he was unable to complete his training; shortly before his twenty-first birthday, he abandoned his medical studies in order to shore up the family's failing

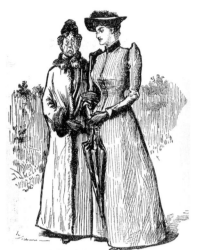

129 George Du Maurier, 'THE IMPORTANCE OF EXTERNALS.', wood engraving, from *Punch*, 9 July 1892.

The captioning reads: "'BUT WHY DON'T YOU SEND FOR DR. MASHER, AUNT JANE? HE'S THE CLEVEREST DOCTOR IN THE WHOLE COUNTY!' 'OH, MY DEAR, I COULDN'T! HE *DRESSES* SO IRRELIGIOUSLY!'"

THE IMPORTANCE OF EXTERNALS.

fortunes, supporting his father (who outlived him) all his adult life.[31]

The great George Du Maurier contributed his first drawing in October 1860. Like Leech, at an early age he too had changed the direction of his career plans, switching from science to painting, and learning his craft at Antwerp and Paris. Introduced to *Punch*'s editor Mark Lemon, he agreed to provide some illustrations for the periodical[32] and, after Leech's death, he joined the staff in 1864.

In Du Maurier's hands the physician came to assume a far more rarefied air, even approximating to that of an aesthete (illus. 129). Better bred than Leech's medical men, the superior profile of Du Maurier's physicians would not be out of place in London's elite drawing-rooms (or drawing-room comedies) – with their debonair looks and nonchalant demeanour there is little in their appearance to suggest that they are not gentlemen to the manor born. Much as depicted in prints such as these, the stereotypical Victorian physician has been described by David Piper as 'bald on top ... but compensating by cultivation of undergrowth lower down. Silk-faced, frock-coat, trousers, gloves, and immaculate top hat, though with no trace of a stethoscope bulge.'[33] Du Maurier reflected and largely endorsed, if gently mocking, the growing social aspirations – or pretensions – of the Victorian physician.

In course of time, and under Du Maurier's influence, the target of *Punch*'s satire shifted from the physician himself – invariably the butt in the Georgian and Regency eras – to the ignorance and obtuseness of the (typically lower-class) patient.[34] Time and again, Du Maurier and others found the common man's incomprehension of a physician's

265

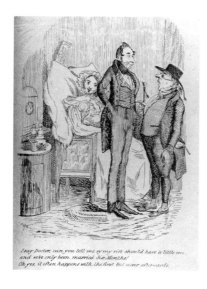

130 This undated engraving, though not a *Punch* cartoon, is indicative of mid-Victorian humour. The captioning reads: "'I say Doctor, can you tell me vy my vife should have a little one, and ve've only been married Six Months!' / "Oh yes, it often happens with the first but never afterwards.'"

diagnosis or advice a subject worthy of his wit (illus. 130). In a hospital scene called *A Lucid Diagnosis*, a gardener is made to say:

> Well Miss, I don't know what they call it; but the young medical gentleman as looked after me, he says:- 'What you've got in your 'ed, he says, 'im as lies in the next bed to you, he've got in 'is hinside.'

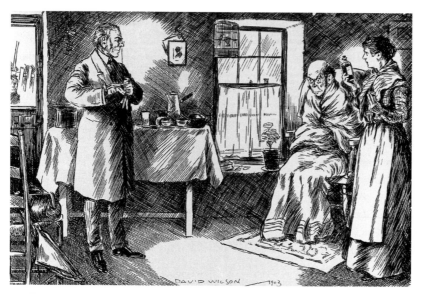

131 David Wilson, wood engraving, from *Punch*, 7 October 1903.
    The dialogue reads: '*Doctor*. "Well, Mrs O'Brien, I hope your husband has taken his Medicine regularly, eh?" / *Mrs. O'Brien*. "Sure, then, Docthor, I've been sorely puzzled. The label says, 'One Pill to be taken three times a day,' and for the life of me I don't see how it can be taken more than *once*!"'

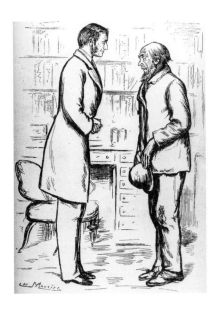

132 George Du Maurier, 'DIAGNOSIS.', wood engraving, from *Punch*, 23 January 1875.

The dialogue reads: 'I CAN TELL YOU WHAT *YOU'RE* SUFFERING FROM, MY GOOD FELLOW! YOU'RE SUFFERING FROM *ACNE*! / *ACKNEY*? WHY, THAT'S JUST WHAT THE *T'OTHER* MEDICAL GENT HE TOLD ME*! I ONLY WISH I'D NEVER BEEN NEAR THE PLACE!'*

Dozens of cartoons in this vein patronized and mocked the ignorance of working-class patients, often rendered doubly stupid as illiterate and illogical Irish or stingy Scots (illus. 131). If Cockneys could equally be represented as vulgar, sometimes they possessed a certain earthy intuition (illus. 132).

Charles Keene joined *Punch* in 1851 and was still providing copy into the 1880s. Like Leech and Du Maurier, he had been earmarked for another career, in his case the law – hence the ambiguous and insecure status of professional men may well have been as close to his heart as it was to Leech. By the age of sixteen he had already developed a love of drawing. Moving to *Punch*, his first signed illustration appeared on 3 June 1854,[35] though it was not until 1860 that he was 'called to the table' to join such dignitaries as Leech, Tenniel (the illustrator of *Alice in Wonderland*) and Thackeray.[36]

Though he relied on others for his jokes, Keene's own renderings of them proved enormously popular, for he had the knack of freezing a humorous moment. In *Mistimed Pleasantry*, another of the perennially popular dentist jokes, the caption has the dentist declaring 'Oh, my dear Sir! There's no necessity to open your mouth so wide. I can do it from the outside easily, I assure you!' Knees locked, with his hands jammed between them, the nervous patient has terror writ large in his eyes. His body bent forward in anticipation, head raised in a 'trust me' fashion, clasping what looks more like a spanner than a piece of dental equipment, the dentist for his part can hardly wait to get his hands on the patient's jaw. The petrified patient is the most common of *Punch*'s dental vignettes.[37] With its psychological insights, there is a marked contrast to the physical coarseness of the dentist jokes of the Georgian era.

'Bred up in the *Punch* tradition', Harry Furniss was employed on the weekly from 1880.[38] While still at school in Ireland he produced, edited and illustrated 'The Schoolboy's Punch' in longhand, in pious homage to the original.[39] Furniss was closer in spirit to his Georgian and Regency predecessors than some of the other *Punch* artists, his views on society and his jibes against specific public figures being quite caustic.[40] In *Doctor Dubitans* a crazed-looking physician blurts out: 'I'm afraid I've given him the wrong stuff,' 'him' being a ghostly infant in the grip of extreme and presumably terminal pain. An ominous grey shadow lurks in the background, terror etched on its face. In this unflattering view, the physician has taken on the appearance of a madman. Furniss was certainly not bound by narrow Victorian convention; his humour and caustic wit were unbridled, and some of his finest caricatures were bitterly resented.[41]

'Already in the foremost rank of humorous draughtsmen of the day',[42] Phil May joined *Punch* at the age of 30 and was offered a position 'at the table' in February 1895.[43] His arrival coincided serendipitously with the new photographic process of reproduction – lucky timing as May was the master of the graphic epigram, and his dynamic lines would have lost a great deal had they been dependent on wood.[44] His subjects were largely taken from the street: urchins, strays, waifs and newspaper sellers. In a typical instance (illus. 133), the caption reads:

> Patient: 'What would you think of a warmer climate for me, Doctor?'

> Doctor: 'Good Heavens, Sir, That's just what I am trying to save you from!'

As can be seen, in stark contrast to Furniss's demented doctor, May's medical man is elegance itself: with his high collar, waistcoat and handkerchief in his coat top pocket, the physician is self-possessed, understated, conservative and quite terrifyingly sound.

The image of the medical man in *Punch* changed considerably from 1841 to 1914. For the first 40 years the artists followed what has been called 'the academic tradition'.[45] Taking the form of portraits, the illustrations were, for the most part, representations of medical men, phenotypically and physiognomically rather as the profession might have wished itself to be seen, if pompous in its postures.[46]

At the same time *Punch* provided a joking and rather conservative running commentary upon developments within the medical profes-

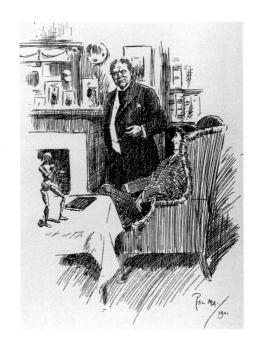

133 Phil May, wood engraving, from *Punch*, 30 October 1901.

The comfortable armchair and artist's mannequin hint at the patient's lifestyle. The captioning reads: *Patient*. 'WHAT WOULD YOU THINK OF A WARMER CLIMATE FOR ME, DOCTOR?' *Doctor*. 'GOOD HEAVENS, SIR, THAT'S JUST WHAT I AM TRYING TO SAVE YOU FROM!'

sion and medical politics. For an instance of that, let us look, very briefly, at just one issue, the emergence of the professional female doctor, against the backdrop of the more general movement for female emancipation.

Though, as indicated in Chapter 7, women had always been engaged in practical healing, in 1800 they were professionally excluded, not least because they were barred from university. Reactionaries warned that young ladies were unfit for higher education: dominated by her ovaries, a woman's place was in the home as wife and mother. Over-exercise of the brain would divert energy from the womb and lead to sterility and hysteria – and anyway, medicine was no profession for a lady!

The first woman to qualify in Britain was Elizabeth Garrett, who exploited various legal loopholes to obtain the diploma of the Society of Apothecaries in 1865, thereby securing enrolment on the Medical Register. Indefatigable in her efforts in pressing for women's acceptance in the profession, by 1870 she had developed an extensive private practice, established St Mary's Dispensary for Women in London, received a medical degree from the University of Paris and married the wealthy James Anderson. She was instrumental in the establishment in 1874 of the London School of Medicine for Women, and through a further bureaucratic oversight was also admitted to the British Medical Association, which did not officially enrol women until 1892.

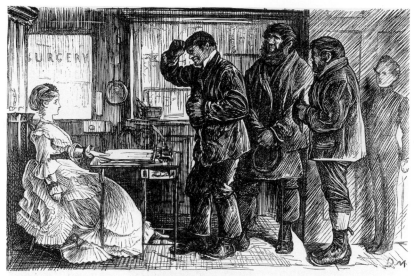

OUR PRETTY DOCTOR.

134 George Du Maurier, 'OUR PRETTY DOCTOR.', wood engraving, from *Punch*, 13 August 1870.

The dialogue reads: '*Dr. Arabella*. "WELL, MY GOOD FRIENDS, WHAT CAN I DO FOR YOU?" / *Bill.* "WELL, MISS, IT'S ALL ALONG O' ME AND MY MATES BEIN'OUT O' WORK, YER SEE, AND WANTIN' TO TURN AN HONEST PENNY HANYWAYS WE CAN; SO, 'AVIN 'EARD TELL'AS *YOU* WAS A RISIN' YOUNG MEDICAL PRACTITIONER, WE THOUGHT AS P'RAPS YOU WOULDN'T MIND JUST A RECOMMENDIN' OF *HUS* AS NURSES."'

The main battleground in the educational war was Edinburgh University, thanks to campaigns waged by Sophia Jex-Blake. After being refused by London University, she was admitted as a student to Edinburgh, matriculating in 1869 with four other female students. But complaints to the University Court led to their being disqualified from graduation and offered as a sop mere 'certificates of proficiency'. Amidst student riots, an appeal against this ruling was first upheld then overturned.

The battling Jex-Blake, who had meanwhile taken her MD in Berne, eventually became licensed through the College of Physicians in Ireland. She opened the London School of Medicine for Women in 1874, and three years later female medical students gained access to clinical experience through the London (later the Royal) Free Hospital. An Act of Parliament in 1876 finally empowered examining bodies to allow women to qualify. Resistance remained strong, however: St Mary's Hospital Medical School in London, which finally let female students in during the crisis of the First World War, later barred them again, since the School prided itself on its rugby team.

Punch offered readers many cartoons featuring the new women

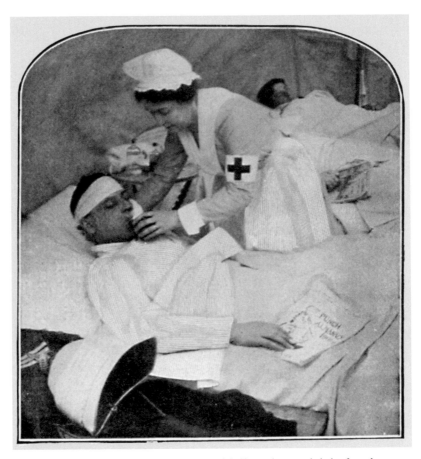

135 'In a field hospital on the Tugela River.', halftone photograph dating from the
Second Boer War, c. 1900.

practitioners (illus. 134). It would be an exaggeration to say that they
were standardly misogynistic or overtly hostile to female practice.
There is no doubt however that the tenor of the cartoons, as in the
example here, was to find the intrusion of the gender element into
medicine, and female practice itself, odd and intrinsically mirthful. By
contrast, the new post-Nightingale nurse could readily be idealized.
She was no threat to professional males, be they doctors or general
readers of *Punch*. No longer was the nurse the terrifying figure as
depicted by Rowlandson or Cruikshank (illus. 135).

In the devoted nurse or general practitioner, the Victorians found or
fantasized medical personnel with whom they could at last feel
comfortable. Jesting Death has virtually been expelled.

Afterword

The chapters of this book have examined the body beliefs and medical practices of early modern England from a distinctive angle, the public representations of them in a variety of media, verbal and visual. My discussions have focused upon perceptions of embodiment; being healthy and falling ill; the symbiotic relations which linked the sick to their medical attendants; and, more broadly, the various occupational incarnations of the healing arts; and they have also glanced at the wider metaphorical and symbolic meanings of health and sickness for society and politics.

The approach used is illuminating and fruitful for many reasons. The cultural conventions of early modern times were highly prescriptive with respect to the comportment and performances of the body, beautiful or ugly, noble or base, sacred or profane, clean or dirty, healthy or sick. As argued in Chapters 2 and 3, in face-to-face pre-industrial times, man was still very largely the measure of all things, created by a God pictured anthropomorphically and patriarchally as a Father, and tellingly as an author or artist. Yet prevailing religio-moral values also disparaged the body, and made its display and demonstration (enactments required, sanctioned and approved in specified social and aesthetic contexts) also matters of potential denigration, dishonour and danger.

Social life involved systems within systems of publicly prescribed rituals and performances, which were explicitly considered dramaturgically as scenes in the play of life, be that tragedy or comedy, satire or farce; all individuals had their prescribed parts to play, their props and togs, in the staging of the ages of man from cradle to grave within the great *theatrum mundi*.[1]

More specifically, the microcosm of medicine itself was a costume drama or a travelling circus, embodied in performance, rhetoric and ritual. Illness had to make itself known, had to become audible and visible; patients adopted what sociologists later called the 'sick role',[2] while it was recognized that the conduct of healing was inseparable from accredited routines and repertoires of therapeutic stage-management by the healing arts, employing the placebo effect.

In a Protestant nation in an age of critical reason, however, theatricality was widely censured – above all by those of a puritan, reformist, or utilitarian temper – as mindless artifice, magic and mumbo–jumbo, an idolatrous infatuation with tawdry tinsel and specious show. And likewise, more narrowly in healing itself, critics loved to unmask and debunk the pomp and circumstance of physic, maintaining that it was all verbosity and vain pretence – indeed that the whole of medicine was, if truth be known, barely better (perhaps even worse) than arrant quackery. Medical men and sympathetic observers might, for their part, counter that the efficaciousness of healing actually, and quite properly, rested on confidence created by words and looks and by the power of suggestion conveyed by solemn utterances and gestures. If medicine worked, where lay the harm if it was, more or less, all a matter of confidence, a suspension of disbelief?

It has further been part of the argument of this book that medicine was particularly perceived as stagy because of developments not merely within the healing arts but integral to the arts themselves. Supplementing the ever popular theatre, that perennial analogue and metaphor for healing,[3] newspapers, magazines, novels, portraits, satirical prints and other media developments bred all manner of images of healing; making, breaking and remaking the identities of patients and practitioners alike. The post-Restoration age brought explosive cultural production; and the consequent proliferation of verbal and visual forms created and reinforced in the public imagination narratives and images of the sick, their healers and healing-related performances. Other offshoots of commercial culture, for instance the spa and the seaside resort, multiplied sites for public medical spectacle. There was much doubling between doctors and men of letters, the sons of Aesculapius and of Apollo; the satirist wielded the scalpel, and literature touted social diagnosis and political cure. 'I pretended, when I first set up, to astrology only; but, I am told, I have deep skill also in medicine,' Mr Spectator tells us:

> Having taken upon me to cure all the distempers which proceed from affections of the mind, I have laboured, since I first kept this public stage, to do all the good I could, and have perfected many cures at my own lodgings; carefully avoiding the common methods of mountebanks, to do their most common operations in sight of the people.[4]

The profusion of such cultural games, and the longevity of certain jokes and tropes which just ran and ran (illus. 136, 137) betoken the fact

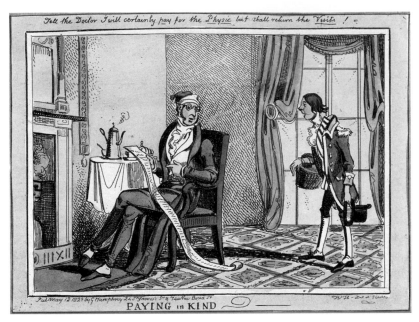

136 William Heath, 'PAYING IN KIND', 1823, etching with watercolour.

The captioning reads: 'Tell the doctor I will certainly pay for the Physic but shall return the Visits!' The same joke appears nearly a century later in the cartoon which follows, though the servant has made way for the wife.

that matters of health and sickness, life and death were close to the bone. I have, however, desisted from speculating as to the nature of the psychological appeal, conscious or subliminal, of what is so often the black comedy of representations of pain, risible patients, repulsive physicians and disgusting treatments. Terror and humour have myriad functions and crisscross in many ways. Not unimportant, in my view, is the likelihood that, in the teeth of the distress and danger of sickness and possible death, the banal familiarity offered by stock narratives, jests, icons and rituals was in itself a source of comfort: forewarned was forearmed. In offering conjectures upon the visual images here presented, I hope at least I haven't been just a latter-day Julep or Apozem, dogmatizing my erroneous readings or missing what was under my nose all along.

It has not been part of my argument in this book, but it may serve as a final suggestion, that certain aspects of the potent early-modern 'theatre of medicine' have faded in more recent times. Medicine, of course, assumes great prominence in modern mass media: the last half-century has brought *Dr Kildare* and *Emergency Ward Ten*, endless Mills and Boon novelettes, the affectionate humour of Richard Gordon's *Doctor in the House* (laddish medical students, in the mould of Bob

274

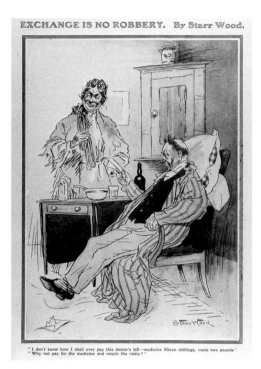

EXCHANGE IS NO ROBBERY. By Starr Wood.

"I don't know how I shall ever pay this doctor's bill—medicine fifteen shillings, visits two pounds"
"Why not pay for the medicine and return the visits?"

137 'EXCHANGE IS NO ROBBERY.', photomechanical reproduction after Starr Wood, from *The Tatler*, 22 March 1911.
The dialogue includes this comment: '"I don't know how I shall ever pay this doctor's bill – medicine fifteen shillings, visits two pounds." / "Why not pay for the medicine and return the visits?"'

Sawyer, always come good in the end), *Dr Finlay's Casebook* and *Casualty*, *ER* and *Chicago Hope*.[5] And, very recently, in the wake of a spate of scandals, particularly that of the mass-murderer GP Harold Shipman, the doctor has once more begun to seem a prime source of danger. But the human body undergoing medicine and surgery is no longer a fundamental template for satire, nor does the doctor any longer assume pride of place in political cartoons as a surrogate for the statesman. The rise to dominance of high-tech hospital medicine has much to do with this – despite the continuing idiom of the 'operating theatre'. To say this is not to imply that medicine itself has been de-ritualized and de-moralized into 'science', merely that modern medicine does not lend itself to the body-centred takes of patients and healers (knife clenched between the teeth) which have formed the core subject matter of this study.

References

Preface

1 Barbara Maria Stafford, *Body Criticism. Imaging the Unseen in Enlightenment Art and Medicine* (Cambridge, MA, 1991), p. 2.

2 A point made in Leonard Shlain's polemical *The Alphabet versus the Goddess. Male Words and Female Images* (London, 1999).

3 One complication, not further addressed, is that alongside the widespread suspicion of *images* has gone a suspicion of *words* too, when perceived to be rhetorical, mere verbiage. Just as words are 'better' than images, so 'reality' is better than 'verbality': see Peter Dear, '*Totius in Verba*: Rhetoric and Authority in the Early Royal Society', *Isis*, LXXVI (1985), pp. 145–61.

4 The best general discussion, though focused on the upper end of the market, is Timothy Clayton, *The English Print, 1688–1802* (New Haven and London, 1997). For portraits, see David Piper, *The English Face*, ed. Malcolm Rogers (London, 1992); Marcia Pointon, *Hanging the Head: Portraiture and Social Formation in Eighteenth-Century England* (New Haven, 1993).

5 There are scores of early Dutch conversation pieces around such themes as the medical consultation or the examination of a young woman for love-sickness; there is no equivalent English tradition: Laurinda S. Dixon, *Perilous Chastity: Women and Illness in Pre-Enlightenment Art and Medicine* (Ithaca, 1995).

6 The interplay of image and text is brought out especially by Ronald Paulson, *Book and Painting: Shakespeare, Milton and the Bible: Literary Texts and the Emergence of English Painting* (Knoxville, 1982); and by Robert Patten, ed., *George Cruikshank: A Revaluation* (Princeton, 1992), pp. 38f.

7 Quotation is of course ubiquitous within culture. A different sort of example is Tobias Smollett's novel *The Life and Adventures of Sir Launcelot Greaves* (1760-2), the story of two lovers incarcerated in a madhouse to prevent their marriage. The novel contains many pages plagiarised from Dr William Battie's *Treatise on Madness* (1758), but Smollett concealed his source.

8 Though for such a possibility see Peter Burke, *Eyewitnessing* (London, 2001).

9 The obsolete assumption that Georgian prints are snapshots of reality is discussed in Roy Porter, 'Capital Art: Hogarth's London', in F. Ogée, ed., *The Dumb Show. Image and Society in the Works of William Hogarth* (Oxford, Studies on Voltaire and the Eighteenth Century, 1997), pp. 47–64; for warnings against accepting medical photographs at face value, see Daniel M. Fox and Christopher Lawrence, *Photographing Medicine: Images and Power in Britain and America Since 1840* (Westport and London, 1988).

10 Roy Porter and Dorothy Porter, *In Sickness and in Health: The British Experience 1650–1850* (London, 1988); Dorothy Porter and Roy Porter, *Patient's Progress: Doctors and Doctoring in Eighteenth-Century England* (Cambridge, 1989); Roy Porter,

Health for Sale: Quackery in England 1650–1850 (Manchester, 1989); *idem, Mind Forg'd Manacles: Madness and Psychiatry in England from Restoration to Regency* (London, 1987). One might add *idem, Doctor of Society: Thomas Beddoes and the Sick Trade in Late Enlightenment England* (London, 1991), which looks at that medical world through the eyes of a radical physician.

11 Roy Porter, *Quacks: Fakers and Charlatans in English Medicine* (Stroud, 2000).

1 Introductory: Framing the Picture

1   The most rewarding discussion for me has been Peter Wagner, *Reading Iconotexts: From Swift to the French Revolution* (London, 1995).

2   For whom see Chap. 7.

3   Francis Doherty, *A Study in Eighteenth-Century Advertising Methods: The Anodyne Necklace* (Lewiston, 1992); Fiona Haslam, *From Hogarth to Rowlandson. Medicine in Art in Eighteenth-Century Britain* (Liverpool, 1996), p. 73.

4   C. J. S. Thompson, *The Quacks of Old London* (London, 1928), p. 312. Rock also figures on an advertising billboard in Hogarth's *Morning* from *The Four Times of the Day*.

5   The contents are very fully discussed in Haslam, *From Hogarth to Rowlandson*, pp. 106 f. Our knowledge of Misaubin has been greatly enlarged by Barry Hoffbrand, 'John Misaubin MD and Licentiate of the College of Physicians: Hogarth's "Quack"', *Journal of the Royal Society of Medicine* (forthcoming).

6   Harold Avery, 'Misaubin and Veron, Butts of the Caricaturists', *International Congress of the History of Medicine (21 Siena, 1968)* (Rome, 1970) vol. 2, pp. 1018–22; Jean Savare, 'Le docteur Misaubin, de Watteau, ou un charlatan français à Londres au XVIIIe siècle', *Revue d'histoire de la pharmacie* (Paris), XVIII (1967), pp. 597–607; Haslam, *From Hogarth to Rowlandson*, pp. 94f. Fielding satirized Misaubin in his play *The Mock Doctor*, first performed in 1732, which he also dedicated to him.

7   For the argument that the very notion of the artist's 'message' is misguided, see Peter Wagner, 'How to (Mis)read Hogarth; Or, Ekphrasis Galore', *1650–1850: Aesthetics, and Inquiries into the Early Modern Era*, II (1996), pp. 203–40.

8   See Roy Porter, ed., *The Popularization of Medicine, 1650–1850* (London, 1992), *passim*.

9   See Roy Porter, '"Expressing Yourself Ill": The Language of Sickness in Georgian England', in P. Burke and R. Porter, eds, *Language, Self and Society: The Social History of Language* (Cambridge, 1991), pp. 276–99; *idem*, 'Reading: A Health Warning', in Robin Myers and Michael Harris , eds, *Medicine, Mortality and the Booktrade* (Winchester, 1998), pp. 131–52. Perhaps the harridan is handing out 'domestic medicine'.

10 Samuel Foote, *The Dramatic Works* (London, 1797), vol. II. The play was first published in 1778.

11 L. G. Stevenson, 'The Siege of Warwick Lane, Together with a Brief History of the Society of Collegiate Physicians 1767–98', *Journal of the History of Medicine*, VII (1952), pp. 105–21; Sir George Clark, *A History of the Royal College of Physicians of London*, 3 vols (Oxford, 1964–72), ii, pp. 562–3.

12 Samuel Foote, *The Devil upon Two Sticks*, in *The Dramatic Works* (London, 1797), vol. II, pp. 324–6, act ii.

13 There certainly was an earlier (1762), but different, offering entitled *The State Quack*, one of scores of attacks on the Scottish Prime Minister, Lord Bute, and on his supposed mistress, George III's mother, the Princess Dowager, portrayed as a falling rope-walker. Bute figured as a mountebank performing in *The Senate, a Farce*.

14 Gillray's *Britannia Between Death and the Doctors* is also reproduced in W. H.

Helfand, 'Medicine and Pharmacy in British Political Prints – the Example of Lord Sidmouth', *Medical History*, XXIX (1985), pp. 375–85. See Chap. 9.

15 Helfand, 'Medicine and Pharmacy in British Political Prints' pp. 375–85; Mortimer Frank, 'Caricature in Medicine', *Bulletin of the Society of Medical History of Chicago*, I (1911–16), pp. 46–57. For Addington see Chap. 9.

16 See Chap. 9.

17 L. Clarkson, *Death, Disease and Famine in Pre-Industrial* England (Dublin, 1975); E. A. Wrigley and R. S. Schofield, *The Population History of England 1541–1871: A Reconstruction* (London, 1981); L. Stevenson, '"New Diseases" in the Seventeenth Century', *Bulletin of the History of Medicine*, XXXIX (1965), pp. 1–21.

18 Anne Hardy, *The Epidemic Streets: Infectious Disease and the Rise of Preventive Medicine, 1856–1900* (Oxford and New York, 1993); Anthony S. Wohl, *Endangered Lives: Public Health in Victorian Britain* (Cambridge, MA, 1983); Roy Porter and G. S. Rousseau, *Gout: The Patrician Malady* (New Haven and London, 1998).

19 F. B. Smith, *The Retreat of Tuberculosis 1850–1950* (London and New York, 1988).

20 Michael MacDonald and Terrence R. Murphy, *Sleepless Souls: Suicide in Early Modern England* (Oxford, 1990).

21 D. Little and G. Kahrl, eds, *The Letters of David Garrick*, 3 vols (London, 1963), II, p. 557; Laurence Sterne, *The Life and Opinions of Tristram Shandy*, ed. Graham Petrie (Harmondsworth, 1967), p. 461.

22 Andrew Wear, *Knowledge and Practice in English Medicine 1550–1680* (Cambridge, 2000); Keith Thomas, *Religion and the Decline of Magic. Studies in Popular Beliefs in Sixteenth- and Seventeenth-Century England* (London, 1971).

23 Charles Webster, ed., *Health, Medicine and Mortality in the Sixteenth Century* (Cambridge, 1979); Margaret Pelling, 'Medical Practice in Early Modern England: Trade or Profession?', in W. Prest, ed., *The Professions in Early Modern England* (London, 1987), pp. 90–128.

24 Far the best explication of this view is to be found in Natsu Hattori, 'Performing Cures: Practice and Interplay in Theatre and Medicine of the English Renaissance', DPhil thesis, University of Oxford, 1995.

25 J.-C. Agnew, *Worlds Apart: The Market and the Theater in Anglo-American Thought, 1550–1750* (Cambridge, 1986); Peter Borsay, 'All the Town's a Stage', in P. Clark, ed., *The Transformation of English Provincial Towns, (1660–1800)* (London, 1985), pp. 228–58; R. Sennett, *The Fall of Public Man* (1976) (London, 1986); D. Barnett, *The Art of Gesture: The Practice and Principles of 18th Century Acting* (Heidelberg, 1987); Peter Burke, *The Historical Anthropology of Early Modern Italy: Essays on Perception and Communication* (Cambridge, 1987); Roy C. Strong, *Splendour at Court: Renaissance Spectacle and Illusion* (London, 1973); M. Byrd, *London Transformed: Images of the City in the Eighteenth Century* (New Haven and London, 1978), p. 63: 'The theater appears prominently – one would say takes a prominent role – in almost every account of eighteenth-century London.' For the need for 'performative' readings, see Fay Bound, 'Emotion in Early Modern England 1660–1760: Performativity and Practice at the Church Courts of York', DPhil thesis, University of York, 2000.

26 Thomas Hobbes, *Leviathan: or, the Matter, Forme and Power of a Commonwealth Ecclesiasticall and Civil*, ed. C. B. Macpherson (Harmondsworth, 1968), p. 6; see discussion in Edward Hundert, 'Performing the Passions in Commercial Society: Bernard Mandeville and the Theatricality of Eighteenth-Century Thought', in Kevin Sharpe and Steven N. Zwicker, eds, *Refiguring Revolutions* (Berkeley, 1998), pp. 142–72.

27 J. Addison and R. Steele, *The Spectator*, ed. Donald Bond, 5 vols (Oxford, 1965),

II, p. 352, Saturday 10 November 1711; Ronald Paulson, *The Beautiful, Novel, and Strange. Aesthetics and Heterodoxy* (Baltimore and London, 1996), pp. 55f., for Addison's image of the stage of life and the persona of being a spectator.

28 Quoted from the 'Autobiographical Notes' in Derek Jarrett, *The Ingenious Hogarth* (London, 1976), pp. 106–7.

29 E. P. Thompson, *The Making of the English Working Class* (London, 1963); *idem*, *Customs in Common* (London, 1991); *idem*, 'Patrician Society, Plebeian Culture', *Journal of Social History*, VII (1973–4), pp. 382–405; Tim Harris, *London Crowds in the Reign of Charles II: Propaganda and Politics from the Restoration until the Exclusion Crisis* (Cambridge, 1990); John Brewer, *The Common People and Politics, 1750–1790* (Cambridge, 1986).

30 I. Veith, *Hysteria: The History of a Disease* (Chicago and London, 1965), p. 151. Galen's apothegm: 'he cures most in whom most are confident' was often quoted: David Harley, 'Rhetoric and the Social Construction of Sickness and Healing', *Social History of Medicine*, XII (1999), pp. 407–36.

31 John Haygarth, *Of the Imagination as a Cause and as a Cure of Disorders of the Body* (Bath, 1800).

32 Hattori, 'Performing Cures', p. 1.

33 An interesting case is Alexander Lesassier, an Edinburgh-trained doctor who recorded (and presumably lived) his life in large measure through the clichés of the sentimental novel, and in part put down his own autobiography in such a novel, the unpublished 'Edward Neville, or the Memoirs of an Orphan': see Lisa Rosner, *The Most Beautiful Man in Existence: The Scandalous Life of Alexander Lesassier* (Philadelphia, 1999).

34 These verses are attributed to David Garrick: see G. S. Rousseau, ed., *Letters and Papers of Sir John Hill* (New York, 1982).

35 Strong, *Splendour at Court*.

36 This viewpoint is stressed in Roger King, 'Curing Toothache on the Stage?: The Importance of Reading Pictures in Context', *History of Science*, XXXIII (1995), pp. 396–416; see also Colin Jones, 'The Great Chain of Buying: Medical Advertisements, the Bourgeois Public Sphere, and the Origins of the French Revolution', *American Historical Review*, CI (1996), pp. 13–40.

37 For the idea of 'pharmakon', both remedy and poison, see Jacques Derrida, *Of Grammatology* (Baltimore, 1974). In satirical prints, the (quack) doctor was often juxtaposed against the (quack) preacher, for instance the Methodist.

38 Sander L. Gilman, *Health and Illness: Images of Difference* (London, 1995); see also Irving Goffman, *Stigma: Notes on the Management of Spoiled Identity* (Harmondsworth, 1968); M. M. Bakhtin, *Rabelais and his World*, trans. H. Iswolsky (Cambridge, MA, 1968).

39 M. Bloch, *The Royal Touch: Sacred Monarchy and Scrofula in England and France* (London, 1973).

40 James Raven, Naomi Tadmore and Helen Small, eds, *The Practice and Representation of Reading in Britain 1500–1900* (Cambridge, 1996), pp. 4f.; John Feather, 'The Power of Print: Word and Image in Eighteenth-Century England', in Jeremy Black, ed., *Culture and Society in Britain 1660–1800* (Manchester, 1997), pp. 51–68.

41 Porter, ed., *The Popularization of Medicine*.

42 Samuel Johnson, 'Preface' to the *Gentleman's Magazine*, 1740, quoted in Geoffrey Alan Cranfield, *The Development of the Provincial Newspaper 1700–1760* (Oxford, 1962), p. 93.

43 C. de Saussure, *A Foreign View of England in 1725–29* (London, 1995), p. 102.

44 Fielding H. Garrison, 'Medicine in *The Tatler*, *Spectator* and *Guardian*', *Bulletin*

of the History of Medicine, II (1934), pp. 477–503; Roy Porter, 'Laymen, Doctors and Medical Knowledge in the Eighteenth Century: The Evidence of the *Gentleman's Magazine*', in Roy Porter, ed., *Patients and Practitioners: Lay Perceptions of Medicine in Pre-Industrial Society* (Cambridge, 1985), pp. 283–314; *idem, Enlightenment: Britain and the Creation of the Modern World* (Harmondsworth, 2000), chap. IV.

45 Ann L. Reitz, 'Sawbones to Savior to Cynic: The Doctor's Relation to Society in English Fiction of the Eighteenth, Nineteenth, and Twentieth Centuries', PhD thesis, University of Cincinnati, 1985; Hattori, 'Performing Cures'.

46 Dror Wahrman, 'National Society, Communal Culture: An Argument about the Recent Historiography of Eighteenth Century Britain', *Social History*, XVII (1992), pp. 43–72; Richard D. Altick, *The English Common Reader* (Columbus, 1957).

47 See Ian Watt, *The Rise of the Novel: Studies in Defoe, Richardson and Fielding* (London, 1957); John J. Richetti, *Popular Fiction before Richardson: Narrative Patterns, 1700–1789* (Oxford, 1969; repr. 1992); Michael McKeon, *The Origins of the English Novel, 1600–1740* (Baltimore, 1987); R. F. Brissenden, *Virtue in Distress: Studies in the Novel of Sentiment from Richardson to Sade* (London, 1974). On self-identification, see Alan Richardson, *Literature, Education, and Romanticism: Reading as Social Practice, 1780–1832* (Cambridge, 1994).

48 To borrow the term used in other contexts by Thomas Laqueur: 'Bodies, Details, and Humanitarian Narrative', in Lynn Hunt, ed., *The New Cultural History* (Berkeley, 1989), pp. 176–204.

49 See Janet Todd, *Sensibility: An Introduction* (London, 1986), p. 90.

50 Thomas Beddoes, *Hygëia: or Essays Moral and Medical, on the Causes Affecting the Personal State of our Middling and Affluent Classes*, 3 vols (Bristol, 1802), vol. 1, essay III, p. 77.

51 Beddoes, *Hygëia*, 1, III, p. 78. On masturbation see J. Stengers and A. Van Neck, *Histoire d'une grande peur: Le masturbation* (Brussels, 1984).

52 Timothy Clayton, *The English Print, 1688–1802* (New Haven and London, 1997).

53 The word comes from the Italian *caricare*, meaning to overload: R. Ashbee, *Caricature* (London, 1928); Frank, 'Caricature in Medicine', pp. 46–57; E. H. Gombrich and E. Kris, *Caricature* (London, 1939); Edward Lucie-Smith, *The Art of Caricature* (London, 1981).

54 Clayton, *The English Print*, p. 232.

55 Kate Arnold-Forster and Nigel Tallis, comps, *The Bruising Apothecary: Images of Pharmacy and Medicine in Caricature* (London, 1989), pp. 4–6; John Geipel, *The Cartoon. A Short History of Graphic Comedy and Satire* (London, 1972); Bevis Hillier, *Cartoons and Caricatures* (London, 1970).

56 Mary Douglas, 'The Construction of the Physician: A Cultural Approach to Medical Fashions', in Susan Budd and Ursula Sharma, eds, *The Healing Bond. The Patient-Practitioner Relationship and Therapeutic Responsibility* (London and New York, 1994), pp. 23–41, p. 25.

57 Roy Porter, *Mind Forg'd Manacles: Madness and Psychiatry in England from Restoration to Regency* (London, 1987; paperback edition, Harmondsworth, 1990).

58 Desmond King-Hele, ed., *The Letters of Erasmus Darwin* (Cambridge, 1981), p. 104. Elsewhere Darwin wrote of the 'infernal Divinities, who visit mankind with diseases': p. 84.

59 Norbert Elias, *The Civilizing Process*, vol. 1, *The History of Manners* (New York, 1978); vol. 2, *Power and Civility* (New York, 1982); vol. 3, *The Court Society* (New York, 1983).

60 See T. G. H. Drake, 'The Medical Caricatures of Thomas Rowlandson', *Bulletin of the History of Medicine*, XII (1942), pp. 323–35; William C. Butterfield, 'The Medical Caricatures of Thomas Rowlandson', *Journal of the American Medical Association*, CCXXIV (1973), pp. 113–7; Ronald Paulson, 'Thomas Rowlandson: His Medical Satire', *Hospital Update* (Oct. 1974), pp. 619–28. More generally on medical cartoons see Jean Avalon, 'Malades, médecins et charlatans dans la caricature anglaise au temps d'Hogarth et de Rowlandson', *Aesculape*, XL (1957), pp. 2–62; W.-H. Hein, *Die Pharmazie in der Karikatur* (Frankfurt-am-Main, 1964); E. Holländer, *Die Karikatur und Satire in der Medizin* (Stuttgart, 1921); W. H. Helfand, *Drugs and Pharmacy in Prints* (Madison, WI, 1967); *idem*, 'Medicine and Pharmacy in French Political Prints', *Pharmacy in History*, XVII (1975), pp. 119–31.

61 See for instance Wagner, *Reading Iconotexts*. Wagner takes issue with the more 'intentionalist' readings offered by Paulson: Wagner, 'How to (Mis)read Hogarth', pp. 203–40.

62 Ronald Paulson, *Representations of Revolution 1789–1820* (New Haven, 1983), the most powerful analysis of the techniques of the comic, the grotesque and the satirical.

63 Mark S. R. Jenner, 'Body, Image, Text in Early Modern Europe', *Social History of Medicine*, XII (1999), pp. 143–54; Roy Porter, 'History of the Body', in Peter Burke, ed., *New Perspectives on Historical Writing* (Cambridge, 1991), pp. 206–32. A fresh article, 'History of the Body Reconsidered', appears in the second edition (Cambridge, 2001), pp. 233–60. Pioneering was Bryan S. Turner, *The Body and Society: Explorations in Social Theory* (Oxford, 1984). See also his 'Recent Developments in the Theory of the Body', in Mike Featherstone, Mike Hepworth and Bryan S. Turner, eds, *The Body. Social Process and Cultural Theory* (London, 1991), pp. 1–35; and 'The Body in Western Society: Social Theory and its Perspectives', in Sarah Coakley, ed., *Religion and the Body* (Cambridge, 1997), pp. 15–41.

64 A turn brilliantly explored in P. Stallybrass and A. White, *The Politics and Poetics of Transgression* (Ithaca, 1986).

65 E. J. Climenson, ed., *Elizabeth Montagu, the Queen of the Blue Stockings: Her Correspondence from 1720–1766*, 2 vols (London, 1906), I, 36.

66 N. D. Jewson, 'Medical Knowledge and the Patronage System in Eighteenth Century England', *Sociology*, VIII (1974), pp. 369–85.

67 Donald G. MacRae, 'The Body and Social Metaphor', in J. Benthall and T. Polhemus, eds, *The Body as a Medium of Expression: An Anthology* (New York, 1975), pp. 59–73.

68 Daniel M. Fox and Christopher Lawrence, *Photographing Medicine: Images and Power in Britain and American Since 1840* (Westport and London, 1988).

2 The Body Grotesque and Monstrous

1 Laurence Sterne, *The Life and Opinions of Tristram Shandy*, ed. Graham Petrie (Harmondsworth, 1967), vol. VII, p. 472.

2 George Lakoff and Mark Johnson, *Metaphors We Live By* (Chicago, 1980). For introductions to body history see Michel Feher, *Fragments for a History of the Human Body*, 3 vols (New York, 1989); David Hillman and Carla Mazzio, eds, *The Body in Parts: Discourses and Anatomies in Early Modern Europe* (London, 1997); Bryan S. Turner, *The Body and Society: Explorations in Social Theory* (Oxford, 1984); Deborah Lupton, *Medicine as Culture: Illness, Disease and the Body in Western Societies* (London, 1994).

3 J. B. Bamborough, *The Little World of Man* (London, 1952); Leonard Barkan, *Nature's Work of Art: The Human Body as Image of the World* (New Haven, 1975);

Michel Foucault, *The Order of Things: An Archaeology of the Human Sciences* (London, 1970).

4 Carolyn Walker Bynum, *Fragmentation and Redemption Essays on Gender and the Human Body in Medieval Religion* (New York, 1991); Miri Rubin, *Corpus Christi. The Eucharist in Late Medieval Culture* (Cambridge, 1991).

5 For shame, see Gail Kern Paster, *The Body Embarrassed: Drama and the Disciplines of Shame in Early Modern England* (Ithaca, 1993).

6 Edward Gibbon, *Memoirs of My Life*, ed. G. A. Bonnard (London, 1966), p. 29.

7 Mary Midgley, 'The Soul's Successors: Philosophy and the "Body"', in Sarah Coakley, ed., *Religion and the Body* (Cambridge, 1997), pp. 53–68.

8 Coakley, ed., *Religion and the Body*; Andrew Louth, 'The Body in Western Catholic Christianity', in Coakley, ed., *Religion and the Body*, pp. 111–30; Piero Camporesi, *The Incorruptible Flesh: Bodily Mutation and Mortification in Religion and Folklore* (Cambridge, 1988); *idem*, *The Fear of Hell: Images of Damnation and Salvation in Early Modern Europe*, trans. Lucinda Byatt (Cambridge, 1991); *idem*, *The Anatomy of the Senses: Natural Symbols in Medieval and Early Modern Italy*, trans. Allan Cameron (Cambridge, 1994); Frank Bottomley, *Attitudes to the Body in Western Christendom* (London, 1979); Peter Brown, *The Body and Society: Men, Women and Sexual Renunciation in Early Christianity* (New York, 1988).

9 Morris Berman, *Coming to our Senses. Body and Spirit in the Hidden History of the West* (New York, 1990).

10 John Milton, *Paradise Lost* (London, 1667), book x, lines 512–21.

11 David Harley, 'The Good Physician and the Godly Doctor: The Exemplary Life of John Tylston of Chester (1663–99)', *The Seventeenth Century*, IX (1994), pp. 93–117.

12 Carol Houlihan Flynn, *The Body in Swift and Defoe* (Cambridge, 1990), pp. 21–2.

13 Philip Stubbes, *Anatomie of Abuses* (London, 1585), ff. 99–99v. Good Puritan as he was, Stubbes disapproved all show and theatricality: Jean-Christophe Agnew, *Worlds Apart: The Market and the Theater in Anglo-American Thought, 1550–1750* (Cambridge, 1986), p. 127.

14 John Donne, *Devotions upon Emergent Occasions*, ed. Anthony Raspa (Montreal, 1975), p. 7, discussed in Jonathan Sawday, *The Body Emblazoned: Dissection and the Human Body in Renaissance Culture* (London, 1995), p. 33; Francis Barker, *The Tremulous Private Body* (London, 1984).

15 Donne, *Devotions upon Emergent Occasions*, p. 52; John Carey, *John Donne: Life Mind and Art* (London, 1981); David Tripp, 'The Image of the Body in the Formative Phases of the Protestant Reformation', in Coakley, ed., *Religion and the Body*, pp. 131–52.

16 From *An Anatomie of the World* (London, 1611): Donne's line is contextualized in V. I. Harris, *All Coherence Gone* (London, 1966).

17 L. M. Beier, 'In Sickness and in Health: A Seventeenth Century Family Experience', in R. Porter, ed., *Patients and Practitioners* (Cambridge, 1985), pp. 101–28, p. 119; Andrew Wear, 'Puritan Perceptions of Illness in Seventeenth-Century England', in R. Porter, ed., *Patients and Practitioners*, pp. 55–99.

18 Sterne, *Tristram Shandy*, pp. 184f.

19 William Shakespeare, 'The Passionate Pilgrim', VIII, in Stanley Wells and Gary Taylor, eds, *The Complete Oxford Shakespeare* (Oxford, 1987), i, 46.

20 Quoted in O. L. Dick, ed., *Aubrey's Brief Lives* (Harmondsworth. 1972), p. 10.

21 Hamlet contemplated 'how a king may go a progress through the guts of a beggar': William Shakespeare, *Hamlet*, Act 4 Scene 3.

22 W. Brockbank and F. Kenworthy, eds, *The Diary of Richard Kay (1716–51) of Baldingstone, near Bury* (Manchester, 1968), p. 20.

23 Sander L. Gilman, *Sexuality: An Illustrated History* (New York, 1989); Margaret

Jane Healy, 'Fictions of Disease: Representations of Bodily Disorder in Early
Modern Writings', PhD thesis, University College London, 1995.

24 E. S. De Beer, ed., *The Diary of John Evelyn*, 6 vols (Oxford, 1955), 9 August 1682.
See Barbara Maria Stafford, *Body Criticism. Imaging the Unseen in Enlightenment
Art and Medicine* (Massachusetts, 1991), p. 341.

25 Sterne, *Tristram Shandy*, p. 557.

26 M. M. Bakhtin, *Rabelais and his World*, trans. H. Iswolsky (Cambridge, MA, 1968);
for explication see P. Stallybrass and A. White, *The Politics and Poetics of
Transgression* (Ithaca, 1986). The cultural anthropology of bodies high and low is
also explored in Mary Douglas, *Natural Symbols: Explorations in Cosmology*
(Harmondsworth, 1973).

27 Bryan S. Turner, 'The Body in Western Society: Social Theory and its
Perspectives', in Coakley, ed., *Religion and the Body*, pp. 15–41. Turner notes that
'medicine is one of the technologies for controlling this dangerous body'.

28 Irving Goffman, *Stigma: Notes on the Management of Spoiled Identity*
(Harmondsworth, 1970), p. 9.

29 Martin Bernal, *Black Athena: The Afroasiatic Roots of Classical Civilization*, vol. I,
The Fabrication of Ancient Greece, 1785–1985 (London, 1987); vol. II, *Greece:
Aryan or Mediterranean? The Archaeological and Documentary Evidence* (London,
1991); Sander Gilman, *On Blackness without Blacks: Essays on the Image of the
Black in Germany* (Boston, MA, 1982).

30 See for instance James Sharpe, *Instruments of Darkness. Witchcraft in England
1550–1750* (London, 1996); Keith Thomas, *Religion and the Decline of Magic:
Studies in Popular Beliefs in Sixteenth and Seventeenth-Century England* (London,
1971).

31 Jane Kromm, 'Studies in the Iconography of Madness, 1600–1900', PhD thesis,
Emory University, 1984; *idem*, 'The Feminization of Madness in Visual
Representation', *Feminist Studies*, XX (1994), pp. 507–35; Sander L. Gilman:
Seeing the Insane: A Cultural History of Madness and Art in the Western World (New
York, 1982); John M. MacGregor, *The Discovery of the Art of the Insane*
(Princeton, 1989).

32 David Piper, 'Take the Face of a Physician', in Gordon Wolstenholme, ed.,
Portraits: The Royal College of Physicians of London, Catalogue II (Amsterdam,
1977), 25–49, p. 25.

33 Natsu Hattori, 'Performing Cures: Practice and Interplay in Theatre and
Medicine of the English Renaissance', DPhil thesis, University of Oxford, 1995,
p. 137.

34 E. L. Griggs, ed., *Collected Letters of Samuel Taylor Coleridge*, 6 vols (Oxford,
1956–68), I, pp. 154, 256.

35 Claude Rawson, *Satire and Sentiment 1660–1830* (Cambridge, 1994).

36 Ronald Paulson, *Representations of Revolution 1789–1820* (New Haven, 1983).

37 For Swift, see Flynn, *The Body in Swift and Defoe*; for Hogarth and literature, see
Ronald Paulson, *Popular and Polite Art in the Age of Hogarth and Fielding* (Notre
Dame and London, 1979); Peter Wagner, *Reading Iconotexts: From Swift to the
French Revolution* (London, 1995).

38 Ronald Paulson, 'Putting out the Fire in her Imperial Majesty's Apartment:
Opposition Politics, Anticlericalism and Aesthetics', *ELH*, LXIII (1996),
pp. 79–107; David Nokes, *Jonathan Swift: A Hypocrite Reversed: A Critical
Biography* (Oxford, 1985), p. 111; Joseph McMinn, *Jonathan's Travels: Swift
and Ireland* (Belfast, 1994).

39 Jonathan Swift, *Gulliver's Travels* (1726) (London, 1954), pp. 284–5. Capable on
Lilliput of taking up twenty or thirty smaller fowl at the end of his knife, Gulliver

teases his captors with his voracious ways, pretending on one occasion, penknife in hand, a readiness to eat the more impudent members of the rabble alive. In turn, Gulliver on Brobdingnag barely escapes being eaten alive by a large infant pacified only by 'the last Remedy', a 'monstrous Breast'.

40 For explanations of female flesh construed as inferior, see Thomas W. Laqueur, *Making Sex* (Cambridge, MA, 1990); Katharine Park and Robert A. Nye, 'Destiny is Anatomy' [essay review of Laqueur, *Making Sex*], *New Republic*, XVIII (1991), pp. 53–7; Mary Russo, *The Female Grotesque: Risk, Excess and Modernity* (New York and London, 1994).

41 'A Beautiful Young Nymph Going to Bed – Written for the Honour of the Fair Sex': Jonathan Swift, *The Complete Poems*, ed. Pat Rogers (London, 1983), pp. 434–55; Stallybrass and White, *The Politics and Poetics of Transgression*, p. 9. For venereal symptoms, see Linda E. Merians, ed., *The Secret Malady. Venereal Disease in Eighteenth-Century Britain and France* (Lexington, 1996).

42 J. A. Sharpe, *Crime and the Law in English Satirical Prints 1600–1832* (Cambridge, 1986); Lionello Puppi, *Torment in Art. Pain, Violence and Martyrdom* (New York, 1991); Richard J. Evans, *Rituals of Retribution. Capital Punishment in Germany, 1600–1987* (Harmondsworth, 1997); Pieter Spierenburg, *The Spectacle of Suffering: Executions and the Evolution of Repression: From a Preindustrial Metropolis to the European Experience* (Cambridge, 1984).

43 E. P. Thompson, *Customs in Common* (London, 1991).

44 M. Foucault, *Discipline and Punish: The Birth of the Prison* (Harmondsworth, 1979); M. Ignatieff, *A Just Measure of Pain: The Penitentiary in the Industrial Revolution, 1750–1850* (London, 1978).

45 Andrea Carlino, *Books of the Body: Anatomical Ritual and Renaissance Learning*, trans. John Tedeschi and Anne C. Tedeschi (Chicago, 2000); Jan C. C. Rupp, 'Matters of Life and Death: The Social and Cultural Conditions of the Rise of Anatomical Theatres, With Special Reference to Seventeenth Century Holland', *History of Science*, XXVIII (1990), pp. 263–87.

46 Hattori, 'Performing Cures', p. 45; Jonathan Sawday, *The Body Emblazoned: Dissection and the Human Body in Renaissance Culture* (London, 1995); Ruth Richardson, *Death, Dissection and the Destitute: A Political History of the Human Corpse* (London, 1987).

47 Fiona Haslam, *From Hogarth to Rowlandson. Medicine in Art in Eighteenth-Century Britain* (Liverpool, 1996), p. 263; Martin Kemp and Marina Wallace, *Spectacular Bodies: The Art and Science of the Human Body. From Leonardo to Now* (Berkeley and Los Angeles, 2000).

48 See the discussion in Ludmilla Jordanova, *Nature Displayed. Gender, Science and Medicine 1760–1820* (London and New York, 1999), p. 185; and Chap. 7.

49 John Bulwer, *Anthropometamorphosis: Man Transform'd: or the Artificial Changeling Historically presented, In the mad and cruel Gallantry, foolish Bravery, ridiculous Beauty, filthy Finenesse, and loathsome Lovelinesse of most Nations, fashioning and altering their Bodies from the mould intended by Nature; with Figures of those Transfigurations. To which artificial and affected Deformations are added, all the Native and Nationall Monstrosities that have appeared to disfigure the Humane Fabrick. With a Vindication of the Regular Beauty and Honesty of Nature. And an Appendix of the Pedigree of the English Gallant* (London, 1653), pp. 18–19; H. J. Norman, 'John Bulwer and his Anthropometamorphosis', in E. Ashworth Underwood, ed., *Science Medicine and History. Essays on the Evolution of Scientific Thought and Medical Practice Written in Honour of Charles Singer*, 2 vols (Oxford, 1953), II, pp. 80–99; see also Dudley Wilson, *Signs and Portents. Monstrous Births from the Middle Ages to the Enlightenment* (London and New York, 1993), p. 123.

50 Bulwer, *Anthropometamorphosis*, p. 20.

51 Londa Schiebinger, 'The Anatomy of Difference: Race and Sex in 18th-Century Science', *Eighteenth-Century Studies*, XXIII (1990), pp. 387–405.

52 Dennis Todd, *Imagining Monsters: Miscreations of the Self in Eighteenth-Century England* (Chicago and London, 1995), pp. 47f.; Laurent Joubert, *Popular Errors*, trans. and ed. Gregory David de Rocher (Tuscaloosa and London, 1989); Wilson, *Signs and Portents*.

53 For a challenging interpretation of Hogarth on Toft, see Paulson, 'Putting out the Fire in her Imperial Majesty's Apartment'. For freaks, see De Beer. ed., *The Diary of John Evelyn*, pp. 197–98; K. Park and L. J. Daston, 'Unnatural Conceptions: The Study of Monsters', *Past and Present*, XCII (1981), pp. 20–54; Richard D. Altick, *The Shows of London: A Panoramic History of Exhibitions, 1600–1862* (Cambridge, MA, 1978); L. Fiedler, *Freaks* (Harmondsworth, 1978).

54 Haslam, *From Hogarth to Rowlandson*, pp. 29f. Note that Mary Toft made a repeat appearance in Hogarth's *A Medley: Credulity, Superstition and Fanaticism*.

55 Aileen Douglas, *Uneasy Sensations. Smollett and the Body* (Chicago and London, 1995), pp. 16–17; G. S. Rousseau, *Enlightenment Borders. Pre- and Post-Modern Discourses, Medical, Scientific* (Manchester and New York, 1991), pp. 182–3; Todd, *Imagining Monsters*, pp. 47f. The Toft scandal opened once again the whole question of the respective roles of the male and female in generation.

56 *Philosophical Transactions*, no. 286 (July–August 1703), vol. 23, p. 1418; Simon Schaffer, 'Natural Philosophy and Public Spectacle in the Eighteenth Century', *History of Science*, XXI (1983), pp. 1–43.

57 Roy Porter, 'John Hunter: A Showman in Society', *The Transactions of the Hunterian Society* (1993–4), pp. 19–24.

58 Porter, 'John Hunter: A Showman in Society'.

59 Gaby Wood, *The Smallest of all Persons Mentioned in the Records of Littleness* (London, 1998).

60 Romans 7:18, 23–4.

61 Rudolph Bell, *Holy Anorexia* (Chicago, 1985); Walker Bynum, *Fragmentation and Redemption: Essays on Gender and the Human Body in Medieval Religion*; idem, *The Resurrection of the Body in Western Christianity, 200–1336* (New York, 1995).

62 Andrew Marvell, 'A Dialogue Between the Soul and Body', in Elizabeth Story Donne, ed., *Andrew Marvell, the Complete Poems* (Harmondsworth, 1972), p. 103, lines 1–4; 19–20; Sawday, *The Body Emblazoned*, p. 21; Rosalie Osmond, *Mutual Accusation: Seventeenth-Century Body and Soul Dialogues in Their Literary and Theological Context* (Toronto, 1990).

63 Marvell, 'A Dialogue Between the Soul and Body', in Donne, ed., *Andrew Marvell, the Complete Poems*, p. 104, lines 31–6; 41–2.

64 *Ibid*, p. 104, lines 11–14; 19–20.

65 Robert A. Erickson, *Mother Midnight: Birth, Sex, and Fate in Eighteenth-Century Fiction (Defoe, Richardson, and Sterne)* (New York, 1986), p. 202; L. Landa, 'The Shandean Homunculus: the Background of Sterne's "Little Gentleman"', in C. Camden, ed., *Restoration and Eighteenth-Century Literature: Essays in Honour of Alan Dugald McKillop* (Chicago, 1963), pp. 49–68; Roy Porter, '"The Whole Secret of Health": Mind, Body and Medicine in *Tristram Shandy*', in John Christie and Sally Shuttleworth, eds, *Nature Transfigured* (Manchester, 1989), pp. 61–84; idem, 'Against the Spleen', in Valerie Grosvenor Myer, ed., *Laurence Sterne: Riddles and Mysteries* (London and New York, 1984), pp. 84–99.

66 Myer, 'Tristram and the Animal Spirits', in Myer, ed., *Laurence Sterne*, pp. 99–112.

67 Aileen Douglas, *Uneasy Sensations. Smollett and the Body* (Chicago, 1995).

68 And additionally 'the Infirmities of others I have treated': see George Cheyne,

The English Malady (1733) ed. Roy Porter (London, 1990); *idem, An Essay on Health and Long Life*, 8th edn (London, 1734 [1724]), p. xvi.

69 Cheyne, *The English Malady*, pp. xvi–xvii.

70 Anita Guerrini, *Obesity and Depression in the Enlightenment: The Life and Times of George Cheyne* (Norman, OK, 2000), p. 135.

71 Cheyne, *The English Malady*, p. 351.

72 Guerrini, *Obesity and Depression in the Enlightenment*, p. 136.

73 Cheyne, *The English Malady*, p. 361.

74 *The Letters of Doctor George Cheyne to Samuel Richardson (1733–1743)*, ed. and intro. Charles F. Mullett (Missouri, 1943), p. 81.

75 Jonathan Swift, *A Tale of a Tub. Written for the Universal Improvement of Mankind ... To Which is added, An Account of a Battel between the Ancient and Modern Books in St. James' Library (A Discourse Concerning the Mechanical Operation of the Spirit. In a Letter to a Friend)* (1704) ed. K. Williams (London, 1975), p.176.

76 Simon Schaffer, 'Regeneration: The Body of Natural Philosophers in Restoration England', in Christopher Lawrence and Steven Shapin, eds, *Science Incarnate – Historical Embodiments of Natural Knowledge* (Chicago and London, 1998), pp. 83–120.

77 G. Becker, *The Mad Genius Controversy* (London and Beverly Hills, 1978). See the discussion of Thomas Carlyle in Chap. 6.

78 P. Linebaugh, 'The Tyburn Riot Against the Surgeons', in E. P. Thompson *et al.*, eds, *Albion's Fatal Tree* (1975) (Harmondsworth, 1977), pp. 65–118.

79 Piero Camporesi, *The Incorruptible Flesh: Bodily Mutation and Mortification in Religion and Folklore* (Cambridge, 1988); Bynum, *Fragmentation and Redemption*.

80 Mark S. R. Jenner, 'Early Modern English Conceptions of "Cleanliness" and "Dirt" as Reflected in the Environmental Regulation of London, c.1530–c.1700', DPhil thesis, Oxford University, 1991.

81 Peter Burke, *Popular Culture in Early Modern Europe* (London, 1978).

82 Bakhtin, *Rabelais and his World;* Veronica Kelly and Dorothea E. von Mücke, eds, *Body & Text in the Eighteenth Century* (Stanford, 1994), p. 6.

83 A. W. Exell, *Joanna Southcott at Blockley and the Rock Cottage Relics* (Shipston-on-Stour, 1977); James K. Hopkins, *A Woman to Deliver Her People: Joanna Southcott and English Millenarianism in an Era of Revolution* (Austin, 1982); Tim Marshall, *Murdering to Dissect: Grave-Robbing, Frankenstein and the Anatomy Literature* (Manchester, 1995), p. 191.

3 The Body Healthy and Beautiful

1 J. D. Bernal, *The World, the Flesh, and the Devil* (London, 1929), 45. Bernal is being playfully earnest.

2 For the harmonious body, wrought in God's image, see Leonard Barkan, *Nature's Work of Art: The Human Body as Image of the World* (New Haven, 1975); H. Baker, *The Dignity of Man: Studies in the Persistence of an Idea* (Cambridge, MA, 1947); J. B. Bamborough, *The Little World of Man* (London, 1952); see also Carol Houlihan Flynn, *The Body in Swift and Defoe* (Cambridge, 1990), p. 15.

3 1 Corinthians 6:19. See also Martin Kemp and Marina Wallace, *Spectacular Bodies: The Art and Science of the Human Body. From Leonardo to Now* (Berkeley and Los Angeles, 2000).

4 F. E. Hutchinson, ed., *The Works of George Herbert* (Oxford, 1941), 'The Temple', p. 91.

5 Cotton Mather, *The Christian Philosopher*, ed. Winton U. Solberg (Urbana and Chicago, 1994), pp. 237–40.

6 Elizabeth Singer Rowe, *Friendship in Death, in Twenty Letters from the Dead to the*

Living, 3rd edn (London, 1733 [1728]), pp. 7f.; . On her reputation, see John J.
Richetti, *Popular Fiction before Richardson: Narrative Patterns 1700–1739*
(Oxford, 1969), pp. 239–61.

7   John Dunton, ed., *The Athenian Gazette*, pp. 1, 29; G. McEwen, *The Oracle of the
Coffee House: John Dunton's Athenian Mercury* (San Marino, CA, 1972).

8   A. Marwick, *Beauty in History: Society, Politics and Personal Appearance c.1500 to
the Present* (London, 1988).

9   Kenneth Clark, *The Nude: A Study of Ideal Art* (Harmondsworth, 1970); Lucy
Gent and Nigel Llewellyn, eds, *Renaissance Bodies: The Human Figure in English
Culture c. 1540–1660* (London, 1990); K. B. Roberts and J. D. W. Tomlinson, *The
Fabric of the Body* (Oxford, 1992); G. Scott, *The Architecture of Humanism*
(London, 1929).

10 Christine Stevenson, *Medicine and Magnificence: British Hospital and Asylum
Architecture 1660–1815* (New Haven and London, 2000); Paul Fussell, *The
Rhetorical World of Augustan Humanism. Ethics and Imagery from Swift to Burke*
(Oxford, 1967); Richard Sennett, *Flesh and Stone: The Body and the City in
Western Civilisation* (London, 1994).

11 John Barrell, *The Political Theory of Painting from Reynolds to Hazlitt: The Body of
the Public* (New Haven, 1986).

12 For this distinction between the naked and the nude, see Clark, *The Nude*.

13 A. Darlington, 'The Teaching of Anatomical Instruction at the Royal Academy of
Arts and the Cultural Consequences of Art-Anatomy Practices, circa 1768–1782',
PhD thesis, University of London, 1991; Fiona Haslam, *From Hogarth to
Rowlandson. Medicine in Art in Eighteenth-Century Britain* (Liverpool, 1996),
p. 278; Deanna Petherbridge, ed., *The Quick and the Dead: Artists and Anatomy*
(London, 1997).

14 Geo. Baglivi, *Practice of Physick* (London, 1704), p. 35.

15 Quoted in Jonathan Sawday, *The Body Emblazoned: Dissection and the Human
Body in Renaissance Culture* (London, 1995), p. 28. For the science and
hermeneutics of particular organs see David Hillman and Carla Mazzio, eds, *The
Body in Parts: Fantasies of Corporeality in Early Modern Europe* (New York and
London, 1997). 'Renes' is roughly the kidneys.

16 Robert Boyle, *The Usefulness of Experimental Natural Philosophy*, in *The Works of
Robert Boyle*, eds, Michael Hunter and Edward B. Davis, 14 vols (London, 1999),
vol. III, p. 266, essay 5.

17 Richard Blackmore, *The Creation: A Philosophical Poem, in Seven Books* (London,
1712), book VI; see Harry M. Solomon, *Sir Richard Blackmore* (Boston, 1980), pp. 128f.

18 Robert A. Erickson, 'William Harvey's *De motu cordis* and "The Republick of
Literature"', in Marie Mulvey Roberts and Roy Porter, eds, *Literature and
Medicine During the Eighteenth Century* (London, 1993), pp. 58–83.

19 Mary Cowling, *The Artist as Anthropologist. The Representation of Type and
Character in Victorian Art* (Cambridge, 1989).

20 M. M. Bakhtin, *Rabelais and his World*, trans. H. Iswolsky (Cambridge, MA, 1968);
Sawday, *The Body Emblazoned*, pp. 19f.; P. Stallybrass and A. White, *The Politics
and Poetics of Transgression* (Ithaca, 1986).

21 Martin Porter, 'English "Treatises on Physiognomy" c. 1500–c. 1780', DPhil
thesis, University of Oxford, 1997; Roy Porter, 'Making Faces: Physiognomy and
Fashion in Eighteenth-Century England', *Etudes Anglaises*, XXXVIII (Oct–Dec.
1985), pp. 385–96; Graeme Tytler, *Physiognomy in the European Novel: Faces and
Fortunes* (Princeton, 1982); Cowling, *The Artist as Anthropologist*.

22 C. C. Hankin, ed., *Life of Mary Anne Schimmelpenninck*, 2 vols (London, 1858), II,
p. 127.

23 This is the finding of Roderick Floud, Kenneth Wachter and Annabel Gregory, *Height, Health and History: Nutritional Status in the United Kingdom, 1750–1980* (Cambridge, 1990).

24 Quoted in Jan Bremmer and Herman Roodenburg, eds, *A Cultural History of Gesture: From Antiquity to the Present Day* (Cambridge, 1991), p. 2.

25 For the dance, see Lucia Dacome, 'Policing Bodies and Balancing Minds: Self and Representation in Eighteenth-Century Britain', PhD thesis, University of Cambridge, 2000, chap. 2. The disappearance of the disciplined body has been dubbed 'genteel Cartesianism': Simon Schaffer, 'Regeneration: The Body of Natural Philosophers in Restoration England', in Christopher Lawrence and Steven Shapin, eds, *Science Incarnate – Historical Embodiments of Natural Knowledge* (Chicago and London, 1998), pp. 83–120. Similar dilemmas attended the pursuit of cleanliness: Georges Vigarello, *Le Propre et le Sale: L'Hygiène du Corps Depuis le Moyen Age* (Paris, 1985; English trans., *Concepts of Cleanliness: Changing Attitudes in France since the Middle Ages*, Cambridge, 1988); Virginia S. Smith, 'Cleanliness: The Development of an Idea and Practice in Britain 1770–1850', PhD thesis, University of London, 1985.

26 C. F. Barrett, ed., *The Diary and Letters of Madame d'Arblay, Author of 'Evelina', 'Cecilia', etc. 1778–1840*, 7 vols (London, 1842–6), II, p. 407.

27 *Ibid.*, ii, p. 407.

28 Anne Hollander, *Seeing Through Clothes* (New York, 1980); Alison Lurie, *The Language of Clothes* (New York, 1981); Ellen Moers, *The Dandy: Brummel to Beerbohm* (London and New York, 1960).

29 *Professional Anecdotes, or ANA of Medical Literature*, 3 vols (London, 1825), p. 182. Her body ended up in the College of Surgeons, where it was destroyed by a German bomb in 1941.

30 E. J. Climenson, ed., *Elizabeth Montagu, the Queen of the Blue Stockings: Her Correspondence from 1720–1766*, 2 vols (London, 1906), II, p. 204; J. A. Home, ed., *Letters and Journals of Lady Mary Coke*, 4 vols (Bath, 1970), III, pp. 385.

31 Ruth Richardson and Brian Hurwitz, 'Jeremy Bentham's Self Image: An Exemplary Bequest for Dissection', *British Medical Journal*, CCVC (1987), pp. 195–8.

32 Simon Schaffer, 'States of Mind: Enlightenment and Natural Philosophy', in G. S. Rousseau, ed., *The Languages of Psyche: Mind and Body in Enlightenment Thought* (Berkeley, Los Angeles and Oxford, 1990), pp. 233–90. Bentham's auto-icon sits in state in University College, London. There were few public statues in London at that time.

33 Thomas W. Laqueur, *Making Sex. Gender and the Body from Aristotle to Freud* (Cambridge, MA, 1990); Londa Schiebinger, *The Mind Has No Sex? Women in the Origins of Modern Science* (Cambridge, MA, 1989).

34 Erickson, 'William Harvey's *De motu cordis* and "The Republick of Literature"', in Roberts and Porter, eds, *Literature and Medicine During the Eighteenth Century*, pp. 58–83; Helkiah Crooke, *Microcosmographia, A Description of the Body of Man, Collected and Translated out of all the Best Authors of Antiquity* (London, 1614), pp. 274–6; Schiebinger, *The Mind Has No Sex?*, p. 184.

35 James Thomson, 'Autumn', in *The Seasons* (London, 1744), pp. 157–8, lines 610–16. For the domestic woman constructed 'in and by print', see Kathryn Shevelow, *Women and Print Culture: The Construction of Femininity in the Early Periodical* (London, 1989), p. 5.

36 Londa Schiebinger, *Nature's Body: Gender in the Making of Modern Science* (Boston, MA, 1993); Hollander, *Seeing Through Clothes*.

37 The fullest discussion is Roy Porter and Lesley Hall, *The Facts of Life: The*

  History of Sexuality and Knowledge from the Seventeenth Century (New Haven, 1994).

38 Desmond King-Hele, *Doctor of Revolution: The Life and Genius of Erasmus Darwin* (London, 1977), p. 240.

39 James Graham, *Lecture on the Generation of the Human Species* (London, 1780), p. 28.

40 *Ibid.*, p. 3.

41 *Ibid.*, p. 42.

42 Arthur Marwick, *Beauty in History. Society, Politics and Personal Appearance c. 1500 to the Present* (London, 1988), p. 187.

43 For background see W. F. Bynum, 'Treating the Wages of Sin: Venereal Disease and Specialism in Eighteenth-Century Britain', in W. F. Bynum and R. Porter, eds, *Medical Fringe and Medical Orthodoxy, 1750–1850* (London, 1987); F. Gunn, *The Artificial Face* (Newton Abbot, 1973); Vigarello, *Le Propre et le Sale: L'Hygiène du Corps Depuis le Moyen Age*; M. Pelling, 'Appearance and Reality: Barber-Surgeons, the Body and Disease', in A. L. Beier and R. Finlay, eds, *London 1500–1700: The Making of the Metropolis* (New York, 1986), pp. 82–112.

44 Leo Kanner, *Folklore of Teeth* (New York, 1928); Roger King, 'Curing Toothache on the Stage?: The Importance of Reading Pictures in Context', *History of Science*, XXXIII (1995), pp. 396–416.

45 British Library 551 a. 171; see discussion in Roy Porter, *Quacks: Fakers and Charlatans in English Medicine* (Stroud, 2000).

46 British Library C112 f. 61.

47 British Library 551 a. 230; 551 a. 148.

48 Porter, *Quacks: Fakers and Charlatans*; British Library 551 a. 96; M. Pelling, 'Appearance and Reality'.

49 Marwick, *Beauty in History*, p. 82.

50 A letter of 1773 to Count Bentinck, printed in J. C. Beaglehole, ed., *The Endeavour Journal of Joseph Banks*, 2 vols (Sydney, 1962), I, p. 275.

51 See discussion in Marwick, *Beauty in History*.

52 A letter of 1773 to Count Bentinck, printed in Beaglehole, ed., *The Endeavour Journal of Joseph Banks*, II, p. 330.

53 *Ibid.*

54 *Ibid.* Note here the striking and rare use of 'luxury' in an approving sense.

55 *Ibid.*

56 *Ibid.*

57 *Ibid.*

58 *Ibid.*

59 *Ibid.*

60 *Ibid.*

61 *Ibid.*

62 *Ibid.*

63 Peter Burke, *The Fabrication of Louis XIV* (New Haven, 1992); Norbert Elias, *The Civilizing Process*, vol. 1, *The History of Manners* (New York, 1978); vol. 2, *Power and Civility* (New York, 1982); vol. 3, *The Court Society* (New York, 1983); Hollander, *Seeing Through Clothes*.

64 H. J. Norman, 'John Bulwer and his Anthropometamorphosis', in E. Ashworth Underwood, ed., *Science, Medicine and History. Essays on the Evolution of Scientific Thought and Medical Practice*, 2 vols (Oxford, 1953), II, pp. 80–99.

65 Bernard Mandeville, *The Fable of the Bees*, ed. P. Harth (Harmondsworth, 1970), p. 151.

66 Philip Carter, *Men and the Emergence of Polite Society, Britain 1660–1800* (Harlow, 2000), chap. iv, pp. 124f.

67 Robert Gittings, ed., *Letters of John Keats* (Oxford, 1970) p. 3, discussed in Roy Porter, 'The Patient's View: Doing Medical History from Below', *Theory and Society*, XIV (1985), pp. 175–98, 192. Keats's sentiment is of course a parody of Falstaff in *Henry IV Part I*, Act 2 Scene 4.

68 R. W. Chapman, ed., *The Letters of Samuel Johnson*, 3 vols (Oxford, 1952), ii, p. 507 (letter 806).

69 M. P. Tilley, ed., *Dictionary of Proverbs in England* (Ann Arbor, 1950), p. 299. See also 'Health is better than wealth'; more hardbitten is 'health without money is half an ague.' For Walter Shandy, see Roy Porter, 'Against the Spleen', in Valerie Grosvenor Myer, ed., *Laurence Sterne: Riddles and Mysteries* (London and New York, 1984), pp. 84–99, p. 86.

70 T. Trotter, *A View of the Nervous Temperament* (London, 1807), pp. xvi, xvii; see also 'Introduction' by Roy Porter to *Thomas Trotter, An Essay on Drunkenness* (London, 1988).

71 Thomas Beddoes, *Hygëia: or Essays Moral and Medical, on the Causes Affecting the Personal State of our Middling and Affluent Classes*, 3 vols (Bristol, 1802), vol. 1, essay III, p. 84.

72 Dryden, from 'To my honour'd Kinsman, John Driden of Chesterton' (1700) in John Sargeaunt, ed., *The Poems of John Dryden* (London, 1959), p. 173, lines 88–93.

73 *Ibid.*, lines 73–4.

74 William Cadogan, *A Dissertation on the Gout* (London, 1771), p. 18.

75 Edwin W. Marrs, ed., *Letters of Charles and Mary Anne Lamb*, 3 vols (Ithaca, 1975–8), II, p. 155; J. Drummond and A. Wilbraham, *The Englishman's Food: A History of Five Centuries of English Diet* (1936) (London, 1957); D. J. Oddy, *The Making of the Modern British Diet* (London, 1976).

76 G. Miller, *Letters of Edward Jenner* (Baltimore, 1983), p. 5.

77 Michael Duffy, *The Englishman and the Foreigner* (Cambridge, 1986). Not until the Regency dandies did bucks aspire to be trim and slim, dieting like Byron on dry biscuits and soda water: L. A. Marchand, ed., *Byron's Letters and Journals*, 12 vols (London, 1973–82).

78 Hankin, ed., *Life of Mary Anne Schimmelpenninck*, I, p. 241.

79 Hillel Schwartz, *Never Satisfied: A Cultural History of Diets, Fantasies and Fat* (New York and London, 1986).

80 Gerald J. Gruman, *A History of Ideas about the Prolongation of Life: The Evolution of Prolongevity Hypotheses to 1800* (Transactions of the American Philosophical Society n.s. 56, pt 9, Philadelphia, 1966); Marie Mulvey Roberts, '"A Physic Against Death": Eternal Life and the Enlightenment – Gender and Gerontology', in Roberts and Porter, eds, *Literature and Medicine During the Eighteenth Century*, pp. 151–67. On weightwatching, see Lucia Dacome, 'Policing Bodies and Balancing Minds: Self and Representation in Eighteenth-Century Britain', PhD thesis, University of Cambridge, 2000.

81 J. Addison and R. Steele, *The Spectator*, ed. Donald Bond, 5 vols (Oxford, 1965), vol. II, no. 195, pp. 263–7, 13 October 1711; Flynn, *The Body in Swift and Defoe*, pp. 50, 47.

82 Her letter concluded with a health PS: 'Dont forget your bathing': Lord Herbert, ed., *Pembroke Papers (1790–1794): Letters and Diaries of Henry, Tenth Earl of Pembroke and His Circle* (London, 1950), II, p. 84; George Cheyne, *An Essay on Health and Long Life* (1724) (8th edn, London, 1734), p. 2; Anita Guerrini, *Obesity and Depression in the Enlightenment: The Life and Times of George Cheyne* (Norman, OK, 2000), pp. 124–5; Carol Houlihan Flynn, 'Running out of Matter: The Body Exercised in Eighteenth Century Fiction', in G. S. Rousseau, ed., *The*

Language of Psyche: Mind and Body in the Enlightenment (Los Angeles, 1990), pp. 147–85.

83 George Cheyne, *The English Malady*, (1733) ed. Roy Porter (London, 1990).

84 Cheyne, *An Essay on Health and Long Life*.

85 James L. Axtell, *The Educational Writings of John Locke: A Critical Edition with Introduction and Notes* (Cambridge, 1968), p. 61.

86 Axtell, *The Educational Writings of John Locke*, p. 134.

87 *Ibid.*, p. 140.

88 Desmond King-Hele, ed., *The Letters of Erasmus Darwin* (Cambridge, 1981), p. 3.

89 Thomas Beddoes, *Essay on the Causes, Early Signs, and Prevention of Pulmonary Consumption for the Use of Parents and Preceptors* (Bristol, 1799), p. 114. For the wider sensibilities of 'anorexia', see Schwartz, *Never Satisfied*; J. J. Brumberg, *Fasting Girls: The Emergence of Anorexia Nervosa as a Modern Disease* (Cambridge, MA, 1988); R. M. Bell, *Holy Anorexia* (Chicago, 1985).

90 David Vaisey, ed., *The Diary of Thomas Turner of East Hoathley* (Oxford, 1984), p. 26.

91 William Godwin, *Enquiry Concerning Political Justice*, (1793) ed. Isaac Kramnick (Harmondsworth, 1985), p. 777.

92 Godwin, *Enquiry Concerning Political Justice*, p. 776.

93 *Ibid.*, p. 730.

94 *Ibid.*, p. 722.

95 For similar dilemmas at the close of the twentieth century see Dorothy Porter, 'The Healthy Body', in Roger Cooter and John Pickstone, eds, *Medicine in the Twentieth Century* (Abingdon, 2000), pp. 201–16.

4 Imagining Disease

1 For what follows see N. D. Jewson, 'The Disappearance of the Sick Man from Medical Cosmology, 1770–1870', *Sociology*, X (1976), pp. 225–44; Mary E. Fissell, 'The Disappearance of the Patient's Narrative and the Invention of Hospital Medicine', in Roger French and Andrew Wear, eds, *British Medicine in an Age of Reform* (London and New York, 1992), pp. 92–109; Roy Porter, 'The Rise of Physical Examination', in W. F. Bynum and Roy Porter, eds, *Medicine and the Five Senses* (Cambridge, 1992), pp. 179–97; Stanley Joel Reiser, *Medicine and the Reign of Technology* (1978) (Cambridge, 1981).

2 H. Brody, *Stories of Sickness* (New Haven, 1987).

3 Bynum and Porter, eds, *Medicine and the Five Senses*, pp. 179–97. It is indicative of the relative importance of the patient's account and the physical examination in traditional medicine that diagnosis was frequently undertaken by letter.

4 Jewson, 'The Disappearance of the Sick Man from Medical Cosmology', pp. 225–44; C. Lawrence, 'Incommunicable Knowledge: Science, Technology and the Clinical Art in Britain, 1850–1914', *Journal of Contemporary History*, XX (1985), pp. 503–20.

5 Michaela Reid, *Ask Sir James* (London, 1987), p. 201.

6 Bettyann Holtzmann Kevles, *Naked to the Bone. Medical Imaging in the Twentieth Century* (New Brunswick, NJ, 1996); Barbara Maria Stafford, *Body Criticism: Imagining the Unseen in Enlightenment Art and Medicine* (Cambridge, MA, 1991).

7 Deuteronomy 28; Elaine Scarry, *The Body in Pain: The Making and Unmaking of the World* (Oxford, 1985).

8 Irving Goffman, *Stigma: Notes on the Management of Spoiled Identity* (Harmondsworth, 1968); idem, *The Presentation of Self in Everyday Life* (Harmondsworth, 1969).

9 Sander L. Gilman, Helen King, Roy Porter, G. S. Rousseau and Elaine Showalter, *Hysteria Beyond Freud* (Berkeley, 1993).

10 Fiona Haslam, *From Hogarth to Rowlandson. Medicine in Art in Eighteenth-Century Britain* (Liverpool, 1996), pp. 132f. Hogarth undertook the task himself gratis. He also contributed a *Good Samaritan*.

11 A point particularly well made in Christine Stevenson, *Medicine and Magnificence: British Hospital and Asylum Architecture 1660–1815* (New Haven and London, 2000).

12 Miles Ogborn, *Spaces of Modernity: London's Geographies, 1680–1780* (New York, 1998).

13 Richard D. Altick, *The Shows of London: A Panoramic History of Exhibitions, 1600–1862* (Cambridge, MA, 1978).

14 Jonathan Andrews, Asa Briggs, Roy Porter, Penny Tucker and Keir Waddington, *The History of Bethlem* (London, 1997), p. 183.

15 Andrews *et al.*, *The History of Bethlem*.

16 Though see Chap. 2.

17 [Anon.], 'Ingenuity of the Gout Stools', *The Times*, 14 July 1962; J. C. Dagnall, 'A Gout Stool', *British Journal of Chiropody*, XXXVI (1971), p. 76. For the quotation, see A. Buzaglo, *A Treatise on the Gout* (London, 1778), p. 4; Roy Porter and G. S. Rousseau, *Gout: The Patrician Malady* (New Haven and London, 1998).

18 For syphilis, see Margaret Jane Healy, 'Fictions of Disease: Representations of Bodily Disorder in Early Modern Writings', PhD thesis, University College London, 1995; Sander Gilman, *Sexuality: An Illustrated History* (New York, 1989).

19 Leon Guilhamet, 'Pox and Malice. Some Representations of Venereal Disease in Restoration and Eighteenth-Century Satire', in Linda E. Merians, ed., *The Secret Malady. Venereal Disease in Eighteenth-Century Britain and France* (Lexington, 1996), pp. 196–212; Gilman, *Sexuality: An Illustrated History*.

20 Merians, ed., *The Secret Malady*, p. 2.

21 Samuel Garth, *The Dispensary* (London, 1699), canto II, pp. 83–84; canto III, pp. 82–3.

22 W. Thompson, *Sickness. A Poem* (London, 1745–6), book I, lines 4–5; pp. 362–5.

23 Erasmus Darwin, *The Temple of Nature; Or, The Origin of Society: A Poem with Philosophical Notes* (London, 1803), pp. 10–11.

24 Susan Sontag, *Illness as Metaphor* (New York, 1978).

25 'An Exact List of Maladies Suffered by the Townsfolk of Chelmsford!', *Chelmsford Chronicle*, January 1765.

26 Wolfgang Born, 'The Nature and History of Medical Caricature', *Ciba Symposia*, VI (1944–5), pp. 1910–24, p. 1920.

27 The print is reproduced in Juanita Burnby, *Caricatures and Comments* (Staines, 1989), p. 16.

28 James Spottiswoode Taylor, *Montaigne in Medicine: Being the Essayist's Comments on Contemporary Physic and Physicians; His Thoughts on Many Material Matters Relating to Life and Death; An Account of His Bodily Ailments and Peculiarities and of His Travels in Search of Health* (London, 1922), p. 109.

29 B. Fitzgerald, ed., *Correspondence of Emily, Duchess of Leinster*, 3 vols (Dublin, 1949–57) I, p. 492.

30 John Wiltshire, *Samuel Johnson in the Medical World. The Doctor and the Patient* (Cambridge, 1991), p. 66. Such bleeding does indeed ease breathing and induce sleep.

31 B. Aldington, *The Strange Life of Charles Waterton 1782–1865* (London, 1948). By way of parallel, William Cowper recounted, with some self-satisfaction, how he

succeeded in yanking out an aching tooth over the dinner table, without so much
as interrupting the meal: J. King and C. A. Ryskamp, eds, *The Letters and Prose
Writings of William Cowper*, 4 vols (Oxford, 1979–84), III, p. 73.

32 A. Fremantle, ed., *The Wynne Diaries*, 3 vols (London, 1935–40), I, p. 143.

33 L. A. Marchand, ed., *Byron's Letters and Journals*, 12 vols (London, 1973–82), XI,
p. 161.

34 Jonathan Swift, *Gulliver's Travels* (1726) (London, 1954), pp. 270–71; Carol
Houlihan Flynn, *The Body in Swift and Defoe* (Cambridge, 1990); S. La Casce,
'Swift on Medical Extremism', *Journal of the History of Ideas*, XXXI (1970),
pp. 599–606.

35 Haslam, *From Hogarth to Rowlandson*, p. 191.

36 Richard Hunter and Ida Macalpine, *Three Hundred Years of Psychiatry:
1535–1860* (London, 1963), p. 328.

37 Joseph Mason Cox, *Practical Observations on Insanity: In Which Some Suggestions
Are Offered Towards an Improved Mode of Treating Diseases of the Mind ... to Which
are Subjoined, Remarks on Medical Jurisprudence as Connected with Diseased
Intellect*, 2nd edn (London, 1806), pp. 137f.; Roy Porter, 'Shaping Psychiatric
Knowledge: The Role of the Asylum', in Roy Porter, ed., *Medicine in the
Enlightenment* (Amsterdam, 1995), pp. 256–73.

38 Cox, *Practical Observations on Insanity*, p. 47. There is a long theoretical tradition
of the advocacy of such therapeutic spectacle, including such renaissance figures
as Du Laurens and Burton; what is interesting about Cox is that he states that he
actually put them into effect.

39 *Ibid.*, p. 55.

40 *Ibid.*, p. 66.

41 *Ibid.*, p. 47.

42 *Ibid.*, p. 48.

43 *Ibid.*, p. 87.

44 *Ibid.*, p. 88.

45 H. B. Anderson, 'Robert Burns, His Medical Friends, Attendants, and
Biographer', *Annals of Medical History*, X (1928), pp. 48–58, p. 55.

46 C. C. Hankin, ed., *Life of Mary Anne Schimmelpenninck*, 2 vols (London, 1858), I,
pp. 6–7.

47 J. C. Jeaffreson, *A Book About Doctors* (London, n.d.), p. 201.

48 Roger King, 'Curing Toothache on the Stage?: The Importance of Reading
Pictures in Context', *History of Science*, XXXIII (1995), pp. 396–416; Colin Jones,
'Pulling Teeth in Eighteenth Century Paris', *Past and Present*, CLXVI (2000),
pp. 99–145; Curt Proskauer, 'The Dentist in Caricature', *Ciba Symposia*, VI
(1944), pp. 1933–48; T. G. H. Drake, 'English Caricatures of Medical Interest',
Ciba Symposia, VI (1944–5), pp. 1925–32, 1947–8.

49 See Proskauer, 'The Dentist in Caricature', pp. 1933–47.

50 Laurence Sterne, *The Life and Opinions of Tristram Shandy*, ed. Graham Petrie
(Harmondsworth, 1967), p. 459.

51 Roy Porter, 'Laymen, Doctors and Medical Knowledge in the Eighteenth
Century: The Evidence of the *Gentleman's Magazine*', in Roy Porter, ed.,
Patients and Practitioners: Lay Perceptions of Medicine in Pre-Industrial Society
(Cambridge, 1985), pp. 283–314; Ralph A. Houlbrooke, *Death, Religion and the
Family in England, 1480–1750* (Oxford, 1998).

52 'When I think of dying, it is always without pain or fear': D. King-Hele, *The
Letters of Erasmus Darwin* (Cambridge, 1981), p. 279: letter 95E, to Richard Lovell
Edgeworth, 15 March 1795; Philippe Ariès, *Western Attitudes Towards Death:
From the Middle Ages to the Present* (Baltimore, 1974); idem, *The Hour of Our*

Death, trans. H. Weaver (London, 1981); *idem, Images of Man and Death*, trans. Janet Lloyd (Cambridge, 1985); Nigel Llewellyn, *The Art of Death: Visual Culture in the English Death Ritual c.1500–c.1800* (London, 1991).

53 Robert Coope, comp., *The Quiet Art. A Doctor's Anthology* (Edinburgh, 1952), p. 176.

54 R. R. Wark, *Rowlandson's Drawings for the English Dance of Death* (San Marino, CA, 1966), pp. 3–27; Aldred Scott Warthin, 'The Physician of the Dance of Death', *Annals of Medical History*, ns II (1930), pp. 351–71, 453–69, 697–710; ns III (1931), pp. 75–109, 134–65. The prints, with accompanying verse by William Combe, were issued monthly, from April 1814 until March 1816.

55 T. G. H. Drake, 'The Medical Caricatures of Thomas Rowlandson', *Bulletin of the History of Medicine*, XII (1942), pp. 323–35, p. 330.

56 Haslam, *From Hogarth to Rowlandson*, p. 292.

5 Prototypes of Practitioners

1 G. Lloyd, ed., *Hippocratic Writings* (Harmondsworth, 1978), p. 67; Robert Baker, 'The History of Medical Ethics', in W. F. Bynum and Roy Porter, eds, *Companion Encyclopedia of the History of Medicine* (London, 1993), pp. 848–83.

2 Andrew Wear, *Knowledge and Practice in English Medicine 1550–1680* (Cambridge, 2000); *idem*, 'Epistemology and Learned Medicine in Early Modern England', in Don Bates, ed., *Knowledge and the Scholarly Medical Traditions* (Cambridge, 1995), pp. 151–74; *idem*, 'Medical Ethics in Early Modern England', in Andrew Wear, Johanna Geyer-Kordesch and Roger French, eds, *Doctors and Ethics: The Earlier Setting of Professional Ethics* (Amsterdam, 1993), pp. 98–130; Margaret Pelling, 'Medical Practice in Early Modern England: Trade or Profession?', in W. Prest, ed., *The Professions in Early Modern England* (London, 1987), pp. 90–128; Harold J. Cook, 'Good Advice and Little Medicine: The Professional Authority of Early Modern English Physicians', *Journal of British Studies*, XXXIII (1994), pp. 1–31.

3 John Securis, *A Detection and Querimonie of the Daily Enormities and Abuses Committed in Physick* (London, 1566), AIII–AIIIv, quoted in Natsu Hattori, 'Performing Cures: Practice and Interplay in Theatre and Medicine in the English Renaissance', DPhil thesis, University of Oxford, 1995, p. 40.

4 Christopher Lawrence, 'Medical Minds, Surgical Bodies: Corporeality and the Doctors', in Christopher Lawrence and Steven Shapin, eds, *Science Incarnate – Historical Embodiments of Natural Knowledge* (Chicago and London, 1998), pp. 156–201, p. 156; for representations of learnedness, see Ludmilla Jordanova, *Defining Features: Scientific and Medical Portraits 1660–2000* (London, 2000).

5 Ben Jonson, *Volpone*, ed. R. Parker (Manchester, 1983), Act 2, Scene 2, p. 152; Roy Porter, *Health for Sale: Quackery in England 1650–1850* (Manchester, 1989), p. 2.

6 In 1518 the King granted a Charter to the body that became the Royal College of Physicians in 1551. An Act of 1540 empowered the Company to ensure the purity of drugs sold by apothecaries.

7 Herbert Silvette, *The Doctor on Stage. Medicine and Medical Men in Seventeenth Century England*, ed. F. Butler (Knoxville, 1967); Hattori, 'Performing Cures'; Wolfgang Born, 'The Nature and History of Medical Caricature', *Ciba Symposia*, VI (1944–5), pp. 1910–24, for the background of medical satire. The comic type of the doctor found a place of refuge on the stage of the *commedia dell'arte* in Italy. The popular improvised comedy with its spirited stock characters flourished in the seventeenth and the early eighteenth centuries. See M. A. Katritzky, 'Was *Commedia dell'arte* Performed by Mountebanks?: *Album amicorum* Illustrations and Thomas Platter's Descriptions of 1598', *Theatre Research International*, XXIII

(1998), pp. 104–25.

8 Graham Everitt, *Doctors and Doctors: Some Curious Chapters in Medical History and Quackery* (London, 1888), pp. 24f. The physician as pedant had long featured in the *Commedia dell'Arte*, offering models for Molière's prating physicians and the asinine doctors in the picaresque novels of Gil Blas and Tobias Smollett (himself a practitioner), where they are duped by their wives and valets while pretending to omniscience. Richard Wilson's *The Cheats* (1662) features a 'physician' who adopts all the cozening devices of empirics, while John Lacy's *The Dumb Lady* (1672) exemplifies the idea that anyone, by wearing the right garb and uttering the right words, might pass as a learned physician: Hattori, 'Performing Cures', p. 174.

9 See Marcia Pointon, *Hanging the Head: Portraiture and Social Formation in Eighteenth-Century England* (New Haven, 1993); Kathleen Adler and Marcia Pointon, eds, *The Body Imaged: The Human Form and Visual Culture Since the Renaissance* (Cambridge, 1993); Renate Burgess, *Portraits of Doctors and Scientists in the Wellcome Institute for the History of Medicine* (London, 1973).

10 David Harley, 'The Good Physician and the Godly Doctor: The Exemplary Life of John Tylston of Chester (1663–99)', *The Seventeenth Century*, LX (1994), pp. 93–117; David Piper, 'Take the Face of a Physician', in Gordon Wolstenholme, ed., *Portraits: The Royal College of Physicians of London, Catalogue II* (Amsterdam, 1977), pp. 25–49.

11 Piper, 'Take the Face of a Physician', pp. 25–49, p. 28; Christopher Lawrence, 'Medical Minds, Surgical Bodies', pp. 156–201, p. 161.

12 C. R. Hone, *The Life of Dr. John Radcliffe 1652–1714: Benefactor of the University of Oxford* (London, 1950), p. 51.

13 R. Cook, *Sir Samuel Garth* (Boston, 1980), p. 42; Christopher Booth, 'Sir Samuel Garth FRS: The Dispensary Poet', *Notes and Records of the Royal Society of London*, XL (1985–86), pp. 125–45. Messenger Monsey imagined a sickbed scene:

> Seven wise physicians lately met,
> To save a wretched sinner;
> Come, Tom, said Jack, pray let's be quick,
> Or I shall lose my dinner.
> Some roared for rhubarb, jalap some,
> And some cried out for Dover;
> Let's give him something, each man said –
> Why e'en let's give him – over.

J. C. Jeaffreson, *A Book About Doctors* (London, n.d.), p. 199. 'Dover' was Dr Dover's Powders, a nostrum designed to purge: K. Dewhurst, *The Quicksilver Doctor. The Life and Times of Thomas Dover* (Bristol, 1957), p. 141.

14 Quoted in Anita Guerrini, *Obesity and Depression in the Enlightenment: The Life and Times of George Cheyne* (Norman, OK, 2000), p. 56. According to Guerrini, this work is by John Woodward.

15 Hone, *Life of Dr. John Radcliffe*, p. 58; William Macmichael, *The Gold-Headed Cane*, ed. with Explanatory and Illustrative Notes and an Essay on William Macmichael, MD, His Life, His Works, and his Editors by Herbert Spencer Robinson (New York, 1932), p. 151.

16 Jeaffreson, *A Book About Doctors*, p. 16.

17 J. Levine, *Dr Woodward's Shield* (Berkeley, 1977), chap. 1, *passim*.

18 John Gay, *Three Hours After Marriage* (London, 1717); see Calhoun Winton, *John Gay and the London Theatre* (Lexington, 1993); David Nokes, *John Gay. A Profession of Friendship* (Oxford, 1995). Woodward was not the first actual doctor to figure on stage: the Tudor Dr Caius appears in Shakespeare's *The Merry Wives*

of Windsor: Hattori, 'Performing Cures', p. 141.

19 Anita Guerrini, '"A Club of Little Villains": Rhetoric, Professional Identity and Medical Pamphlet Wars', in Marie Mulvey Roberts and Roy Porter, eds, *Literature and Medicine During the Eighteenth Century* (London, 1995), pp. 226–44.

20 Roy Porter, 'William Hunter: A Surgeon and a Gentleman', in W. F. Bynum and Roy Porter, eds, *William Hunter and the Eighteenth Century Medical World* (Cambridge, 1985), pp. 7–34, p. 26.

21 Levine, *Dr Woodward's Shield*, p. 16. For later medical duellists see F. L. M. Pattison, *Granville Sharpe Pattison: Anatomist and Antagonist* (Edinburgh, 1987).

22 The apothecaries maintained that the 1542 Act, 'The Quack's Charter', entitled them to give advice to patients as long as they charged only for the drugs they dispensed.

23 Diagnosis by horoscope, part of traditional medicine, was discredited by the late seventeenth century.

24 Samuel Garth, *The Dispensary* (London, 1699), canto III, p. 31.

25 *Ibid.*, canto V, p. 54.

26 *Ibid.*, canto VI, p. 81.

27 *Ibid.*, canto I, p. 10.

28 *Ibid.*, canto VI, p. 75.

29 R. Cook, *Sir Samuel Garth* (Boston, 1980), p. 77.

30 J. Addison and R. Steele, *The Spectator*, ed. Donald Bond, 5 vols (Oxford, 1965), no. 21, 24 March 1711, vol. i, p. 90.

31 Garth, *The Dispensary*, canto iv, p. 42.

32 Cook, *Sir Samuel Garth*, p. 78.

33 *Ibid.*, p. 16; Harry M. Solomon, *Sir Richard Blackmore* (Boston, 1980).

34 Roy Porter, 'John Woodward: A Droll Sort of Philosopher', *Geological Magazine*, CXVI (1979), pp. 395–417; David Nokes, *John Gay. A Profession of Friendship* (Oxford, 1995), p. 245.

35 *Professional Anecdotes, or ANA of Medical Literature*, 3 vols (London, 1825), I, p. 245. William Stukeley noted Mead's 'decrepit amours', and the Reverend Edmund Pyle simultaneously accused and exculpated him by remarking that the President of the Royal Society, Martin Folkes, was the 'most foolishly and beastly vicious in the wenching way of any body I every heard of, – a good deal beyond Dr Mead': Roy Porter, 'A Touch of Danger: The Man-Midwife as Sexual Predator', in G. S. Rousseau and R. Porter, eds, *Sexual Underworlds of the Enlightenment* (Manchester, 1988), pp. 206–32, p. 210.

36 Laurence Sterne, *The Life and Opinions of Tristram Shandy*, ed. Graham Petrie (Harmondsworth, 1967), p. 43.

37 Hone, *Life of Dr. John Radcliffe*, p. 57.

38 *Professional Anecdotes, or ANA of Medical Literature*, I, p. 229.

39 For the alleged irreligion of doctors, see Philip K. Wilson, *Surgery, Skin and Syphilis: Daniel Turner's London (1667–1741)* (Amsterdam and Atlanta, GA, 1999), p. 100. A 1707 issue of *The Weekly Comedy* claimed that 'Physicians ... are generally accounted atheists'. That term was loosely bandied about, however, as a term of abuse.

40 Harold Cook, *The Decline of the Old Medical Regime in Stuart London* (Ithaca, 1986).

41 The apothecaries gained the legal right to act as advisers, in addition to dispensing, following the Rose Case verdict in 1703: Harold J. Cook, 'The Rose Case Reconsidered: Physicians, Apothecaries and the Law in Augustan England', *Journal of the History of Medicine*, XLV (1990), pp. 527–55.

42 Roy Porter, 'William Hunter: A Surgeon and a Gentleman', pp. 7–34; N. D. Jewson, 'Medical Knowledge and the Patronage System in Eighteenth Century

England', *Sociology*, VIII (1974), pp. 369–85.

43 For professional optimism, see Penelope Corfield, *Power and the Professions in Britain 1700–1850* (London, 1995); G. Holmes, *Augustan England: Professions, State and Society, 1680–1730* (London, 1982). For secularization, see Roy Porter, *Enlightenment: Britain and the Creation of the Modern World* (Harmondsworth, 2000), chap. IX.

44 See for instance the career of Sir John Colbatch: Harold J. Cook, 'Sir John Colbatch and Augustan Medicine: Experimentalism, Character and Entrepreneurialism', *Annals of Science*, XLVII (1990), pp. 475–505. Colbatch was a regular but he marketed nostrums and sold himself energetically.

45 Ann L. Reitz, 'Sawbones to Savior to Cynic: The Doctor's Relation to Society in English Fiction of the Eighteenth, Nineteenth, and Twentieth Centuries', PhD thesis, University of Cincinnati, 1985, p. 53; see also Leo Braudy, *The Frenzy of Renown* (Oxford, 1987).

46 Eric S. Rump, ed., *The Comedies of William Congreve* (Harmondsworth, 1985), p. 333.

47 Peter Stallybrass and Allon White, *The Politics and Poetics of Transgression* (Ithaca, 1986), pp. 100f.; Warren Chernaik, *Sexual Freedom in Restoration Literature* (Cambridge, 1995).

48 R. Campbell, *The London Tradesman: Being a Compendious View of All the Trades, Professions, Arts, Both Liberal and Mechanic, now Practised in the Cities of London and Westminster* (London, 1747), p. 41; Phillis Cunnington and Catherine Lucas, *Occupational Costume in England* (London, 1967); James Laver, *A Concise History of Costume* (London, 1969). The 'mercenary colleges' the author would have had in mind were St Andrews and Aberdeen.

49 Lawrence, 'Medical Minds, Surgical Bodies', pp. 156–201, p. 170. On wigs, see David Piper, *The English Face* (London, 1992), p. 102.

50 Lawrence, 'Medical Minds, Surgical Bodies', pp. 156–201, p. 170.

51 Porter, 'William Hunter: A Surgeon and a Gentleman', pp. 7–34, p. 29.

52 Reitz, 'Sawbones to Savior to Cynic', p. 246; for a visual comparison see Peter Wagner, 'The Satire on Doctors in Hogarth's Graphic Works', in Roberts and Porter, eds, *Literature and Medicine During the Eighteenth Century*, pp. 200–25.

53 Reitz, 'Sawbones to Savior to Cynic', p. 259.

54 *Ibid.*, p. 260.

55 The 'famous empyrick' was Joshua Ward: *ibid.*, p. 260.

56 Dorothy Porter and Roy Porter, *Patient's Progress: Doctors and Doctoring in Eighteenth-Century England* (Cambridge, 1989), p. 119.

57 Porter and Porter, *Patient's Progress*, p. 125.

58 Addison and Steele, *The Spectator*, ed. Bond, no. 21 (24 March 1711), p. 90.

59 K. Garlick and A. Macintyre, eds, *The Diary of Joseph Farington*, 16 vols (New Haven, 1978–9), II, p. 477.

60 F. Bamford, ed., *Dear Miss Heber* (London, 1936), p. 168.

61 'Dress', according to Lord Chesterfield, was 'a very foolish thing': 'and yet it is a very foolish thing for a man not to be well dressed, according to his rank and way of life'. A letter to his son, 19 November 1745: Lord Chesterfield, *Letters to His Son*, 2 vols (London, 1774), letter LXXIV, vol. i, p. 183; Quentin Bell, *On Human Finery* (London, 1992), p. 18.

62 Lawrence, 'Medical Minds, Surgical Bodies', pp. 156–201; *idem*, 'Democratic, Divine and Heroic: The History and Historiography of Surgery', in Christopher Lawrence, ed., *Medical Theory, Surgical Practice: Studies in the History of Surgery* (London, 1992), pp. 1–47.

63 Roy Porter, 'The Rise of Physical Examination', in W. F. Bynum and Roy Porter, eds, *Medicine and the Five Senses* (Cambridge, 1992), pp. 179–97.

64 Rob Iliffe, 'Isaac Newton: Lucatello Professor of Mathematics', in C. Lawrence and S. Shapin, eds, *Science Incarnate – Historical Embodiments of Natural Knowledge* (Chicago and London, 1998), pp. 121–55; Steven Shapin, 'The Philosopher and the Chicken: On the Dietetics of Disembodied Knowledge', in Lawrence and Shapin, eds, *Science Incarnate*, pp. 21–50.

65 Campbell, *The London Tradesman*, p. 42; Lawrence, 'Medical Minds, Surgical Bodies', in Lawrence and Shapin, eds, *Science Incarnate*, pp. 156–201, p. 169.

66 T. J. Pettigrew, *Memoirs of the Life and Writings of the Late John Coakley Lettsom*, 3 vols (London, 1817), I, p. 21.

67 *Ibid.*, II, p. 53.

68 William Cole, quoted in Ernest Heberden, *William Heberden: Physician of the Age of Reason* (London, 1989), p. 61.

69 John Wiltshire, *Samuel Johnson in the Medical World. The Doctor and the Patient* (Cambridge, 1991), p. 92; Heberden, *William Heberden*.

70 Steven Shapin, ' "The Mind Is Its Own Place": Science and Solitude in Seventeenth-Century England', *Science in Context*, IV (1991), pp. 191–218; Harold J. Cook, 'The New Philosophy and Medicine in Seventeenth-Century England', in David C. Lindberg and Robert S. Westman, eds, *Reappraisals of the Scientific Revolution* (Cambridge, 1990), pp. 397–436. The Renaissance scholar was meant to assume a melancholy disposition, because that was a sign of both asceticism and genius. In his *Anatomy of Melancholy*, Burton devoted a section to this phenomenon and entitled it 'Love of Learning, or overmuch Study. With a Digression of the Misery of Schollers, and why the Muses are Melancholy': study made a man melancholy.

71 Dress and demeanour were regarded as of great importance. Adam Smith wrote of the young nobleman that 'His air, his manner, his deportment, all mark that elegant and graceful sense of his own superiority which those who are born to inferior stations can hardly ever arrive at.' Quoted in Jan Bremmer and Herman Roodenburg, eds, *A Cultural History of Gesture: From Antiquity to the Present Day* (Cambridge, 1991), p. 7; see also Penelope Byrde, *The Male Image: Men's Fashion in Britain 1300–1970* (London, 1979).

72 See Porter, 'William Hunter: A Surgeon and a Gentleman', pp. 7–34.

73 Richard H. Mead, *In the Sunshine of Life: a Biography of Dr. Richard Mead 1673–1754* (Philadelphia, 1974); A. Zuckerman, 'Dr Richard Mead (1673–1754): a Biographical Study', PhD thesis, University of Illinois, 1965; Ludmilla Jordanova, *Defining Features*, p. 27; Macmichael, *The Gold-Headed Cane*, p. 148. Mead had a library of over 10,000 volumes. Having established a lucrative practice in London, he indulged his enthusiasm for classical learning by gradually amassing an impressive collection of books, manuscripts, statuary, coins, gems and drawings. At his Great Ormond Street house, he held regular levées at which persons with suitable introductions were welcomed and shown round the exhibits. For images of gentility, see Anna Bryson, 'The Rhetoric of Status; Gesture, Demeanour and the Image of the Gentleman in Sixteenth- and Seventeenth-Century England', in Lucy Gent and Nigel Llewellyn, eds, *Renaissance Bodies: The Human Figure in English Culture c. 1540–1660* (London, 1990), pp. 136–53; Fenella Childs, 'Prescriptions for Manners in Eighteenth Century Courtesy Literature', DPhil thesis, University of Oxford, 1984.

74 C. H. Brock, 'The Happiness of Riches', in Bynum and Porter, eds, *William Hunter*, pp. 35–56.

75 Pettigrew, *Memoirs of the Life and Writings of the Late John Coakley Lettsom*, I, p. 118; Roy Porter, 'John Coakley Lettsom and "The Highest and Most Divine Profession, that can Engage Human Intellect" ', *Transactions of the Medical*

Society of London (1996), pp. 22–34.

76 Anthony Ashley Cooper, 3rd Earl of Shaftesbury, *Characteristicks of Men, Manners, Opinions, Times*, 2 vols, ed. Philip Ayres (Oxford, 1999), 'Miscellany', III. chap. I; ''Tis the persecuting Spirit has rais'd the *bantering* one': 'Sensus Communis', section 4, vol. I, p. 43.

77 Anthony, 3rd Earl of Shaftesbury, 'Miscellany', III, in *Characteristicks of Men, Manners, Opinions, Times*, II, chap. I, p. 206. L. E. Klein, *Shaftesbury and the Culture of Politeness: Moral Discourse and Cultural Politics in Early Eighteenth-Century England* (Cambridge, 1994), p. 34.

78 Addison and Steele, *The Spectator*, I, no. 10, p. 54.

79 'Of Essay Writing', in *David Hume, Selected Essays*, ed. and intro. Stephen Copley and Andrew Edgar (Oxford, 1993), p. 2.

80 Macmichael, *The Gold-Headed Cane*, p. 107.

81 Levine, *Dr Woodward's Shield*, p. 10.

82 Macmichael, *The Gold-Headed Cane*, p. 24; Levine, *Dr Woodward's Shield*, p. 10; Hone, *Life of Dr. John Radcliffe.*

83 George Cheyne, *The English Malady*, (1733) ed. Roy Porter (London, 1990), p. 326; Bernard Mandeville, *The Fable of the Bees*, ed. P. Harth (Harmondsworth, 1970), p. 35.

84 Cheyne, *The English Malady*, p. 326; Guerrini, *Obesity and Depression*, pp. 5, 59.

85 Maureen McNeil, *Under the Banner of Science: Erasmus Darwin and His Age* (Manchester, 1987). Mandeville said that the way to get on as a young doctor was to shine as a man of letters: 'shew your self a Scholar, write a Poem, either a good one, or a long one; Compose a *Latin* Oration, or do but Translate something out of that Language with your Name on it. If you can do none of all these, Marry into a good Family': quoted in Guerrini, *Obesity and Depression*, p. 56. Doctors hobnobbed with men of letters: Dr John Arbuthnot was part of the Scriblerus Circle. Pope wrote:

> I'll do what Mead and Cheselden advise
> To keep these limbs, and to preserve these eyes.

Pope's couplet is discussed in G. S. Rousseau and Marjorie Hope Nicolson, *This Long Disease My Life: Alexander Pope and the Sciences* (Princeton, 1968), p. 9.

86 Porter, *Enlightenment: Britain and the Creation of the Modern World*, chs IV and VII.

87 R. Hingston Fox, *Dr John Fothergill and His Friends: Chapters in Eighteenth Century Life* (London, 1919), p. 32.

88 Macmichael, *The Gold-Headed Cane*, p. 107.

89 K. Coburn, ed., *The Letters of Sara Hutchinson from 1800–1835* (London, 1954), p. 272.

90 Macmichael, *The Gold-Headed Cane*; Fiona Haslam, *From Hogarth to Rowlandson. Medicine in Art in Eighteenth-Century Britain* (Liverpool, 1996), p. 20.

91 Thomas Gisborne, *An Enquiry into the Duties of Men in the Higher and Middle Classes of Society in Great Britain, Resulting from their Respective Stations, Professions and Employments*, 2 vols (London, 1794), II, p. 132.

6 Profiles of Patients

1 Tobias Smollett, *The Expedition of Humphry Clinker* (1771) ed. A. Ross (Harmondsworth, 1967), Matthew Bramble to Doctor Lewis, p. 187.

2 The corollary of this is that, in those times, lower-class patients got only restricted access, if any, to superior physicians. See N. D. Jewson, 'Medical Knowledge and the Patronage System in Eighteenth Century England', *Sociology*, VIII (1974), pp. 369–85; *idem*, 'The Disappearance of the Sick Man from Medical Cosmology, 1770–1870', *Sociology*, X (1976), pp. 225–44; Mary E. Fissell, 'The Disappearance

of the Patient's Narrative and the Invention of Hospital Medicine', in Roger French and Andrew Wear, eds, *British Medicine in an Age of Reform* (London and New York, 1992), pp. 92–109; Roy Porter, 'The Patient's View: Doing Medical History from Below', *Theory and Society*, XIV (1985), pp. 175–98.

3 Samuel Taylor Coleridge, *Table Talk*, in *The Collected Works of Samuel Taylor Coleridge* (London, 1990), vol. XIV, ed. Carl Woodring, p. 106.

4 Thomas Beddoes, *A Letter to the Right Honourable Sir Joseph Banks ... on the Causes and Removal of the Prevailing Discontents, Imperfections, and Abuses, in Medicine* (London, 1808), p. 115.

5 See G. Thomas Couser, *Recovering Bodies. Illness, Disability, and Life Writing* (Wisconsin, 1997); Dorothy Porter and Roy Porter, *Patient's Progress: Doctors and Doctoring in Eighteenth-Century England* (Cambridge, 1989); Roy Porter and Dorothy Porter, *In Sickness and in Health: The British Experience 1650-1850* (London, 1988); Lucinda McCray Beier, *Sufferers and Healers: The Experience of Illness in Seventeenth-Century England* (London, 1987); Joan Lane, '"The Doctor Scolds Me": The Diaries and Correspondence of Patients in Eighteenth Century England', in Roy Porter, ed., *Patients and Practitioners: Lay Perceptions of Medicine in Pre-Industrial Society* (Cambridge, 1985), pp. 204–48.

6 H. W. Robinson and W. Adams, eds, *The Diary of Robert Hooke (1672–1680)* (London, 1935), pp. 17–18.

7 R. Latham and W. Matthews, eds, *The Diary of Samuel Pepys*, 11 vols (London, 1970–83), vol. iv, p. 39, 9 February 1663; Beier, *Sufferers and Healers*.

8 Mary E. Fissell, 'Readers, Texts and Contexts: Vernacular Medical Works in Early Modern England', in Roy Porter, ed., *The Popularization of Medicine* (London and New York, 1992), pp. 72–96; C. J. Lawrence, 'William Buchan: Medicine Laid Open', *Medical History*, XIX (1975), pp. 20–35.

9 B. Haley, *The Healthy Body and Victorian Culture* (Cambridge, MA, 1978).

10 John Brewer and Roy Porter, eds, *Consumption and the World of Goods in the 17th and 18th Centuries* (London and New York, 1993); Roy Porter, 'The Patient in England, c.1660–c.1800', in Andrew Wear, ed., *Medicine in Society* (Cambridge, 1992), pp. 91–118.

11 J. Timbs, *Doctors and Patients; or Anecdotes of the Medical World and Curiosities of Medicine* (London, 1876), p. 360; M. P. Tilley, ed., *Dictionary of Proverbs in England* (Ann Arbor, 1950).

12 D. Little and G. Kahrl, eds, *The Letters of David Garrick*, 3 vols (London, 1963), II, p. 743.

13 David Vaisey, ed., *The Diary of Thomas Turner of East Hoathley* (Oxford, 1984), p. 105.

14 Charles E. Mullett, ed. and intro., *The Letters of Dr. George Cheyne to the Countess of Huntingdon* (San Marino, CA, 1940); *idem*, ed., *The Letters of Doctor George Cheyne to Samuel Richardson (1733–1743)* (Missouri, 1943); Anita Guerrini, *Obesity and Depression in the Enlightenment: The Life and Times of George Cheyne* (Norman, OK, 2000).

15 Mullett, ed. and intro., *The Letters of Dr. George Cheyne to the Countess of Huntingdon*, pp. 59–60; Carol Houlihan Flynn, 'Running out of Matter: The Body Exercised in Eighteenth Century Fiction', in G. S. Rousseau, ed., *The Language of Psyche: Mind and Body in the Enlightenment* (Los Angeles, 1990), pp. 147–85.

16 Mullett, ed. and intro., *The Letters of Dr. George Cheyne to the Countess of Huntingdon*, p. 59. Note that Cheyne speaks about buying the horse: evidently it was a commercial speculation.

17 See discussion in Guerrini, *Obesity and Depression*.

18 *Gentleman's Magazine*, II (1732), p. 769; William Macmichael, *The Gold-Headed Cane*, ed. with Explanatory and Illustrative Notes and an Essay on William Macmichael, MD, His Life, His Works, and his Editors by Herbert Spencer Robinson (New York, 1932), p. 183.

19 R. W. Chapman, ed., *Jane Austen's Letters to Her Sister Cassandra & Others* (London, 1952), p. 426.

20 T. G. H. Drake, 'The Medical Caricatures of Thomas Rowlandson', *Bulletin of the History of Medicine*, XII (1942), pp. 323–35, p. 324.

21 C. F. Barrett , ed., *The Diary and Letters of Madame d'Arblay, Author of 'Evelina', 'Cecilia', etc. 1778–1840*, 7 vols (London, 1842–6), I, p. 292.

22 Thomas Beddoes, *Hygëia: or Essays Moral and Medical, on the Causes Affecting the Personal State of our Middling and Affluent Classes*, 3 vols (Bristol, 1802) vol. I essay II, p. 23; I essay II, p. 25.

23 George Eliot, *Middlemarch* (Harmondsworth, 1965), pp. 116–7.

24 Roy Porter, 'The Patient in England, c. 1660–c. 1800', pp. 91–118. The hypochondriac was largely seen as male. The female analogue was the hysteric. The culture of the early modern hysterical woman has been studied, with particular reference to Netherlandish paintings, in Laurinda S. Dixon, *Perilous Chastity: Women and Illness in Pre-Enlightenment Art and Medicine* (Ithaca, 1995). See also Sander L. Gilman, Helen King, Roy Porter, G. S. Rousseau and Elaine Showalter, *Hysteria Beyond Freud* (Berkeley, 1993); Mark Micale, *Approaching Hysteria. Disease and its Interpretations* (Princeton, 1995).

25 B. Mandeville, *A Treatise of the Hypochondriack and Hysterick Diseases*, 2nd edn (London, 1730) (reprinted Hildesheim: George Olms Verlag, 1981), 49; see also Roy Porter, 'Reading: A Health Warning', in Robin Myers and Michael Harris, eds, *Medicine, Mortality and the Booktrade* (Winchester, 1998), pp. 131–52.

26 Joseph Addison and Richard Steele, *The Spectator*, ed. Donald Bond, 5 vols (Oxford, 1965), I, pp. 105–6.

27 J. M. Adair, *Essays on Fashionable Diseases* (London, 1790), p. 95; Steven Shapin, 'The Philosopher and the Chicken: On the Dietetics of Disembodied Knowledge', in Christopher Lawrence and Steven Shapin, eds, *Science Incarnate – Historical Embodiments of Natural Knowledge* (Chicago and London, 1998), pp. 21–50.

28 Adair, *Essays on Fashionable Diseases*, p. 95.

29 J. Hill, *Hypochondriasis* (London, 1756), p. 24.

30 Quoted in A. M. Ingram, *Boswell's Creative Gloom* (London, 1982), p. 104.

31 Quoted in R. Hunter and I. Macalpine, *Three Hundred Years of Psychiatry 1535–1860* (London, 1963), p. 312.

32 Mullett, ed. and intro., *The Letters of Dr. George Cheyne to the Countess of Huntingdon*.

33 Aphra Behn, *Sir Patient Fancy* (London, 1678), Act 3 Scene 1, in J. Todd, ed., *The Works of Aphra Behn*, vol. VI: *The Plays* (London, 1996), p. 31.

34 Behn, *Sir Patient Fancy*, Act 2 Scene 2, p. 30; see Natsu Hattori, 'Performing Cures: Practice and Interplay in Theatre and Medicine of the English Renaissance', DPhil thesis, University of Oxford, 1995, p. 84.

35 John Wiltshire, *Jane Austen and the Body: 'The Picture of Health'* (Cambridge, 1992), p. 200.

36 Jane Austen, *Sanditon*, ed. M. Drabble (Harmondsworth, 1974), p. 174.

37 Austen, *Sanditon*, p. 175. On the fashion for biliousness, see Roy Porter, 'Biliousness' in W. F. Bynum, ed., *Gastroenterology in Britain* (London: Occasional Publications 3, 1997), pp. 7–28; for nervousness, see *idem*, '"Expressing Yourself Ill": The Language of Sickness in Georgian England', in P. Burke and R. Porter, eds, *Language, Self and Society: The Social History of*

Language (Cambridge, 1991), pp. 276–99.

38 Austen, *Sanditon*, p. 175. For self-medication see Porter and Porter, *Patient's Progress*, chaps 1–4.

39 Austen, *Sanditon*, pp. 202–3.

40 For documentation of what follows, see Roy Porter, 'Biliousness' pp. 7–28.

41 George M. Gould, *Biographic Clinics: The Origin of the Ill-health of De Quincey, Carlyle, Darwin, Huxley and Browning* (London, 1903), p. 44.

42 *Ibid.*, p. 54. Carlyle's use of 'nicotine' is rather early.

43 *Ibid.*, p. 54.

44 *Ibid.*, p. 64.

45 *Ibid.*, p. 49.

46 *Ibid.*, p. 54.

47 Edwin W. Marrs, Jr, ed., *The Letters of Thomas Carlyle to his Brother, Alexander, with Related Family Letters* (Cambridge, MA, 1968), p. 591.

48 Anne Hunsaker Hawkins, *Reconstructing Illness: Studies in Pathography* (West Lafayette, 1993); illuminating is Oliver Sacks, *A Leg to Stand On* (London, 1984). For the Augustan refusal to mythologize illness in this way, see G. S. Rousseau and Marjorie Hope Nicolson, *This Long Disease My Life: Alexander Pope and the Sciences* (Princeton, 1968).

49 Tobias Smollett, *Humphry Clinker* pp. 65–66; Fiona Haslam, *From Hogarth to Rowlandson. Medicine in Art in Eighteenth-Century Britain* (Liverpool, 1996), pp. 174f.

50 Janet Browne, 'I Could have Retched All Night: Charles Darwin and His Body, in Early Victorian England', in Christopher Lawrence and Steven Shapin, eds, *Science Incarnate – Historical Embodiments of Natural Knowledge* (Chicago and London, 1998), pp. 240–87; *idem*, 'Spas and Sensibilities: Darwin at Malvern', in Roy Porter, ed., *The Medical History of Waters and Spas* (London: Medical History, Supplement 10, 1990), pp. 102–13.

51 A. Barbeau, *Life and Letters at Bath in the Eighteenth Century*, ed. A. Dobson (London, 1904), p. 92; Barbara Brandon Schnorrenberg, 'Medical Men of Bath', *Studies in Eighteenth Century Culture*, XIII (1984), pp. 189–203; Aileen Douglas, *Uneasy Sensations. Smollett and the Body* (Chicago, 1995).

52 Fielding H. Garrison, 'Medicine in *The Tatler, Spectator* and *Guardian*', *Bulletin of the History of Medicine*, II (1934), pp. 477–503.

53 Schnorrenberg, 'Medical Men of Bath', pp. 189–203; Brigitte Mitchell and John Penrose, eds, *Letters from Bath, 1766–67* (Gloucester, 1983), p. 35.

54 Mitchell and Penrose, eds, *Letters from Bath, 1766–67*, p. 35.

55 Christopher Anstey, *The New Bath Guide: or Memoirs of the B-n-r-d Family, in a Series of Poetical Epistles* (1801), ed. Peter Wagner (Hildesheim, Zurich and New York, 1989); Smollett, *Humphry Clinker*; G. S. Rousseau, *Tobias Smollett: Essays of Two Decades* (Edinburgh, 1982); Barbeau, *Life and Letters at Bath in the Eighteenth Century*; Phyliss Hembry, *The English Spa 1560–1815: A Social History* (London, 1990).

56 Anstey, *The New Bath Guide*, letter II, p. 14.

57 Haslam, *From Hogarth to Rowlandson*, p. 181; Schnorrenberg, 'Medical Men of Bath', p. 196.

58 Tobias Smollett, *Peregrine Pickle* (1751) (Oxford, 1983); Schnorrenberg, 'Medical Men of Bath', p. 195.

59 Thomas Beddoes, *Manual of Health: or, the Invalid Conducted Safely Through the Seasons* (London, 1806), p. 330.

60 Beddoes, *A Letter to the Right Honourable Sir Joseph Banks*, p. 102.

61 Beddoes, *Manual of Health*, p. 331.

62 Beddoes, *A Letter to the Right Honourable Sir Joseph Banks*, p. 104; Mary E.
Fissell, *Patients, Power, and the Poor in Eighteenth-Century Bristol* (Cambridge,
1991).

63 Beddoes, *Manual of Health*, p. 332.

64 *Ibid.*, p. 333.

65 *Ibid.*, p. 335.

66 *Ibid.*, p. 337.

67 Quoted in R. S. Downie, ed., *The Healing Arts. An Oxford Illustrated Anthology*
(Oxford, 1994), p. 155.

68 Quoted in Miriam Bailin, *The Sickroom in Victorian Fiction: The Art of Being Ill*
(Cambridge, 1994), p. 6.

69 H. Martineau, *Life in the Sick-Room: Essays by an Invalid* (2nd edn, London,
1854).

70 Bailin, *The Sickroom*.

7 Outsiders and Intruders

1 For the Scots, see Ivan Waddington, *The Medical Profession in the Industrial
Revolution* (Dublin, 1984); C. J. Lawrence, 'Medicine as Culture: Edinburgh and
the Scottish Enlightenment', PhD thesis, University of London, 1984; Lisa
Rosner, *Medical Education in the Age of Improvement: Edinburgh Students and
Apprentices, 1760–1826* (Edinburgh, 1990).

2 I. S. L. Loudon, *Medical Care and the General Practitioner 1750–1850* (Oxford,
1986); Anne Digby, *Making a Medical Living: Doctors and Patients in the English
Market for Medicine, 1720–1911* (Cambridge, 1994). For the Continent, see Mary
Lindemann, *Health and Healing in Seventeenth- and Eighteenth-Century Germany*
(Baltimore, 1996); Matthew Ramsey, *Professional and Popular Medicine in France,
1770–1830. The Social World of Medical Practice* (Cambridge, 1988); Lawrence
Brockliss and Colin Jones, *The Medical World of Early Modern France* (Oxford,
1997).

3 Sir Z. Cope, *The History of the Royal College of Surgeons of England* (London,
1959); for a new look at the history of surgery, see Christopher Lawrence,
'Democratic, Divine and Heroic: The History and Historiography of Surgery',
in Christopher Lawrence, ed., *Medical Theory, Surgical Practice: Studies in the
History of Surgery*, (London, 1992), pp. 1–47.

4 Lord Herbert, ed., *Pembroke Papers (1790–1794): Letters and Diaries of Henry,
Tenth Earl of Pembroke and His Circle* (London, 1950), II, p. 318.

5 Christopher Lawrence, 'Medical Minds, Surgical Bodies: Corporeality and the
Doctors', in Christopher Lawrence and Steven Shapin, eds, *Science Incarnate –
Historical Embodiments of Natural Knowledge* (Chicago and London, 1998),
pp. 156–201.

6 Tobias Smollett, *Roderick Random* (1748) (Oxford, 1979), p. 86; Joan Druett,
Rough Medicine: Surgeons at Sea in the Age of Sail (New York, 2000), pp. 8of.;
Aileen Douglas, *Uneasy Sensations. Smollett and the Body* (Chicago, 1995).

7 Smollett, *Roderick Random*, p. 139.

8 *Ibid.*, p. 149.

9 *Ibid.*, p. 158.

10 For the following see J. Oppenheimer, *New Aspects of John and of William Hunter*
(London, 1946); Roy Porter, 'John Hunter: A Showman in Society', *The
Transactions of the Hunterian Society* (1993–4), pp. 19–24; *idem*, 'William Hunter:
A Surgeon and a Gentleman', in W. F. Bynum and Roy Porter, eds, *William Hunter
and the Eighteenth Century Medical World* (Cambridge, 1985), pp. 7–34; L. S.
Jacyna, 'Images of John Hunter in the Nineteenth Century', *History of Science*,

xxi (1983), pp. 85–108.

11 S. Paget, *John Hunter* (London, 1897), p. 126.

12 Jacyna, 'Images of John Hunter in the Nineteenth Century', pp. 85–108.

13 Lawrence and Shapin, eds, *Science Incarnate*, p. 193; see more broadly Lawrence, 'Democratic, Divine and Heroic', pp. 1–47.

14 Sir Samuel Garth, *The Dispensary* (London, 1699), canto ii, p. 19; Juanita G. L. Burnby, *A Study of the English Apothecary from 1660 to 1760* (London: *Medical History*, Supplement No. 3, 1983); W. H. Helfand, 'The Apothecary Caricatured', *Journal of the American Pharmaceutical Association*, ns II (1962), pp. 52–3.

15 Sir George Clark, *A History of the Royal College of Physicians of London*, 3 vols (Oxford, 1964–72); Harold Cook, *The Decline of the Old Medical Regime in Stuart London* (Ithaca, 1986).

16 R. Campbell, *The London Tradesman: Being a Compendious View of All the Trades, Professions, Arts, Both Liberal and Mechanic, now Practised in the Cities of London and Westminster* (London, 1747), p. 64; I. S. L. Loudon, *Medical Care and the General Practitioner*; Penelope Corfield, *Power and the Professions in Britain 1700–1850* (London, 1995); G. Holmes, *Augustan England: Professions, State and Society, 1680–1730* (London, 1982); Anne Digby, *Making a Medical Living: Doctors and Patients in the English Market for Medicine, 1720–1911* (Cambridge, 1994).

17 For assessment see Johanna Geyer-Kordesch, 'Women and Medicine', in W. F. Bynum and Roy Porter, eds, *Companion Encyclopedia of the History of Medicine* (London, 1993), pp. 884–910. For an instance, see Richard Aspin, 'Who Was Elizabeth Okeover?', *Medical History*, XLIV (2000), pp. 531–40.

18 D. Gibson, ed., *A Parson in the Vale of White Horse* (Gloucester, 1982), p. 132: 'Sangrado' was a fictional doctor notorious for his bloodletting.

19 *Professional Anecdotes, or ANA of Medical Literature*, 3 vols (London, 1825), p. 126.

20 See James Beresford, *The Miseries of Human Life*, new edn (London, 1806), pp. 252–3; and Chap. 1.

21 Ludmilla Jordanova, *Nature Displayed. Gender, Science and Medicine 1760–1820* (Longman, 1999), p. 23.

22 Aldred Scott Warthin, 'The Physician of the Dance of Death', *Annals of Medical History*, ns ii (1930), pp. 351–71, 453–69, 697–710; ns III (1931), pp. 75–109, 134–65.

23 Fiona Haslam, *From Hogarth to Rowlandson. Medicine in Art in Eighteenth-Century Britain* (Liverpool, 1996), p. 16.

24 Quoted in J. Oppenheimer, *New Aspects of John and of William Hunter* (London, 1946), p. 115.

25 John Beresford, ed., *The Diary of a Country Parson: The Rev. James Woodforde, 1758–1802*, 5 vols (Oxford, 1978–81), I, pp. 184–5.

26 See N. Steneck, 'Greatrakes the Stroker: The Interpretations of Historians', *Isis*, LXXIII (1982), pp. 160–77.

27 David Gentilcore, *Healers and Healing in Early Modern Italy* (Manchester, 1998).

28 Haslam, *From Hogarth to Rowlandson*, p. 249.

29 Christine Hillam, ed., *The Roots of Dentistry* (London, 1990); *idem*, *Brass Plate and Brazen Impudence: Dental Practice in the Provinces 1755–1855* (Liverpool, 1991); Roger King, 'Curing Toothache on the Stage?: The Importance of Reading Pictures in Context', *History of Science*, XXXIII (1995), pp. 396–416.

30 D. Sprott, ed., *1784* (London, 1984), pp. 48–9.

31 Haslam, *From Hogarth to Rowlandson. Medicine in Art in Eighteenth-Century Britain*, p. 247; J. A. Donaldson, 'A Rowlandson Caricature. ["Transplanting of

Teeth"]', *British Dental Journal*, CIV (1958), p. 6.

32 Haslam, *From Hogarth to Rowlandson*, p. 246.

33 Robert Burton, *The Anatomy of Melancholy* (1621), ed. D. Floyd and P. Jordan-Smith (New York, 1948), p 390.

34 George Crabbe, *The Borough: A Poem* (London, 1810), pp. 95–6.

35 Roy Porter, 'The Language of Quackery in England', in P. Burke and Roy Porter, eds, *The Social History of Language* (Cambridge, 1987), pp. 73–103; *idem, Quacks: Fakers and Charlatans in English Medicine* (Stroud, 2000).

36 C. J. S. Thompson, *The Quacks of Old London* (New York, 1993), p. 74.

37 William Schupbach, 'Sequah: An English American Medicine Man in 1890', *Medical History*, XXIX (1985), pp. 272–317.

38 J. Crellin, 'Dr James's Fever Powder', *Transactions of the British Society for the History of Pharmacy*, I (1974), pp. 136–43.

39 Quoted in Thompson, *The Quacks of Old London*, p. 125.

40 M. H. Nicolson, 'Ward's Pill and Drop and Men of Letters', *Journal of the History of Ideas*, 29 (1968), pp. 173–96; Haslam, *From Hogarth to Rowlandson*, p. 61.

41 Nicolson, 'Ward's Pill and Drop and Men of Letters', p. 196. Horace Walpole recommended James's powders 'for cough, for gout, for smallpox, for everything'; Henry Fielding wrote of Ward's medicines, 'The powers of Mr. Ward's remedies want indeed no unfair puff of mine to give them credit.'

42 Haslam, *From Hogarth to Rowlandson*, p. 62f, where the painting is reproduced. A well-known copyist, Bardwell drew on some of the characters from Hogarth's *The Pool of Bethesda* at St Bartholomew's Hospital.

43 John Taylor, *History of the Travels and Adventures* (London, 1761), p. 22. For a fuller account of Taylor's career, see Porter, *Quacks: Fakers and Charlatans in English Medicine*, chap. IV, esp. pp. 67ff.

44 For what follows on Graham see R. Porter, 'The Politics of James Graham', *British Journal for Eighteenth Century Studies*, V (1982), pp. 201–6; *idem*, 'Sex and the Singular Man: the Seminal Ideas of James Graham', *Studies on Voltaire & the Eighteenth Century*, CCXXVIII (1984), pp. 3–24. There is a fine collection of Graham's newspaper advertisements in the Wellcome Library for the History and Public Understanding of Medicine, MS 73143; some were reproduced in F. Grose, *A Guide to Health, Beauty, Riches and Honour* (London, 1796).

45 James Graham, *A Sketch, or Short Description of Dr Graham's Medical Apparatus* (London, 1780), p. 53.

46 Haslam, *From Hogarth to Rowlandson*, p. 201.

47 Henry Angelo, *The Reminiscences of Henry Angelo* (London, 1904), II, pp. 61–2.

48 Roy Porter, '"I Think Ye Both Quacks": The Controversy between Dr Theodor Myersbach and Dr John Coakley Lettsom', in W. F. Bynum and Roy Porter, eds, *Medical Fringe and Medical Orthodoxy, 1750–1850* (London, 1986), pp. 56–78.

49 Thompson, *The Quacks of Old London*, p. 345.

50 *Ibid*, p. 344.

51 W. F. Bynum and Roy Porter, eds, *Medical Fringe and Medical Orthodoxy, 1750–1850*, 'Introduction', pp. 1–4.

52 See Paget, *John Hunter*, p. 165.

53 James R. Missett, '"Mercury and His Advocates Defeated, or Vegetable Intrenchment". An Engraving by Thomas Rowlandson, 1789. New Haven, Yale Medical Library. Clements C. Fry Collection', *Journal of the History of Medicine*, XXII (1967), p. 413.

54 See Norman B. Gwyn, 'An Interpretation of the Hogarth Print "The Arms of the Company of Undertakers"', *Bulletin of the History of Medicine*, VIII (1940), pp. 115–277.

55 *Gentleman's Magazine*, 1731, quoted in R. Hambridge, 'Empiricomany, or an Infatuation in Favour of Empiricism, or Quackery', in S. Soupel and R. A. Hambridge, eds, *Literature and Science, and Medicine* (Los Angeles, 1982), pp. 47–102, p. 76.

8 Professional Problems

1 J. Ayres, ed., *Paupers and Pig Killers: The Diary of William Holland, a Somerset Parson 1799–1818* (Gloucester, 1984), p. 24.

2 K. Garlick and A. Macintyre, eds, *The Diary of Joseph Farington*, 16 vols (New Haven, 1978–9), III, p. 819.

3 C. Severn, ed., *Diary of the Rev. John Ward* (London, 1839), p. 119.

4 E. L. Griggs, ed., *Collected Letters of Samuel Taylor Coleridge*, 6 vols (Oxford, 1956–68), I, pp. 154, 256.

5 Penelope Corfield, *Power and the Professions in Britain 1700–1850* (London, 1995); G. Holmes, *Augustan England: Professions, State and Society, 1680–1730* (London, 1982).

6 Harold Cook, *The Decline of the Old Medical Regime in Stuart London* (Ithaca, 1986).

7 L. G. Stevenson, 'The Siege of Warwick Lane, Together with a Brief History of the Society of Collegiate Physicians 1767–98', *Journal of the History of Medicine*, VII (1952), pp. 105–21.

8 D. Little and G. Kahrl, eds, *The Letters of David Garrick*, 3 vols (London, 1963), II, p. 451.

9 B. Mandeville, *A Treatise of the Hypochondriack and Hysterick Diseases* (2nd edn, London, 1730; reprinted, Hildesheim: George Olms Verlag, 1981), pp. 31f. For an instance, see Anita Guerrini, '"A Club of Little Villains": Rhetoric, Professional Identity and Medical Pamphlet Wars', in Marie Mulvey Roberts and Roy Porter, eds, *Literature and Medicine during the Eighteenth Century* (London and New York, 1993), pp. 226–44.

10 Alexander Pope, *Moral Essays*, Epistle III, line 1, in J. Butt, ed., *The Poems of Alexander Pope* (London, 1965), p. 570.

11 Garlick and Macintyre, eds, *The Diary of Joseph Farington*, IX, p. 3221.

12 Philip K. Wilson, *Surgery, Skin and Syphilis: Daniel Turner's London (1667–1741)* (Amsterdam, 1999), pp. 93–4.

13 *Ibid.*, p. 93.

14 W. R. LeFanu, ed., *Betsy Sheridan's Journal* (London, 1960), p. 138; Richard Hunter and Ida Macalpine, *George III and the Mad Business* (London, 1969).

15 F. L. M. Pattison, *Granville Sharpe Pattison: Anatomist and Antagonist* (Edinburgh, 1987); for Dr Andrew Marshal as a duellist, see *Professional Anecdotes, or ANA of Medical Literature*, 3 vols (London, 1825), I, p. 43.

16 Thomas Middleton, *Fair Quarrell*, Act 4, quoted in Herbert Silvette, *The Doctor on Stage. Medicine and Medical Men in Seventeenth Century England*, ed. F. Butler (Knoxville, 1967), p. 269; Peter Burke and Roy Porter, eds, *Languages and Jargons: Contributions to a Social History of Language* (Cambridge, 1995).

17 Henry Fielding, *The History of the Adventures of Joseph Andrews* (1742), in *Joseph Andrews Preceded by Shamela* (London, 1973), book i, p. 40.

18 Thomas Dekker, *Wonder of a Kingdome*, Act 4; John Wilson, *Belphagor*, Act 4, quoted in Silvette, *The Doctor on Stage*, p. 269; see also Thomas Spaulding Willard, 'John Wilson's Satire of Hermetic Medicine', in Roberts and Porter, eds, *Literature and Medicine During the Eighteenth Century*, pp. 136–50.

19 Dorothy Porter and Roy Porter, *Patient's Progress: Doctors and Doctoring in Eighteenth-Century England* (Cambridge, 1989), p. 128.

20 Quoted in Porter and Porter, *Patient's Progress*, p. 129. The practice is discussed in

Chap. 5.

21 Ayres, ed., *Paupers and Pig Killers*, p. 260; Anne Digby, *Making a Medical Living: Doctors and Patients in the English Market for Medicine, 1720–1911* (Cambridge, 1989).

22 Bernard Mandeville, *The Fable of the Bees*, ed. P. Harth (Harmondsworth, 1970), p. 65.

23 Matthew Prior, *Alma*, canto III, line 97, quoted in Porter and Porter, *Patient's Progress*, p. 57. 'Bill' has the double sense of prescription and invoice.

24 Andrew James Symington, 'Of Physicians and their Fees', in William Andrews, FRHS, ed., *The Doctor in History, Literature, Folk-Lore, etc.* (Hull and London, 1896), pp. 252–83.

25 Quoted in Tim Marshall, *Murdering to Dissect: Grave-Robbing, Frankenstein and the Anatomy Literature* (Manchester, 1995), p. 2. Dr Frankenstein was not a practising physician.

26 Thomas Beddoes, *Letter to Erasmus Darwin, M. D., on a New Method of Treating Pulmonary Consumption and Some Other Diseases Hitherto Found Incurable* (Bristol, 1793) p. 4; Roy Porter, *Health for Sale: Quackery in England 1650–1850* (Manchester, 1989), pp. 187f.

27 Beddoes, *Letter to Erasmus Darwin, M. D.*, p. 4.

28 Thomas Beddoes, *Manual of Health: or, the Invalid Conducted Safely Through the Seasons* (London, 1806), p. 416.

29 Seamus Deane, *The French Revolution and Enlightenment in England 1789–1832* (Cambridge, MA, 1988); Norton Garfinkle, 'Science and Religion in England, 1790–1800: The Critical Response to the Work of Erasmus Darwin', *Journal of the History of Ideas*, XVI (1955), pp. 376–88.

30 David Knight, *Humphry Davy: Science & Power* (Oxford, 1992), p. 30.

31 *Ibid.*, p. 30.

32 A. J. Wright, 'Humphrey [sic] Davy's Small Circle of Bristol Friends', *Bulletin of Anesthesia History*, XV (July 1997), pp. 16–20, p. 18.

33 Simon Schaffer, 'States of Mind: Enlightenment and Natural Philosophy', in G. S. Rousseau, ed., *The Languages of Psyche: Mind and Body in Enlightenment Thought* (Berkeley, CA and Oxford, 1990), pp. 233–90, p. 246.

34 Discussed in A. Lothian-Short, 'Pharmaceutical Caricatures', in *Die Vortrage d. Hauptversammlung in Dubrovnik 1959, Stuttgart, Veröffentlichungen d. Intern. Gesellschaft f. Geschichte d. Pharmazie*, 1960, pp. 89–96; R. Burgess, 'Humphry Davy or Friedrich Accum: A Question of Identification', *Medical History*, XVI (1972), pp. 290–93.

35 Fiona Haslam, *From Hogarth to Rowlandson. Medicine in Art in Eighteenth-Century Britain* (Liverpool, 1996), p. 241.

36 See D. Baxby, 'Gillray's "Cowpock" Caricature', *Society for the Social History of Medicine Bulletin*, XXI (1977), p. 60; A. W. Russell, 'Ye Cow-Pock, Gillray and Social Medicine – a Note on Gillray's Caricature of Jenner and the "New Inoculation"', *Society for the Social History of Medicine Bulletin*, XX (1977), pp. 17–22; G. Miller, *The Adoption of Inoculation for Smallpox in England and France* (London, 1957). For Perkins, see Chap. 4.

37 Porter and Porter, *Patient's Progress*, p. 171.

38 Luke Davidson, 'Raising up Humanity: The Introduction of Resuscitation into Late Eighteenth Century Britain (a cultural history)', DPhil thesis, University of York, 2001.

39 Marshall, *Murdering to Dissect*, p. 6. A further echo can be heard during the post mortem, conducted by Dr Thomas Southwood Smith at Grainger's Anatomy Theatre in June 1832, of Jeremy Bentham, when the dead philosopher's features

were dramatically irradiated by a thunderstorm and 'rendered almost vital by the reflection of the lightning playing over them': Ruth Richardson and Brian Hurwitz, 'Jeremy Bentham's Self Image: An Exemplary Bequest for Dissection', *British Medical Journal*, CCVC (1987), pp. 195–8.

40 Mary Shelley, *Frankenstein* (1818) (Oxford, 1993); Stephen Bann, ed., *Frankenstein, Creation and Monstrosity* (London, 1994); Jon Turney, *Frankenstein's Footsteps: Science, Genetics and Popular Culture* (New Haven and London, 1998).

41 P. Linebaugh, 'The Tyburn Riot Against the Surgeons', in E. P. Thompson *et al.*, eds, *Albion's Fatal Tree* (1975) (Harmondsworth, 1977), pp. 65–118.

42 Roy Porter, 'Laymen, Doctors and Medical Knowledge in the Eighteenth Century: The Evidence of the Gentleman's Magazine', in Roy Porter, ed., *Patients and Practitioners: Lay Perceptions of Medicine in Pre-Industrial Society* (Cambridge, 1985), pp. 283–314, p. 306.

43 Robert Southey, *The Poetical Works of Robert Southey* (London, 1845), p. 457; Ruth Richardson, *Death, Dissection and the Destitute: A Political History of the Human Corpse* (London, 1987); *idem*, '"Trading Assassins" and the Licensing of Anatomy', in Roger French and Andrew Wear, eds, *British Medicine in an Age of Reform* (London, 1991), pp. 74–91; Marshall, *Murdering to Dissect*.

44 Haslam, *From Hogarth to Rowlandson*, p. 281.

45 Walter Jerrold, ed., *The Complete Poetical Works of Thomas Hood* (London, 1906), p. 77. Bell and Carpue were amongst the leading anatomy school owners; Sir Astley Cooper was the most eminent surgeon in London.

46 Richardson, *Death, Dissection and the Destitute*.

47 [E. J.], *The Surprize or the Gentleman turn'd Apothecary* (London, 1739).

48 [Anon.], *A Letter to a Physician in the Country on Animal Magnetism* (London, 1786), p. 31. 'Crisis' was a medical term of art meaning the turning point in a bout of sickness.

49 Roy Porter, 'A Touch of Danger: The Man-Midwife as Sexual Predator', in G. S. Rousseau and R. Porter (eds), *Sexual Underworlds of the Enlightenment* (Manchester, 1988), pp. 206–32; C. H. Brock, *William Hunter, 1718–1783* (Glasgow, 1983).

50 For the contemporary 'trials for adultery' sources, see Porter, 'A Touch of Danger: The Man-Midwife as Sexual Predator', pp. 206–32.

51 J. Donnison, *Midwives and Medical Men: A History of Interprofessional Rivalries and Women's Rights* (London, 1977); Adrian Wilson, *The Making of Man-Midwifery: Childbirth in England 1660–1770* (London, 1995).

52 E. Nihell, *A Treatise on the Art of Midwifery* (London, 1760).

53 Haslam, *From Hogarth to Rowlandson*, p. 222; Robert A. Erickson, *Mother Midnight: Birth, Sex, and Fate in Eighteenth-Century Fiction (Defoe, Richardson, and Sterne)* (New York, 1986); Ludmilla Jordanova, *Nature Displayed. Gender, Science and Medicine 1760–1820* (London and New York, 1999), pp. 23–5.

54 George Crabbe, *The Village and Other Poems* (Edinburgh, 1838), p. 22.

55 Frank Nicholls, *The Petition of the Unborn Babes to the Censors of the Royal College of Physicians of London* (London, 1751), p. 6.

56 Philip Thicknesse, *Man Midwifery Analyzed* (London, 1764).

57 Quoted in *ibid.*, p. 28.

58 *Ibid.*, p. 17.

59 *Ibid.*, pp. 15, 10. 'Touch' was of course slang for sexual intercourse.

60 [Anon.], *The Man Midwife Unmasqu'd* (London, 1738), canto III, p. 3.

61 *Ibid*, p. 5.

62 Haslam, *From Hogarth to Rowlandson*, p. 222; Jordanova, *Nature Displayed*, p. 23;

Jason S. Zielonka, '"A Man-Midwife". Etching, Hand Coloured, by S. W. Fores, London, 1793. New Haven, Yale Medical Library, Clements C. Fry Collection', *Journal of the History of Medicine*, XXX (1975), p. 259; Porter, 'A Touch of Danger: The Man-Midwife as Sexual Predator', pp. 206–32.

63 Porter, 'A Touch of Danger: The Man-Midwife as Sexual Predator', pp. 206–32.

64 Karen Louise Harvey, 'Representations of Bodies and Sexual Difference in Eighteenth-Century English Erotica', PhD thesis, University of London, 1999.

65 Thomas Percival, *Medical Ethics; or, A Code of Institutes and Precepts Adapted to the Professional Conduct of Physicians and Surgeons* (Manchester, 1803); Robert Baker, 'Deciphering Percival's Code', in Robert Baker, Dorothy Porter and Roy Porter, eds, *The Codification of Medical Morality*, vol. 1 (Dordrecht/Boston/London, 1993), pp. 179–212; *idem*, 'The History of Medical Ethics', in W. F. Bynum and Roy Porter, eds, *Companion Encyclopedia of the History of Medicine* (London, 1993), pp. 848–83; Lisbeth Haakonssen, *Medicine and Morals in the Enlightenment: John Gregory, Thomas Percival and Benjamin Rush* (Amsterdam, 1997); Mary E. Fissell, 'Innocent and Honorable Bribes: Medical Manners in Eighteenth-Century Britain', in Robert Baker, Dorothy Porter and Roy Porter, eds, *The Codification of Medical Morality*, vol. I, pp. 19–46.

66 George Birkbeck-Hill, *Boswell's Life of Johnson* (Oxford, 1934), vol. IV, p. 306: 13 June 1784.

67 Roy Porter, 'Thomas Gisborne: Physicians, Christians, and Gentlemen', in Andrew Wear, Johanna Geyer Kordesch and Roger French, eds, *Doctors and Ethics: The Historical Setting of Professional Ethics* (Amsterdam, 1993), pp. 253–74.

68 Percival, *Medical Ethics*, pp. 91, 71.

9 The Medical Politician and the Body Politic

1 Mark Jenner, 'Scatology, Coprophagia, and Political Cannibalism: The Rump and the Body Politic in Restoration England', *Past and Present* (forthcoming); H. M. Atherton, 'The British Defend their Constitution in Political Cartoons and Literature', *Studies in Eighteenth Century Culture*, II (1982), pp. 3–31; Roy Porter and G. S. Rousseau, *Gout: The Patrician Malady* (New Haven and London, 1998); Roy Porter, 'Gout: Framing and Fantasizing Disease', *Bulletin of the History of Medicine*, LXVIII (1994), pp. 1–28.

2 John of Salisbury, *Policraticus*, ed. Cary J. Nederman (Cambridge, 1990), p. 67; Jacques Le Goff, 'Head or Heart? The Political Use of Body Metaphors in the Middle Ages', in M. Feher, ed., *Fragments for a History of the Human Body*, 3 vols (New York, 1989), III, pp. 12–27; see also Ernst H. Kantorowicz, *The King's Two Bodies: A Study in Medieval Political Theology* (Princeton, NJ, 1957).

3 Thomas Vicary, *The Surgions Directorie for Young Practitioners* (London, 1651), p. 21; Leonard Barkan, *Nature's Work of Art: The Human Body as Image of the World* (New Haven, 1975); E. M. Tillyard, *The Elizabethan World Picture* (London, 1943).

4 Robert Burton, *The Anatomy of Melancholy*, ed. Floyd Dell and Paul Jordan Smith (New York, 1927), p. 134.

5 William Harvey, *An Anatomical Disputation Concerning the Movement of the Heart and Blood in Living Creatures*, translated and with notes by Gweneth Whitteridge (Oxford, 1976), p. 3; see Robert A. Erickson, 'William Harvey's *De motu cordis* and "The Republick of Literature"', in Marie Mulvey Roberts and Roy Porter, eds, *Literature and Medicine During the Eighteenth Century* (London, 1993), pp. 58–83; Philippa Berry, *Of Chastity and Power: Elizabethan Literature and the Unmarried Queen* (London, 1989); Paul Hammond, 'The King's Two Bodies:

Representations of Charles II', in Jeremy Black and Jeremy Gregory, eds, *Culture, Politics and Society in Britain, 1660–1800* (Manchester, 1991), pp. 13–48; J. N. Figgis, *The Divine Right of Kings* (New York, 1965).

6 Roy Porter, *Enlightenment: Britain and the Creation of the Modern World* (Harmondsworth, 2000), chap. 8.

7 Adam Smith, *An Inquiry into the Nature and Causes of the Wealth of Nations*, ed. R. H. Campbell, A. S. Skinner and W. B. Todd, 2 vols (Oxford, 1976), vol. II, pp. 673–4; for the congruence of physiological and social metaphors in free-market thinking, see Anne Marcovich, 'Concerning the Continuity between the Image of Society and the Image of the Human Body: An Examination of the Work of the English Physician J. C. Lettsom 1746–1815', in P. Wright and A. Treacher, eds, *The Problem of Medical Knowledge* (Edinburgh, 1982), pp. 69–87.

8 Smith, *An Inquiry into the Nature and Causes of the Wealth of Nations*, vol. II, pp. 673–4; Sara E. Melser and Kathryn Norberg, *From the Royal to the Republican Body Incorporating the Political in Seventeenth- and Eighteenth-Century France* (Berkeley, 1997); Dorinda Outram, *The Body and the French Revolution. Sex, Class and Political Culture* (New Haven, 1989).

9 E. H. Gombrich, 'The Cartoonist's Armory', in *Meditations on a Hobby Horse* (London, 1963), pp. 127–42.

10 A point well made in Martin Kemp and Marina Wallace, *Spectacular Bodies: The Art and Science of the Human Body. From Leonardo to Now* (Berkeley and Los Angeles, 2000).

11 George Lakoff and Mark Johnson, *Metaphors We Live By* (Chicago, 1980).

12 Gombrich, 'The Cartoonist's Armory', pp. 127–42.

13 John Brewer, *The Common People and Politics, 1750–1790s* (Cambridge, 1986); H. M. Atherton, *Political Prints in the Age of Hogarth. A Study of the Ideographic Representation of Politics* (Oxford, 1974); Michael Duffy, *The Englishman and the Foreigner* (Cambridge, 1986); M. Dorothy George, *English Political Caricature 1793–1832: A Study of Opinion and Propaganda*, 2 vols (Oxford, 1967); *idem*, *Hogarth to Cruikshank: Social Change in Graphic Satire* (London, 1967); *idem* and F. G. Stephens, *Catalogue of Political and Personal Satires … in the British Museum to 1832*, 12 vols (London, 1870–1954).

14 The links between laughter and aggression have been explored this century, notably in Freud's notion of humour sublimating impermissible desires. For subversion, see P. Stallybrass and A. White, *The Politics and Poetics of Transgression* (Ithaca, 1986).

15 Ronald Paulson, *Hogarth*, vol. 1, *The 'Modern Moral Subject'*, vol. 2, *High Art and Low, 1732–1750*, vol. 3, *Art and Politics, 1750–1764* (Cambridge, 1993).

16 The Napoleonic Wars everywhere gave caricature a more serious tone. Goya's *Disasters of War* developed from the often satiric *Proverbios* and *Caprichos* (his attacks on customs and manners and on Spanish Catholic bigotry).

17 Brewer, *The Common People and Politics, 1750–1790s*. Before the nineteenth century, such traditions of political prints were essentially English. See W. H. Helfand, 'Medicine and Pharmacy in French Political Prints', *Pharmacy in History*, XVII (1975), pp. 119–31; *idem*, *Medicine and Pharmacy in American Political Prints (1765–1870)* (Madison, WI, 1978); *idem* and S. Rocchietta, *Medicina e farmacia nelle caricature politiche Italiane 1848–1914* (Rome, 1982).

18 George Rudé, *The Crowd in History* (New York, 1964); E. P. Thompson, *Customs in Common* (London, 1991).

19 Peter D. G. Thomas, *The American Revolution* (Cambridge, 1986), pl. 46; Paul Langford, *Walpole and the Robinocracy* (Cambridge, 1986), pl. 67, pl. 99 and *passim*.

20 Vincent Carretta, *George III and the Satirists From Hogarth to Byron* (Athens, GA,

and London, 1990), p. 297.

21 Benjamin Franklin, *Poor Richard's Almanack* (1744), quoted in Dorothy Porter and Roy Porter, *Patient's Progress: Doctors and Doctoring in Eighteenth-Century England* (Cambridge, 1989), p. 54.

22 Richard van Dülmen, *Theatre of Horror. Crime and Punishment in Early Modern Germany* (Cambridge, 1990).

23 Thomas, *The American Revolution*, pl. 19; J. G. L. Burnby, *Caricatures and Comments* (Staines, 1989).

24 Fiona Haslam, *From Hogarth to Rowlandson. Medicine in Art in Eighteenth-Century Britain* (Liverpool, 1996), p. 288.

25 Ruth Richardson, *Death, Dissection and the Destitute: A Political History of the Human Corpse* (London, 1987).

26 H. T. Dickinson, *Caricatures and the Constitution* (Cambridge, 1986), pl. 145.

27 Draper Hill, *Mr Gillray the Caricaturist* (London, 1965); Ronald Paulson, *Representations of Revolution 1789–1820* (New Haven, 1983).

28 Brewer, *The Common People and Politics, 1750–1790s*, p. 15.

29 W. H. Helfand, 'John Bull and his Doctors', *Veröffentlichungen der Internationalen Gesellschaft für Geschichte der Pharmazie*, xxviii (1966), pp. 131–42 is splendid.

30 Carretta, *George III and the Satirists From Hogarth to Byron*, p. 125; *English Caricature 1620 to the Present: Caricaturists and Satirists, Their Art, Their Purpose and Influence* (London, 1984), p. 95.

31 Duffy, *The Englishman and the Foreigner*, pl. 132; Atherton, 'The British Defend their Constitution in Political Cartoons and Literature', pp. 3–31.

32 George Cruikshank, 'Radical Quacks Giving a New Constitution to John Bull', in Dickinson, *Caricatures and the Constitution*, pl. 118.

33 Cruikshank's 'The Mountebanks, or Opposition Show Box', is reproduced in Helfand, 'John Bull and his Doctors', p. 139.

34 'The State Quack' is reproduced in Brewer, *The Common People and Politics, 1750–1790s*, pl. 101.

35 Quoted and illustrated in Burnby, *Caricatures and Comments*, p. 7.

36 Gillray, *Doctor Sangrado Curing John Bull of Repletion*, reproduced in W. H. Helfand, 'Medicine and Pharmacy in British Political Prints – the Example of Lord Sidmouth', *Medical History*, xxix (1985), pp. 375–85.

37 W. H. Helfand, 'Medicine and Pharmacy in British Political Prints – the Example of Lord Sidmouth', pp. 375–85.

38 Edgell Rickword, *Radical Squibs & Loyal Ripostes Satirical Pamphlets of the Regency Period, 1819–1821 Illustrated by George Cruikshank and Others* (Bath, 1972), pp. 103–4.

39 William Hone, *The Political House that Jack Built* (London, 1819).

40 See John Derry, *Charles James Fox* (London, 1972). Widely lampooned for his self-proletarianization, Charles James Fox claimed that 'Sayers' caricatures had done him more mischief than the debates in Parliament.'

41 For models for this print see Chap. 4.

42 Dickinson, *Caricatures and the Constitution*, pl. 52; William Schupbach, 'John Monro MD and Charles James Fox: Etching by Thomas Rowlandson', *Medical History*, xxvii (1983), pp. 80–83.

43 Sander L. Gilman, *Seeing the Insane* (New York, 1982); see Haslam, *From Hogarth to Rowlandson*, p. 153.

10 Victorian Developments

 1 See generally Roger French and Andrew Wear, eds, *British Medicine in an Age of Reform* (London, 1992); Christopher Lawrence, *Medicine in the Making of Modern*

Britain, 1700–1920 (London and New York, 1994); W. F. Bynum, *Science and the Practice of Medicine in the Nineteenth Century* (New York, 1994); and, in particular, Adrian Desmond, *The Politics of Evolution: Morphology, Medicine and Reform in Radical London* (Chicago, 1989).

2 *Lancet* (1835–6), II, p. 57.

3 For the following discussion of Morison see W. H. Helfand, 'James Morison and his Pills. A Study of the Nineteenth Century Pharmaceutical Industry', *Transactions of the British Society for the History of Pharmacy*, I (1974), pp. 101–35 and Roy Porter, *Health for Sale: Quackery in England 1650–1850* (Manchester, 1989), chap. VIII.

4 *Lancet* (1836–7), II, p. 130.

5 *Ibid.*, p. 130.

6 W. H. Helfand, 'James Morison and his Pills', pp. 101–35.

7 For this and what follows see Ivan Waddington, *The Medical Profession in the Industrial Revolution* (Dublin, 1984); I. S. L. Loudon, *Medical Care and the General Practitioner 1750–1850* (Oxford, 1986); Peter Bartrip, *Themselves Writ Large. The British Medical Association 1832–1966* (London, 1996).

8 Anne Digby, *The Evolution of British General Practice 1850–1948* (Oxford, 1999); *idem, Making a Medical Living: Doctors and Patients in the English Market for Medicine, 1720–1911* (Cambridge, 1994).

9 W. E. Houghton, *The Victorian Frame of Mind 1830–1870* (New Haven, 1957).

10 E. S. Turner, *Call the Doctor* (London, 1958), p. 202.

11 M. Faith McLellan, 'Images of Physicians in Literature: From Quacks to Heroes', *Lancet*, vol. 348 (17 August) 1996, pp. 458–60.

12 Harriet Martineau, *Deerbrook* (1838) (London, 1892), p. 26. See the discussion in Ann L. Reitz, 'Sawbones to Savior to Cynic: The Doctor's Relation to Society in English Fiction of the Eighteenth, Nineteenth, and Twentieth Centuries', PhD thesis, University of Cincinnati, 1985.

13 George Eliot, *Middlemarch* (1871–2) (Harmondsworth, 1965); W. J. Harvey, 'The Intellectual Background of the Novel: Casaubon and Lydgate', in Barbara Hardy, *Middlemarch: Critical Approaches to the Novel* (New York, 1967), pp. 25–38.

14 W. J. Harvey, 'The Intellectual Background of the Novel: Casaubon and Lydgate', in Hardy, *Middlemarch*, pp. 25–38, p. 35.

15 Eliot, *Middlemarch*, p. 204.

16 *Ibid.*, 206.

17 *Ibid.*, p. 835.

18 Penelope Corfield, *Power and the Professions in Britain 1700–1850* (London, 1995), p. 140.

19 The following draws upon the researches of Gertrude Mae Prescott, 'Fame and Photography, Portrait Publications in Great Britain, 1856–1900', PhD dissertation, University of Texas at Austin, 1985; see also Daniel M. Fox and Christopher Lawrence, *Photographing Medicine: Images and Power in Britain and America Since 1840* (Westport and London, 1988).

20 David Piper, 'Take the Face of a Physician', in Gordon Wolstenholme, ed., *Portraits: The Royal College of Physicians of London, Catalogue II* (Amsterdam, 1977), pp. 25–49.

21 For ethical debate at the time, see P. W. J. Bartrip, *Mirror of Medicine: A History of the BMJ* (Oxford, 1990).

22 Sir St Clair Thomson, 'Some Medical Celebrities of the Victorian Age as Depicted in the Cartoons of Vanity Fair', *The Medical Press and Circular*, CCI (1939), pp. 84–96.

23 E. H. Gombrich and E. Kris, *Caricature* (London, 1939), p. 20.

24 R. G. G. Price, *A History of Punch* (London, 1957), p.20.

25 Richard D. Altick, 'Punch's First Ten Years: The Ingredients of Success', *Journal of Newspaper and Periodical History*, VII (1991), pp. 5–16.

26 Harold Herd, *The March of Journalism. The Story of the British Press from 1622 to the Present Day* (London, 1952), p. 209; Susan and Asa Briggs, eds, *Cap and Bell, Punch's Chronicle of English History in the Making, 1841–61* (London, 1972), see Chap. II, 'The Scope of Reform', pp. 75–94.

27 M. H. Spielmann, *The History of 'Punch'* (London, 1895), p. 409.

28 Richard D. Altick, *Punch: The Lively Youth of a British Institution, 1841–1851* (Columbus, 1997), pp. 129, 250.

29 'John Leech', *Dictionary of National Biography*, vol. XI (1909), p. 830; Graham Everitt, *English Caricaturists and Graphic Humourists of the Nineteenth Century* (London, 1893); W. Feaver and A. Gould, *Masters of Caricature: From Hogarth to Scarfe and Levine* (London, 1981); June Rose, *The Drawings of John Leech* (London, 1950); Henry R. Viets, 'John Leech and the London Medical Student of 1842', *New England Journal of Medicine*, CCLXXX (1969), pp. 79–84.

30 Susan and Asa Briggs, eds, *Cap and Bell, Punch's Chronicle of English History in the Making, 1841–61*, XXVI.

31 Rose, *Drawings of John Leech*, 10.

32 Derek Pepys Whiteley, *George Du Maurier. His Life and Work* (London, 1948), p. 22; C. C. Hoyer Millar, *George Du Maurier and Others* (London, 1937).

33 Piper, 'Take the Face of a Physician', in Wolstenholme, ed., *Portraits: The Royal College of Physicians of London, Catalogue II*, 25–49, p. 44.

34 Wolfgang Born, 'The Nature and History of Medical Caricature', *Ciba Symposia*, VI (1944–5), pp. 1910–24.

35 'Charles Keene', *Dictionary of National Biography*, vol. X (1908), p. 1190.

36 Gordon N. Ray, *Thackeray. The Uses of Adversity. 1811–1846* (London, 1955); idem, *Thackeray. The Age of Wisdom. 1847–1863* (London, 1958); Andrew Sanders, 'Thackeray and Punch, 1842–1847', *Journal of Newspaper and Periodical History*, VII (1991) pp. 17–24.

37 Curt Proskauer, 'The Dentist in Caricature', *Ciba Symposia*, VI (1944), pp. 1933–48: 'The chief and inexhaustible subjects of the dental caricaturist are the fear and pain of the unhappy and unfortunate patient.'

38 Spielmann, *The History of 'Punch'*, p. 549.

39 *Ibid.*, p. 550.

40 John Geipel, *The Cartoon. A Short History of Graphic Comedy and Satire* (London, 1972), p. 86.

41 Spielmann, *The History of 'Punch'*, p. 553.

42 *Ibid.*, p. 568.

43 Shane Leslie, *Edward Tennyson Reed 1860–1933* (London, 1957), p. 56.

44 Spielmann, *The History of 'Punch'*, p. 367.

45 James Thorpe, *English Illustration: The Nineties* (London, 1935), pp. 251–2.

46 For the more recent history see Derek Pepys Whiteley, 'Bernard Partridge and Punch', *Image: A Periodical of the Visual Arts*, Autumn (1952), pp. 48–59.

Afterword

1 Jens Lachmund and Gunnar Stollberg, 'The Doctor, His Audience, and the Meaning of Illness. The Drama of Medical Practice in the Late 18th and Early 19th Centuries', in Jens Lachmund and Gunnar Stollberg, eds, *The Social Construction of Illness: Illness and Medical Knowledge in Past and Present* (Stuttgart, 1992), pp. 53–66.

2 Talcott Parsons, 'The Sick Role and the Role of the Physician Reconsidered',

Milbank Memorial Fund, Health and Society, LIII (1975), pp. 257–78.

3 Natsu Hattori, 'Performing Cures: Practice and Interplay in Theatre and Medicine in the English Renaissance', DPhil thesis, University of Oxford, 1995.

4 Quoted in Fielding H. Garrison, 'Medicine in *The Tatler*, *Spectator* and *Guardian*', *Bulletin of the Institute of the History of Medicine*, II (1934), pp. 477–503, p. 488. See also John F. Sena, 'Smollett's Matthew Bramble and the Tradition of the Physician–Satirist', *Papers on Language & Literature*, XI (1975), pp. 380–96.

5 Anne Karpf, *Doctoring the Media: The Reporting of Health and Medicine* (London, 1988); Peter E. Dans, *Doctors in the Movies. Boil the Water and Just Say Aah*, (Bloomington, 2000).

Select Bibliography

On images and their interpretation:

Burke, Peter, *Eyewitnessing* (London, 2001)
Gilman, Sander L., *Seeing the Insane* (New York, 1982)
—, *Health and Illness: Images of Difference* (London, 1995)
Haslam, Fiona, *From Hogarth to Rowlandson. Medicine in Art in Eighteenth-Century Britain* (Liverpool, 1996)
Jordanova, Ludmilla, *Defining Features: Scientific and Medical Portraits 1660–2000* (London, 2000)
Kemp, Martin, and Marina Wallace, *Spectacular Bodies: The Art and Science of the Human Body. From Leonardo to Now* (Berkeley and Los Angeles, 2000)
Lawrence, Christopher and Steven Shapin, eds, *Science Incarnate – Historical Embodiments of Natural Knowledge* (Chicago and London, 1998)
Paulson, Ronald, *Book and Painting; Shakespeare, Milton, and the Bible; Literary Texts and the Emergence of English Painting* (Knoxville, 1982)
—, *Representations of Revolution 1789–1820* (New Haven, 1983)
—, *The Beautiful, Novel, and Strange. Aesthetics and Heterodoxy* (Baltimore and London, 1996)
Pointon, Marcia, *Hanging the Head: Portraiture and Social Formation in Eighteenth-Century England* (New Haven, 1993)
Wagner, Peter, *Reading Iconotexts: From Swift to the French Revolution* (London, 1995)

On the historical context of early modern England: disease, medicine and print culture:

Agnew, J.-C., *Worlds Apart: The Market and the Theater in Anglo-American Thought, 1550–1750* (Cambridge, 1986)
Altick, Richard D., *The Shows of London: A Panoramic History of Exhibitions, 1600–1862* (Cambridge, MA, 1978)
Bakhtin, M. M., *Rabelais and his World*, trans. H. Iswolsky (Cambridge, MA, 1968)
Clarkson, L., *Death, Disease and Famine in Pre-Industrial England* (Dublin, 1975)
Gittings, C., *Death, Burial and the Individual in Early Modern England* (London, 1984)
Hattori, Natsu, 'Performing Cures: Practice and Interplay in Theatre and Medicine in the English Renaissance', DPhil thesis, University of Oxford, 1995
Houlbrooke, Ralph A., *Death, Religion and the Family in England, 1480–1750* (Oxford, 1998)
Jordanova, Ludmilla, *Nature Displayed. Gender, Science and Medicine 1760–1820* (London and New York, 1999)
Lawrence, Christopher, *Medicine in the Making of Modern Britain, 1700–1920* (London and New York, 1994)

Paster, Gail Kern, *The Body Embarrassed: Drama and the Disciplines of Shame in Early Modern England* (Ithaca, 1993)

On the history of the body, base and beautiful:

Bottomley, Frank, *Attitudes to the Body in Western Christendom* (London, 1979)
Bremmer, Jan, and Herman Roodenburg, eds, *A Cultural History of Gestures From Antiquity to the Present Day* (Cambridge, 1991)
Clark, Kenneth, *The Nude: A Study of Ideal Art* (Harmondsworth, 1970)
Feher, M., ed., *Fragments for a History of the Human Body*, vol. 3 (New York, 1989)
Flynn, Carol Houlihan, *The Body in Swift and Defoe* (Cambridge, 1990)
Porter, Roy, 'History of the Body Reconsidered', in Peter Burke, ed., *New Perspectives on Historical Writing*, 2nd edn (Cambridge, 2001), pp. 233–60
Stafford, Barbara Maria, *Body Criticism: Imagining the Unseen in Enlightenment Art and Medicine* (Cambridge, MA, 1991)
Turner, Bryan S., *The Body and Society: Explorations in Social Theory* (Oxford, 1984)

On doctors, and the history of the medical profession:

Arnold–Forster, Kate and Nigel Tallis, comps, *The Bruising Apothecary: Images of Pharmacy and Medicine in Caricature* (London, 1989)
Burnby, Juanita G. L., *A Study of the English Apothecary from 1660 to 1760* (*Medical History*, Supplement No. 3, London, 1983)
Corfield, Penelope, *Power and the Professions in Britain 1700–1850* (London, 1995)
Hillam, Christine, *Brass Plate and Brazen Impudence: Dental Practice in the Provinces 1755–1855* (Liverpool, 1991)
Lawrence, Christopher, *Medicine in the Making of Modern Britain, 1700–1920* (London and New York, 1994)
Loudon, I. S. L., *Medical Care and the General Practitioner 1750–1850* (Oxford, 1986)
Wear, Andrew, *Knowledge and Practice in English Medicine 1550–1680* (Cambridge, 2000)

On patients, and patient / doctor relations:

Bailin, Miriam, *The Sickroom in Victorian Fiction: The Art of Being Ill* (Cambridge, 1994)
Beier, Lucinda McCray, *Sufferers and Healers: The Experience of Illness in Seventeenth-Century England* (London, 1987)
Brody, H., *Stories of Sickness* (New Haven, 1987)
Duden, Barbara, *Geschichte unter der Haut* (Stuttgart, 1987), trans. as *The Woman Beneath the Skin. A Doctor's Patients in Eighteenth-Century Germany*, by Thomas Dunlap (Cambridge, MA, 1991)
Fissell, Mary E., *Patients, Power, and the Poor in Eighteenth-Century Bristol* (Cambridge, 1991)
Gilman, Sander L., *Health and Illness: Images of Difference* (London, 1995)
Hembry, Phyliss, *The English Spa 1560–1815: A Social History* (London, 1990)
Lane, Joan, '"The Doctor Scolds Me": The Diaries and Correspondence of Patients in Eighteenth Century England', in Roy Porter, ed., *Patients and Practitioners: Lay Perceptions of Medicine in Pre-Industrial Society* (Cambridge, 1985), pp. 204–48
Porter, Dorothy, and Roy Porter, *Patient's Progress: Doctors and Doctoring in Eighteenth-Century England* (Cambridge, 1989)
Porter, Roy, and Dorothy Porter, *In Sickness and in Health: The British Experience 1650–1850* (London, 1988)

On quacks and the fringe:

Bynum, W. F., and Roy Porter, eds, *Medical Fringe and Medical Orthodoxy, 1750–1850* (London, 1987)
Porter, Roy, *Health for Sale: Quackery in England 1650–1850* (Manchester, 1989)
Thompson, C. J. S., *The Quacks of Old London* (London, 1928)

On medical images in political cartoons:

Atherton, H. M., *Political Prints in the Age of Hogarth. A Study of the Ideographic Representation of Politics* (Oxford, 1974)
Brewer, John, *The Common People and Politics, 1750–1790s* (Cambridge, 1986)
Burnby, Juanita, *Caricatures and Comments* (Staines, 1989)
Carretta, Vincent, *George III and the Satirists From Hogarth to Byron* (Athens, GA, and London, 1990)
Duffy, Michael, ed., *The English Satirical Print, 1600–1832*, 7 vols (Cambridge, 1986)
Feaver, W., and A. Gould, *Masters of Caricature: From Hogarth to Scarfe and Levine* (London, 1981)
George, M. D., *British Museum Catalogue of Political and Personal Satires*, 11 vols (London, 1870–1954)
—, *From Hogarth to Cruikshank: Social Change in Graphic Satire* (London, 1967)

On Victorian developments:

Altick, Richard D., *The English Common Reader* (Columbus, 1957)
—, *Punch: The Lively Youth of a British Institution, 1841–1851* (Columbus, 1997)
Digby, Anne, *Making a Medical Living: Doctors and Patients in the English Market for Medicine, 1720–1911* (Cambridge, 1994)
—, *The Evolution of British General Practice 1850–1948* (Oxford, 1999)
Donnison, J., *Midwives and Medical Men: A History of Interprofessional Rivalries and Women's Rights* (London, 1977)
Fox, Daniel M., and Christopher Lawrence, *Photographing Medicine: Images and Power in Britain and America Since 1840* (New York, Westport, CT and London, 1988)
Haley, B., *The Healthy Body and Victorian Culture* (Cambridge, MA, 1978)
Waddington, Ivan, *The Medical Profession in the Industrial Revolution* (Dublin, 1984)

Photographic Acknowledgements

The author and publishers wish to express their thanks to the following sources of illustrative material and/or permission to reproduce it: Victoria Art Gallery, Bath and North East Somerset Council/Bridgeman Art Library: 85; © copyright The British Museum, London: 8, 47, 55, 109–10, 112, 114, 116–18; by kind permission of the Royal College of Physicians, London: 73; Royal College of Surgeons of England: 40; Photography, Illustration and Audiovisual Centre, University College, London: 46. All other photographs are courtesy of the Wellcome Library, London.

Index

Figures in *italics* indicate illustration numbers.